1994
YEAR BOOK OF
HEMATOLOGY®

Statement of Purpose

The YEAR BOOK Service

The YEAR BOOK series was devised in 1901 by practicing health professionals who observed that the literature of medicine and related disciplines had become so voluminous that no one individual could read and place in perspective every potential advance in a major specialty. In the final decade of the 20th century, this recognition is more acutely true than it was in 1901.

More than merely a series of books, YEAR BOOK volumes are the tangible results of a unique service designed to accomplish the following:

- to *survey* a wide range of journals of proven value
- to *select* from those journals papers representing significant advances and statements of important clinical principles
- to provide *abstracts* of those articles that are readable, convenient summaries of their key points
- to provide *commentary* about those articles to place them in perspective.

These publications grow out of a unique process that calls on the talents of outstanding authorities in clinical and fundamental disciplines, trained literature specialists, and professional writers, all supported by the resources of Mosby, the world's preeminent publisher for the health professions.

The Literature Base

Mosby subscribes to nearly 1,000 journals published worldwide, covering the full range of the health professions. On an annual basis, the publisher examines usage patterns and polls its expert authorities to add new journals to the literature base and to delete journals that are no longer useful as potential YEAR BOOK sources.

The Literature Survey

The publisher's team of literature specialists, all of whom are trained and experienced health professionals, examines every original, peer-reviewed article in each journal issue. More than 250,000 articles per year are scanned systematically, including title, text, illustrations, tables, and references. Each scan is compared, article by article, to the search strategies that the publisher has developed in consultation with the 270 outside experts who form the pool of YEAR BOOK editors. A given article may be reviewed by any number of editors, from one to a dozen or more, regardless of the discipline for which the paper was originally published. In turn, each editor who receives the article reviews it to determine whether or not the article should be included in the YEAR BOOK. This decision is based on the article's inherent quality, its probable usefulness to readers of that YEAR BOOK, and the editor's goal to represent a balanced picture of a given field in each volume of the YEAR BOOK. In addition, the editor indicates when to include figures and tables from the article to help the YEAR BOOK reader better understand the information.

Of the quarter million articles scanned each year, only 5% are selected for detailed analysis within the YEAR BOOK series, thereby assuring readers of the high value of every selection.

The Abstract

The publisher's abstracting staff is headed by a physician-writer and includes individuals with training in the life sciences, medicine, and other areas, plus extensive experience in writing for the health professions and related industries. Each selected article is assigned to a specific writer on this abstracting staff. The abstracter, guided in many cases by notations supplied by the expert editor, writes a structured, condensed summary designed so that the reader can rapidly acquire the essential information contained in the article.

The Commentary

The YEAR BOOK editorial boards, sometimes assisted by guest commentators, write comments that place each article in perspective for the reader. This provides the reader with the equivalent of a personal consultation with a leading international authority—an opportunity to better understand the value of the article and to benefit from the authority's thought processes in assessing the article.

Additional Editorial Features

The editorial boards of each YEAR BOOK organize the abstracts and comments to provide a logical and satisfying sequence of information. To enhance the organization, editors also provide introductions to sections or individual chapters, comments linking a number of abstracts, citations to additional literature, and other features.

The published YEAR BOOK contains enhanced bibliographic citations for each selected article, including extended listings of multiple authors and identification of author affiliations. Each YEAR BOOK contains a Table of Contents specific to that year's volume. From year to year, the Table of Contents for a given YEAR BOOK will vary depending on developments within the field.

Every YEAR BOOK contains a list of the journals from which papers have been selected. This list represents a subset of the nearly 1,000 journals surveyed by the publisher and occasionally reflects a particularly pertinent article from a journal that is not surveyed on a routine basis.

Finally, each volume contains a comprehensive subject index and an index to authors of each selected paper.

The 1994 Year Book Series

Year Book of Allergy and Clinical Immunology: Drs. Rosenwasser, Borish, Gelfand, Leung, Nelson, and Szefler

Year Book of Anesthesia and Pain Management: Drs. Tinker, Abram, Kirby, Ostheimer, Roizen, and Stoelting

Year Book of Cardiology®: Drs. Schlant, Collins, Engle, Gersh, Kaplan, and Waldo

Year Book of Chiropractic: Dr. Lawrence

Year Book of Critical Care Medicine®: Drs. Rogers and Parrillo

Year Book of Dentistry®: Drs. Meskin, Currier, Kennedy, Leinfelder, Berry, and Roser

Year Book of Dermatologic Surgery: Drs. Swanson, Glogau, and Salasche

Year Book of Dermatology®: Drs. Sober and Fitzpatrick

Year Book of Diagnostic Radiology®: Drs. Federle, Clark, Gross, Madewell, Maynard, Sackett, and Young

Year Book of Digestive Diseases®: Drs. Greenberger and Moody

Year Book of Drug Therapy®: Drs. Lasagna and Weintraub

Year Book of Emergency Medicine®: Drs. Wagner, Burdick, Davidson, McNamara, and Roberts

Year Book of Endocrinology®: Drs. Bagdade, Braverman, Poehlman, Kannan, Landsberg, Molitch, Morley, Odell, Rogol, Ryan, and Nathan

Year Book of Family Practice®: Drs. Berg, Bowman, Davidson, Dietrich, and Scherger

Year Book of Geriatrics and Gerontology®: Drs. Beck, Reuben, Burton, Small, Whitehouse, and Goldstein

Year Book of Hand Surgery®: Drs. Amadio and Hentz

Year Book of Hematology®: Drs. Spivak, Bell, Ness, Quesenberry, and Wiernik

Year Book of Infectious Diseases®: Drs. Keusch, Wolff, Barza, Bennish, Gelfand, Klempner, and Snydman

Year Book of Infertility®: Drs. Mishell, Lobo, and Sokol

Year Book of Medicine®: Drs. Rogers, Bone, Cline, O'Rourke, Greenberger, Utiger, Epstein, and Malawista

Year Book of Neonatal and Perinatal Medicine®: Drs. Klaus and Fanaroff

Year Book of Nephrology: Drs. Coe, Favus, Henderson, Kashgarian, Luke, Myers, and Curtis

Year Book of Neurology and Neurosurgery®: Drs. Bradley and Crowell

Year Book of Neuroradiology: Drs. Osborn, Eskridge, Grossman, and Harnsberger

Year Book of Nuclear Medicine®: Drs. Hoffer, Gore, Gottschalk, Rattner, Zaret, and Zubal

Year Book of Obstetrics and Gynecology®: Drs. Mishell, Kirschbaum, and Morrow

Year Book of Occupational and Environmental Medicine: Drs. Emmett, Frank, Gochfeld, and Hessl

Year Book of Oncology®: Drs. Simone, Longo, Ozols, Steele, Glatstein, and Bosl

Year Book of Ophthalmology®: Drs. Laibson, Adams, Augsburger, Benson, Cohen, Eagle, Flanagan, Nelson, Rapuano, Reinecke, Sergott, and Wilson

Year Book of Orthopedics®: Drs. Sledge, Poss, Cofield, Frymoyer, Griffin, Hansen, Johnson, Simmons, and Springfield

Year Book of Otolaryngology–Head and Neck Surgery®: Drs. Paparella and Holt

Year Book of Pain: Drs. Gebhart, Haddox, Jacox, Payne, Rudy, and Shapiro

Year Book of Pathology and Clinical Pathology®: Drs. Gardner, Bennett, Cousar, Garvin, and Worsham

Year Book of Pediatrics®: Dr. Stockman

Year Book of Plastic, Reconstructive, and Aesthetic Surgery: Drs. Miller, Cohen, McKinney, Robson, Ruberg, and Whitaker

Year Book of Podiatric Medicine and Surgery®: Dr. Kominsky

Year Book of Psychiatry and Applied Mental Health®: Drs. Talbott, Frances, Breier, Meltzer, Perry, Schowalter, and Yudofsky

Year Book of Pulmonary Disease®: Drs. Bone and Petty

Year Book of Rheumatology: Drs. Sergent, LeRoy, Meenan, Panush, and Reichlin

Year Book of Sports Medicine®: Drs. Shephard, Drinkwater, Eichner, Sutton, Torg, Col. Anderson, and Mr. George

Year Book of Surgery®: Drs. Copeland, Deitch, Eberlein, Howard, Luce, Ritchie, Seeger, Souba, and Sugarbaker

Year Book of Thoracic and Cardiovascular Surgery: Drs. Ginsberg, Lofland, and Wechsler

Year Book of Transplantation: Drs. Ascher, Hansen, and Strom

Year Book of Ultrasound: Drs. Merritt, Babcock, Carroll, Goldstein, and Mittelstaedt

Year Book of Urology®: Drs. Gillenwater and Howards

Year Book of Vascular Surgery®: Dr. Porter

1994

The Year Book of HEMATOLOGY®

Editor

Jerry L. Spivak, M.D.

Professor of Medicine and Oncology, Division of Hematology, Department of Medicine, The Johns Hopkins University School of Medicine

Associate Editors

William R. Bell, M.D.

Professor of Medicine, Radiology, and Nuclear Medicine, Division of Hematology, Department of Medicine, The Johns Hopkins University School of Medicine, The Edythe Harris Lucas—Clara Lucas Lynn Professor in Hematology

Paul M. Ness, M.D.

Director, Blood Bank, Department of Pathology, The Johns Hopkins University School of Medicine; Principal Officer, American Red Cross Blood Services, Greater Chesapeake and Potomac Regions

Peter J. Quesenberry, M.D.

Director, Cancer Center, University of Massachusetts, Worcester

Peter H. Wiernik, M.D.

Gutman Professor and Chairman, Department of Oncology, Montefiore Medical Center; Director, Division of Medical Oncology, Albert Einstein College of Medicine; Associate Director for Clinical Research, Albert Einstein Cancer Center

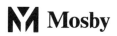 Mosby

St. Louis Baltimore Boston Chicago London Madrid Philadelphia Sydney Toronto

Vice President and Publisher, Continuity Publishing: Kenneth H. Killion
Sponsoring Editor: Nancy Puckett
Illustrations and Permissions Coordinator: Bernadette R. Bauer
Manager, Literature Services: Edith M. Podrazik, R.N.
Senior Information Specialist: Terri Santo, R.N.
Information Specialist: Nancy Dunne, R.N.
Senior Medical Writer: David A. Cramer, M.D.
Senior Project Manager: Max F. Perez
Production Editor: Wendi Schnaufer
Senior Production Assistant: Sandra Rogers
Production Assistant: Rebecca Nordbrock
Proofroom Manager: Barbara M. Kelly

1994 EDITION
Copyright © December 1993 by Mosby-Year Book, Inc.

Printed in the United States of America
Composition by International Computaprint Corporation
Printing/binding by Maple-Vail

Mosby, Inc.
11830 Westline Industrial Drive
St. Louis, MO 63146

Editorial Office:
Mosby, Inc.
200 North LaSalle St.
Chicago, IL 60601

International Standard Serial Number: 0882-5998
International Standard Book Number: 0-8151-8127-2

Table of Contents

Journals Represented

Mosby subscribes to and surveys nearly 1,000 U.S. and foreign medical and allied health journals. From these journals, the Editors select the articles to be abstracted. Journals represented in this YEAR BOOK are listed below.

Acta Paediatrica
American Heart Journal
American Journal of Clinical Pathology
American Journal of Hematology
American Journal of Kidney Diseases
American Journal of Medicine
Americal Journal of Obstetrics and Gynecology
American Journal of Physiology
American Journal of Surgery
American Journal of Surgical Pathology
American Surgeon
Annals of Epidemiology
Annals of Internal Medicine
Annals of Surgery
Annals of Thoracic Surgery
Archives of Dermatology
Archives of Disease in Childhood
Archives of Internal Medicine
Archives of Pathology and Laboratory Medicine
Atherosclerosis
Blood
Bone Marrow Transplantation
British Journal of Cancer
British Journal of Surgery
British Medical Journal
Cancer
Cancer Research
Cell
Circulation
Diabete et Metabolisme
Epilepsia
European Journal of Cancer
European Journal of Haematology
Experimental Hematology
Fertility and Sterility
Gut
Hepatology
International Journal of Cancer
International Journal of Epidemiology
Journal of Bone and Joint Surgery (American Volume)
Journal of Bone and Joint Surgery (British Volume)
Journal of Clinical Investigation
Journal of Clinical Oncology
Journal of Clinical Pathology
Journal of Experimental Medicine
Journal of Immunology
Journal of Internal Medicine
Journal of Pediatrics
Journal of Thoracic and Cardiovascular Surgery
Journal of Trauma

Journal of Urology
Journal of the American Academy of Dermatology
Journal of the American Medical Association
Journal of the National Cancer Institute
Lancet
Leukemia
Medicine
Mount Sinai Journal of Medicine (New York)
Nature
New England Journal of Medicine
Obstetrics and Gynecology
Pediatrics
Proceedings of the National Academy of Sciences
Science
Stroke
Surgery, Gynecology and Obstetrics
Thrombosis and Haemostasis
Transfusion
Vox Sanguinis

STANDARD ABBREVIATIONS

The following terms are abbreviated in this edition: acquired immunodeficiency syndrome (AIDS); central nervous system (CNS); colony-forming unit (CFU); colony-stimulating factor (CSF); computed tomography (CT); electrocardiography (ECG); erythropoietin (EPO); granulocyte colony-stimulating factor (G-CSF); granulocyte-macrophage colony-stimulating factor (GM-CSF); human immunodeficiency virus (HIV); human T cell lymphotropic virus (HTLV); interleukin (IL); magnetic resonance (MR) imaging (MRI); polymerase chain reaction (PCR); red blood cell (RBC); von Willebrand factor (vWF); white blood cell (WBC).

Introduction

As I prepare this edition of the YEAR BOOK OF HEMATOLOGY, I am keenly aware of the ancient Chinese imprecation, "May you live in interesting times." Hematologists have recently survived an assault (CLIA 88) on our role, in specific, as laboratory directors, and we can anticipate another attack on a wider front, not only from the presidential task force on health-care reform, but also from the general public, on our role in general as subspecialists. On a more parochial level, I have been informed by one self-proclaimed authority that hematology is a dying subspecialty, while the demise of the "clinical investigator" is a constant lament amongst our academic leadership. I'm not sure that I agree with any of this.

Taking a broader perspective, I think the French were correct: *"Plus ça change, plus c'est la meme chose,"* which, freely translated, means "It's déjà vu all over again." To substantiate this, one need only go back 20 years, at which time there was sufficient government pressure in the form of monetary incentives that a former president of Johns Hopkins University was interested in converting its highly specialized medical institution to a primary-care facility; fortunately, wiser heads prevailed. Along the same lines, it is instructive to compare the geometric volume of the 1972 ASH meeting's abstract book with that of the 1992 edition. The change is fivefold, reflecting an increase in abstract submissions from 371 to 2,139 (and the use of cheaper paper). Indeed, in terms of absolute volume, the 1992 ASH abstract book is only 17% smaller than the greater Baltimore metropolitan area telephone directory. Therefore, I think that not only is hematology a robust subspecialty but, also, that the demise of the clinical investigator is greatly exaggerated.

My confidence in making such statements about hematology in specific and clinical investigation in general derives from having just put together the 1994 edition of the YEAR BOOK OF HEMATOLOGY, in which you will find evidence that clinical investigation is being vigorously and innovatively pursued using all the tools that modern biology can muster. For specific examples, it is appropriate to start with sickle cell anemia, the first "molecular disease." I am impressed with the congruency of clinical research on this disorder. In the 1993 edition, we featured a large prospective study on the natural history of renal disease in sicklers; this year, we learn (Abstract 1–16) that enalapril can reduce proteinuria in some of these patients, and that this might provide a means for preventing progression of the nephropathy. Articles from 1993 and this year (Abstract 1–17) on osteonecrosis and arthroplasty strongly suggest that early detection and aggressive intervention may be more effective than late-stage arthroplasty. Stroke has also received careful scrutiny with the identification of predictive factors (Abstract 1–18), a new noninvasive screening technique (Abstract 1–19), and a modified transfusion protocol (Abstract 1–20). Of course, the most exciting news is the ability of butyrate (Abstract 1–22) to stimulate synthesis of hemoglobin F. This may prove to be an observation of immense clinical importance.

The Cooperative Study of Sickle Disease represents a model of how the careful investigation of the natural history of a disease can improve its clinical management, and Abstract 1-27 serves as such a model for Gaucher's disease. Gene transfer is at the forefront of medical research—not only with respect to its novelty, but also with respect to its therapeutic potential. Given its cost when applicable, it's important to be certain that it has a meaningful role. Abstract 1-27 explodes a number of myths about adult Gaucher's disease and allows one to view the role of various types of therapy in the proper perspective. More such studies of other, similar chronic metabolic disorders are clearly indicated.

The therapeutic indications for recombinant EPO continue to widen with its approval for use in anemic patients with cancer who are receiving chemotherapy. More importantly, recognition that the allogeneic leukocytes acquired by blood transfusion can reactivate latent HIV (Abstract 2-49) means that the hormone has a more important role in the management of anemic HIV-infected patients than previously recognized. It is obvious that the most important role of EPO is to provide the benefits of blood transfusion without transfusing blood. *In this role, it is always cost-effective.* If you doubt this statement, please read the information on the adverse effects of transfusion in the section on Transfusion Medicine, which features articles on transfusion-related graft-vs.-host disease, infection, impaired wound healing, and cancer recurrence.

Other areas of major interest in the Transfusion Medicine section of this year's edition of the YEAR BOOK include the role of leukocyte depletion and autologous transfusion, both preoperatively and intraoperatively. Platelet-activating factor–like activity generated in stored blood (Abstract 5-1) may be responsible for some of the adverse effects of transfusion therapy, and the problem of blood contamination by *Yersinia enterocolitica,* a cold-growing organism, continues to undergo scrutiny (Abstract 5-2). Leukocyte depletion may also influence alloimmunization by platelet concentrates (Abstract 5-15), but its timing is still a matter of debate.

I suspect that low-molecular-weight heparin will displace tissue plasminogen activator as the most scrutinized therapeutic factor in the area of coagulation. Now approved for use in this country, Abstracts 3-48, 3-49, 3-50, and 3-51 suggest that the exact role of this form of heparin is not entirely delineated. In this regard, antithrombin III is also available therapeutically, but its use is now being questioned (Abstract 3-37). Of course, the manner in which we use such standard anticoagulants as heparin (Abstract 3-52) and warfarin (Abstract 3-55) is also changing. Abstract 3-59 suggests that heparin may also be useful in preventing posttransplant veno-occlusive disease.

I was intrigued by the observations that valproate, an old nemesis from the neurosurgical intensive care unit because of its platelet effects, can induce type I von Willebrand's disease (Abstract 3-21), whereas parvovirus B19 in factor VIII concentrates is resistant to viricidal measures

(Abstract 3–24). Finally, splenic irradiation has been resurrected as a treatment for refractory immune thrombocytopenia (Abstract 3–7). The data, as is usual in this situation, are difficult to interpret because the patients were exposed to other therapies.

The treatment options for patients with low-grade lymphoid malignancies have definitely been widened by the approval of fludarabine and 2-deoxychloroadenosine (2-CDA) (Abstracts 4–35, 4–36, and 4–38). Although most reports have been blissful, the number of observed serious, deep-seated infections with opportunistic organisms is troubling, as is the potential for global marrow suppression. *Primum non nocere* should still be the guiding principle here. The prognostic usefulness of β_2-microglobulin has been widened to include adult acute lymphocytic leukemia (Abstract 4–86), whereas the combination of C-reactive protein (a marker for IL-6 production) and β_2-microglobulin appear to be useful in determining disease activity in patients with multiple myeloma (Abstract 4–30).

This year's guest essayist is my colleague Paul Bray, who has written an excellent review on platelet glycoproteins IIb and IIIa. I chose this topic because of the biological importance of the integrins. You will also find 2 related articles in this issue of the YEAR BOOK that deal with the molecular basis of Glanzmann's thrombasthenia (Abstract 3–1) and the management of infants with this disorder at the time of their delivery (Abstract 3–6).

Hematopoietic stem-cell research continues to evolve at a rapid pace, generally at the expense of existing dogma. A particularly exciting example of this phenomenon was the identification of a hematopoietic stem cell capable of reconstituting the hematopoietic progenitor cell compartment and the hematopoietic microenvironment (Abstract 2–1). This may be the hematologic equivalent of astronomy's Big Bang theory for the origin of the universe; for "chicken and egg" purists, evidently the stroma forms first. Additional interesting studies of fetal stem-cell behavior (Abstracts 2–2 and 2–3) suggest ways in which stem cell manipulation in utero might be exploited for gene therapy. I also want to call your attention to studies establishing endogenous growth factor overproduction as a cause of clinical disease (Abstracts 2–14 and 2–19), as well as data concerning the toxicity of G-CSF (Abstract 4–8) and GM-CSF (Abstracts 4–54 and 4–79). The latter observations are particularly sobering.

In closing, I want to note the passing of Dudley Jackson this past December. Hematology has lost a talented and dedicated physician, and many of us a teacher, colleague, and friend. Finally, after 12 years as Chief of Hematology at Johns Hopkins, I have been succeeded by my colleague, Chi Dang. I hope that you will join me in wishing him every success. This year, because of deficiencies in our convention center, you will not have the pleasure of visiting Baltimore. Instead, Saint Louis will be the venue for the annual ASH congregation. To paraphrase the song, I look forward to meeting all of you there.

Jerry L. Spivak, M.D.

1 Red Blood Cells

Introduction

I have been in academic medicine long enough to expect the unexpected, and this year provides no exceptions to my expectations. For example, examination of EPO receptor messenger RNA (mRNA) expression using PCR has revealed the presence of 3 forms of this receptor: soluble, full length, and truncated (Abstract 1-2). The discovery of a soluble form of the EPO receptor was not really unexpected given that other members of the superfamily of hematopoietic growth factor receptors are also expressed in a soluble form. Its function, of course, remains to be identified. The discovery of a truncated form, however, was a surprise, and the possibility that expression of this receptor is developmentally regulated is of great interest. In addition, evidence of constitutive expression of EPO by the testes and the brain with inducible upregulation by hypoxia was also unexpected, at least to me (Abstract 1-3). I have always labored under the notion that EPO was not only a highly conserved protein but also a highly focused one. Because data will be forthcoming showing that neuronal cells express the EPO receptor, a new dimension to this ligand-receptor complex may be introduced. Of course, in addition to hypoxia, EPO production seems to be regulated by various cytokines with IL-1α and β, and transforming growth factor-β and tumor necrosis factor impairing production and IL-6 enhancing it (Abstract 1-4). This probably partially explains the pathogenesis of the anemia associated with chronic infection or inflammatory disorders. I was also intrigued by the observation that hyperviscosity impairs EPO production (Abstract 1-6), because it has long been recognized that erythrocytosis downregulates EPO production even if the red cells cannot deliver oxygen. Clearly, EPO research continues to uncover new and interesting observations.

The molecular basis for hereditary ovalocytosis, a common abnormality in the Far East, has been elucidated by several groups and involves a mutation causing both increased rigidity of the red cell protein band 3 and an associated impairment of its anion transport capacity (Abstract 1-9). Malaria parasites do not like the mutation either, which accounts for its prevalence. A genetic basis for X-linked sideroblastic anemia is also now at hand and involves a mutation that impairs the binding of pyridoxal 5'-phosphate by δ-aminolevulinic acid (Abstract 1-10).

For the sake of our patients, I was pleased to learn that cyclosporine A alone may be as effective as antithymocyte globulin and methylprednisolone in the treatment of severe aplastic anemia, particularly since the latter therapy was associated with a high incidence of fatal infections (Abstract 1–11). For those predisposed to use antithymocyte globulin and methylprednisolone, apparently a low dose is as efficacious as a very high dose, although any dose seems to be accompanied by some toxicity. As usual, anecdotal claims about the effectiveness of various growth factors in the treatment of aplastic anemia keep appearing, but also, as usual, adequate proof for these claims is invariably lacking.

Sickle cell disease occupies more space than usual this year, but more important information about this "old" and enigmatic disease keeps appearing. Importantly, a retrospective study of the natural history of hip arthroplasty (Abstract 1–15) has yielded disappointing results with a high rate of infection and mechanical failure. An acute decrease in hematocrit may be predictive of stroke in young patients (Abstract 1–18), and transcranial ultrasound (Abstract 1–19) may also be predictive of patients at risk for stroke. Furthermore, exchange transfusion can precipitate neurologic events in some patients. Abstract 1–20, which deals with the management of sickle cell pain, should be required reading for everyone who deals with sickle cell patients, and Abstract 1–22, dealing with the use of butyrate to stimulate hemoglobin F synthesis, may represent a real therapeutic breakthrough for the hemoglobinopathies, but obviously larger clinical trials are necessary.

In addition to forementioned, I want to call attention to other important articles on sickle cell disease that, for reasons of space, we could not abstract. As part of the Cooperative Study of Sickle Cell Disease, West et al. (1) have published a steady-state laboratory profile of sickle cell disease that should prove useful clinically. Chen et al. (2) remind us that patients with sickle cell disease can get pernicious anemia, which concomitant folic therapy can mask, and iron overload can be a cause of hypothyroidism (as well as hypoparathyroidism) in patients with sickle cell anemia. In children, sleep apnea–associated hypoxia can complicate sickle cell disease (3).

With better diagnostic reagents, there has been more interest in the evaluation of erythrocytosis, and Abstract 1–24 provides the first evidence for a genetic abnormality linked to the EPO receptor. Finally, I want to bring Abstract 1–27 to your attention because this nice study of the natural history of Gaucher's disease dispels some myths and brings a new perspective to its therapeutic strategies.

Jerry L. Spivak, M.D.

References

1. West MS, et al: *J Clin Epidemiol* 45:893, 1992.
2. Chen MC, et al: *South Med J* 85:215, 1992.
3. Samuels MP, et al: *Arch Dis Child* 67:925, 1992.

Erythropoiesis and Erythropoietin

Changes in Cell Surface Antigen Expressions During Proliferation and Differentiation of Human Erythroid Progenitors

Okumura N, Tsuji K, Nakahata T (Shinshu Univ Hosp; Shinshu Univ School of Medicine, Matsumoto, Japan)

Blood 80:642–650, 1992

1–1

Introduction.—Differentiating hematopoietic cells undergo various functional and structural changes, including differential expression of antigenic determinants. The expression of antigenic determinants on a human erythroid cell lineage was monitored during proliferation and differentiation.

Methods.—Mononuclear cells were obtained from umbilical cord blood samples. After culturing for 24–36 hours, 3,264 individual cells were micromanipulated into secondary culture dishes. From this population of cells, 2,218 cell doublets were obtained and cytochemical and immunologic characterization was initiated. Colonies formed from 1,994 doublets, producing 1,211 erythroid bursts, 133 macrophage, 117 eosinophil, 81 megakaryocyte, 76 neutrophil, 43 basophil, and 333 mixed colonies.

Results.—All paired daughter and granddaughter cells stained positive for acid phosphatase. Most paired daughter cells forming erythroid burst-forming units expressed platelet glycoprotein (GP)IIb (CD41b) and GPIIb/IIIa complexes, but they were negative for GPIIIa (table). These paired daughter cells also immunoreacted with anti–HLA-DR and antitransferrin receptor antibodies. However, they failed to stain for CD34 or CD33. Blood group A antigens and CD36 antigens were first found at the 32–64 cell stage (Fig 1-1). Glycophorin A was first expressed at the 128–256 cell stage, when proerythroblasts were first identified. Hemoglobin-α was the last major protein expressed.

Conclusion.—Various cell surface antigens have been identified that are sequentially expressed during differentiation of erythroid precursors. However, further studies are needed to understand the physiologic significance of these changes.

▶ This article is remarkable not only for the technical excellence required for its successful performance but also for its information. Okumura and colleagues have performed a real service in timing the expression of specific proteins during erythroid cell development. Of particular interest is the observation that erythroid burst-forming units express platelet GPIIb/IIIa, which might reflect their origin from a bipotent progenitor cell, or this GP complex could have a role in erythroid progenitor cell adhesion to the extracellular matrix.—J.L. Spivak, M.D.

Cell Surface Antigen Expression in Descendants of Erythroid Burst-Forming Units

Days in Secondary Culture	No. of Cells	Cell Surface Antigen Expression (%)								
		CD34	CD33	CD41b	HLA-DR	CD71	CD36	GPA	BG-A	HGBα
1	2	0 (23) †	0 (15)	73.9 (23)	83.3 (18)	72.2 (18)	0 (4)	ND	ND	ND
2	4	0 (26)	0 (22)	16.7 (12)	79.2 (24)	95.0 (20)	0 (26)	ND	ND	ND
3	8-16	ND	0 (13)	3.3 (61)	56.3 (32)	100 (25)	0 (7)	ND	ND	ND
4	32-64	ND	ND	0 ± 0‡	2.9 ± 2.2	100 ± 0	90.7 ± 3.3	ND	8.8 ± 9.8	ND
5	80-128	ND	ND	0 ± 0	0 ± 0	100 ± 0	97.2 ± 4.8	0 ± 0	10.0 ± 17.3	0 ± 0
6	128-256	ND	ND	0 ± 0	ND	100 ± 0	96.6 ± 5.9	74.0 ± 21.0	20.8 ± 36.0	0 ± 0
7	>256	ND	ND	0 ± 0	ND	100 ± 0	99.4 ± 1.0	83.7 ± 7.1	18.1 ± 7.8	4.0 ± 6.9
8	>256	ND	ND	0 ± 0	ND	100 ± 0	99.8 ± 0.4	96.7 ± 2.3	40.8 ± 11.2	79.0 ± 9.5
11	>256	ND	ND	0 ± 0	ND	96.7 ± 2.2	84.9 ± 12.3	100 ± 0	84.3 ± 3.1	98.0 ± 2.6
14	>256	ND	ND	0 ± 0	ND	64.2 ± 20.5	55.7 ± 6.4	100 ± 0	82.0 ± 4.4	100 ± 0

* Abbreviations: GPA, glycophorin A; BG-A, blood group A; HGBα, hemoglobin-α; ND, not done.
† Number of cells examined (pooled data).
‡ Mean ± SD of triplicate experiments.
(Courtesy of Okumura N, Tsuji K, Nakahata T: Blood 80:642-650, 1992.)

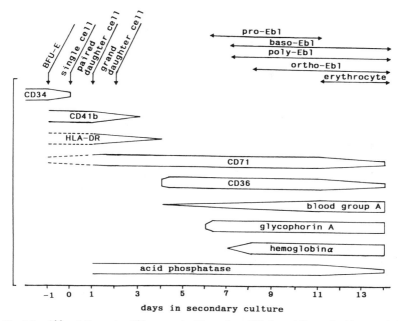

Fig 1–1.—*Abbreviations: pro-Ebl,* proerythroblasts; *baso-Ebl,* basophilic erythroblasts; *poly-Ebl,* polychromatophilic erythroblasts; *ortho-Ebl,* orthochromatic erythroblasts. Schematic representation of cell surface antigen expression in erythroid lineage cells. *Dotted lines* represent the positive HLA-DR and CD71 antigens on erythroid burst-forming units previously reported. (Courtesy of Okumura N, Tsuji K, Nakahata T: *Blood* 80:642–650, 1992.)

A Truncated Erythropoietin Receptor That Fails to Prevent Programmed Cell Death of Erythroid Cells

Nakamura Y, Komatsu N, Nakauchi H (Inst of Physical and Chemical Research, Koyadai, Tsukuba, Japan)
Science 257:1138–1141, 1992   1–2

Background.—Erythropoietin influences erythroid progenitors in the bone marrow through binding to an EPO receptor (EPOR). Three forms of EPOR have been discovered, 2 of them isolated by screening a complementary DNA library from an EPO-dependent megakaryoblastoid cell line. One of these forms represents full-length receptor (EPOR-F) identical to that isolated from erythroid and liver cell lines. The other is a soluble form of receptor lacking the transmembrane and cytoplasmic portions. A third form of receptor resulted from replicating messenger RNAs from normal human bone marrow mononuclear cells in the reverse transcriptase PCR. It lacks most of the cytoplasmic region because of alternative splicing. The truncated form of receptor is termed EPOR-T.

Receptor Function.—Erythropoietin receptor-T was found to be the most prevalent receptor form in early-stage erythroid progenitors, whereas EPOR-F was the most prevalent form in late-stage progenitor cells. Erythropoietin receptor-T is able to transduce a mitogenic signal, but cells transfected with the truncated form of receptor were more likely to undergo programmed cell death than those that expressed EPOR-F. In the presence of excess EPO, the transfectants proliferated equally.

Interpretation.—Erythroid progenitor cells in different stages respond differently to EPO. Most early-stage cells expressing EPOR-T may die of apoptosis, whereas late-stage progenitors expressing EPOR-F may live and differentiate into mature erythrocytes. This mechanism may ensure a large reservoir of late-stage progenitors that can be rapidly mobilized in the event of sudden bleeding or hypoxia.

▶ Ah, the magic of PCR! This interesting article excellently illustrates how research can advance our knowledge unexpectedly. As the authors note, the EPOR was initially cloned by Alan D'Andrea from a murine erythroleukemia cell line. Because the genomic EPOR isolated from human cells was similar to that cloned from this transformed mouse cell line, it was tacitly assumed that there was a single form of the receptor. However, in screening a complementary DNA library from a megakaryoblastoid cell line, Nakamura et al. identified not only the expected full-length receptor but also a soluble form of the receptor lacking the transmembrane and cytoplasmic domain. This in itself, although interesting, is not surprising because other members of the hematopoietic growth factor receptor superfamily also have soluble forms, for example, G-CSF, IL-6, and stem cell factor. The physiologic significance of these soluble receptors is still under scrutiny, although the soluble IL-6 receptor is capable of activating its target cells after binding to its ligand. More importantly, using reverse transcriptase PCR on messenger RNA from normal human marrow cells, the authors unexpectedly discovered a third form of the EPOR. This receptor, thanks to a 95–base pair insert that contains a stop codon, has only 56 amino acids, plus those encoded by the insert, and is missing the additional 200 amino acids that compose the cytoplasmic domain of the full-length receptor.

In screening early and late marrow progenitors, the truncated receptor was most abundant in the former. Additionally, this receptor apparently is less sensitive to EPO, and at low concentrations of the hormone, cells primarily expressing the truncated receptor are subject to apoptosis (programmed cell death).

These are exciting observations because they provide an efficient mechanism for the control of erythropoiesis. It is implied that normally, at the low concentrations of the hormone present in the plasma, most of the earliest erythroid progenitor cells will not propagate, but with hypoxia and elevated EPO levels, this early progenitor cell pool will proliferate, expanding the total erythroid progenitor cell population. However, there are some caveats to all this. First, the astute reader will note that Okumura et al. (Abstract 1–1) indicate that CD34+ was not necessarily synonymous with erythroid differentiation, so it is not totally established that only, or even any early, erythroid progenitors express the truncated receptor. Second, it is unclear why the truncated receptor, if it has the same affinity as the normal full-length receptor and is present in the same copy number, is able to function more efficiently only at higher concentrations of EPO. Because the only in vitro studies were done with a transfected IL-3–dependent cell line and not normal cells, these questions remain unanswered.

This research reminds us to take nothing for granted. Transformed cell lines play a crucial role in basic research, but, eventually, observations made with these cells must be tested in normal cells.—J.L. Spivak, M.D.

Feedback Modulation of Renal and Hepatic Erythropoietin mRNA in Response to Graded Anemia and Hypoxia

Tan CC, Eckardt K-U, Firth JD, Ratcliffe PJ (John Radcliffe Hosp, Oxford, England; Univ of Regensburg, Germany)
Am J Physiol 263:474F–481F, 1992   1–3

Background.—In normal conditions, the kidney is the major source of EPO. However, previous studies have shown that other organs (e.g., the liver) may also contribute significant amounts of EPO during anemia or hypoxia. This regulation of EPO production is achieved through control of EPO messenger RNA (mRNA). The levels of EPO mRNA in rats subjected to normobaric hypoxia or hemorrhagic anemia were examined.

Methods.—Messenger RNA levels were measured in adult male Sprague-Dawley rats using radiolabeled probes in a ribonuclease protection assay. Levels of RNA were visualized on polyacrylamide gels, and the RNA bands were then counted in a liquid scintillation counter. The rats were exposed to graded levels of hypoxia consisting of 14%, 11%, 9%, or 7.5% oxygen. Other experimental groups were venesected of 10.5, 8, 5, or 2.5 mL of blood, which was replaced with normal saline.

Results.—Significant amounts of EPO mRNA were detected in the kidney and testes, and lesser amounts were found in the lung, liver, and brain of unstimulated rats (table). However, no mRNA was found in the small or large intestine, stomach, muscle, salivary gland, or bone marrow of unstimulated rats. After exposure to severe hypoxia, hepatic and renal mRNA levels increased by 200-fold. At 11% oxygen, the liver contributed only 2% of total EPO mRNA, but at 7.5% oxygen, the liver supplied 33% of the total mRNA. The liver also played a significant role in the anemic response, contributing 18% of the mRNA when 2.5 mL of blood was removed and increasing to 37% after venesection of 10.5 mL of blood.

Conclusion.—The liver is the major extrarenal source of EPO during hypoxic stimulation; contributions by other organs are insignificant. Fur-

Quantitation of EPO mRNA by Liquid Scintillation Counting in Unstimulated Animals

Organ	Rat	EPO mRNA Band		Average Background		d	Net EPO mRNA, ccpm	EPO mRNA/μg Total RNA, $\times 10^{-4}$	Total Organ RNA, μg	Total Organ EPO mRNA
		Raw count	ccpm	Raw count	ccpm					
Kidney	1	1,101	23.6	263	5.7	23.0	17.9	1.2	3,700	0.4
	2	1,631	35.3	383	8.3	27.8	27.0	1.8	3,740	0.7
	3	710	15.2	263	5.7	14.3	9.5	0.7	3,800	0.3
	4	810	17.6	342	7.4	13.8	10.2	0.7	4,040	0.3
	5	1,820	39.4	295	6.4	33.2	33.0	2.2	3,680	0.8
	6	1,271	27.5	291	6.3	24.8	21.2	1.3	3,800	0.5
Liver	1	287	6.2	253	5.5	1.5	NQ		45,200	NQ
	2	281	6.1	262	5.7	0.8	NQ		34,000	NQ
	3	254	5.5	268	5.8		NQ		44,030	NQ
	4	334	7.2	288	6.2	1.8	NQ		42,540	NQ
	5	294	6.4	277	6.0	0.7	NQ		41,850	NQ
	6	324	7.0	311	6.7	0.5	NQ		40,730	NQ
Testes	4	541	21.4	322	12.8	7.5	8.6	0.4	4,250	0.16
	5	565	22.3	305	12.2	8.8	10.1	0.4	3,900	0.17
	6	415	16.4	253	10.2	6.3	6.2	0.3	4,400	0.13

Abbreviation: NQ, not quantifiable by scintillation counting.

Note: Counting was performed for 3,600 seconds for each sample (raw count), allowing computation of corrected counts obtained per minute (*ccpm*), corrected for the half-life of decay of ^{32}P calculated from activity date of radioactivity used for labeling the riboprobe. Average background values were obtained from the average counts of gel fragments excised from above and below protected EPO mRNA band. $d = (c_1 - c_2) \div \sqrt{(c_1 - c_2)}$, where c_1 and c_2 are the raw counts for sample and background, respectively; values of $d > 1.96$ indicate statistically significant difference at a 95% confidence level. After subtraction of background, net EPO mRNA levels (ccpm) were divided by the quantity of total RNA analyzed, and the value is expressed relative to the EPO mRNA count in the external standard for the corresponding gel, which was assigned an arbitrary value of 1.

(Courtesy of Tan CC, Eckardt K-U, Firth JD, et al: *Am J Physiol* 263:474F–481F, 1992.)

thermore, the liver responds to the whole physiologic range of hemorrhagic anemia (at least in the rat).

▶ Harry Truman defined an expert as someone who does not want to learn anything new because he would no longer be an expert. Anyone who studies the biology of EPO, as this abstract indicates, can never afford to be an expert. Tan et al. used a ribonuclease protection assay to measure the relative contributions of the liver and kidneys with respect to EPO mRNA levels in response to hypoxia. Interestingly, when this technique was applied to other tissues, both the testes and brain constitutively expressed EPO mRNA that could be upregulated by hypoxia. The authors have made similar observations with respect to the lung and spleen. Whether there is a common cell type shared amongst these organs similar to the EPO-producing interstitial cell of the liver and kidneys is unknown. Nor is it clear what local trophic functions EPO might have outside the bone marrow.—J.L. Spivak, M.D.

Effect of Inflammatory Cytokines on Hypoxia-Induced Erythropoietin Production

Faquin WC, Schneider TJ, Goldberg MA (Brigham and Women's Hosp, Boston)
Blood 79:1987–1994, 1992   1–4

Background.—Serum EPO levels often are reduced in patients with various infectious, inflammatory, and malignant conditions, and recombinant human EPO is able to partially or completely correct anemia in patients whose EPO response is blunted. Some inflammatory cytokines are produced in disorders associated with anemia of chronic disease. These factors may, in turn, suppress the bone marrow response to EPO and, thereby, contribute to anemia.

Objective and Methods.—The effects of several inflammatory cytokines of EPO production were examined using the human hepatoma (Hep3B) cell line, which regulates EPO production physiologically in response to hypoxia. The cytokines studied included IL-1α, IL-1β, and IL-6; transforming growth factor-β; and tumor necrosis factor-α (TNF-α).

Findings.—Hypoxia-induced EPO production was inhibited by as much as 89% in a dose-dependent manner, by IL-1α, IL-1β, and TNF-α (Fig 1–2). In contrast, IL-6 promoted EPO production by hypoxically stimulated cells (Fig 1–3). In combination, the effects of the cytokines were approximately additive. The reduced EPO production seen with IL-1α and TNF-α in combination was reversed by IL-6. Exposure of Hep3B cells to either IL-1α or TNF-α reduced levels of EPO messenger RNA.

Conclusion.—Inflammatory cytokines may influence EPO production in vivo and, thereby, have a significant role in the development of ane-

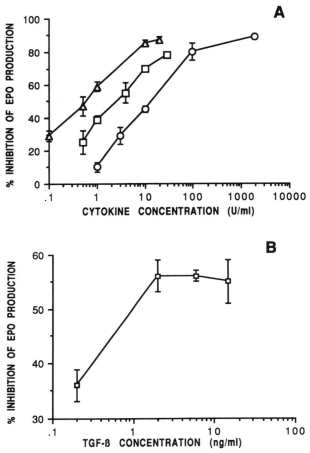

Fig 1–2.—Dose-response inhibition of hypoxia-induced EPO production by IL-1α, IL-1β, TNF-α, and transforming growth factor-β (TGF-β). Hep3B cells were grown to confluency in 100-mm tissue culture dishes and incubated under hypoxic conditions (1% oxygen) for 24 hours in triplicate with varying concentrations of (**A**) IL-1α (*square*), IL-1β (*triangle*), TNF-α (*circle*), or (**B**) TGF-β. At the conclusion of each experiment, the culture medium was collected and stored at −70°C until assayed in duplicate by radioimmunoassay for EPO. Values shown represent the mean percentage inhibition of hypoxia-induced EPO production ± 1 SD. (Courtesy of Faquin WC, Schneider TJ, Goldberg MA: *Blood* 79:1987–1994, 1992.)

mia in chronically ill patients. The mechanisms involved are uncertain, but cytokines could alter EPO messenger RNA levels at several points in the regulatory pathway. The levels of cytokines that inhibit stimulated EPO production in vitro are within the range of plasma levels described in several chronic disorders.

▶ It is well established that the production of EPO is blunted in the presence of inflammatory, infectious, or neoplastic disorders. The mechanism for this

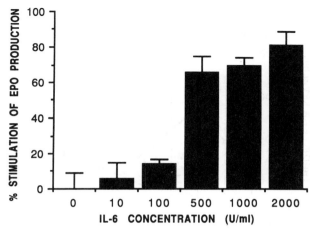

Fig 1–3.—Dose-response stimulation of hypoxia-induced EPO production by IL-6. Confluent 100-mm plates of Hep3B cells were incubated in triplicate for 24 hours with hypoxic conditions and varying concentrations of IL-6. Culture media was collected and assayed in duplicate by radioimmunoassay for EPO. Values represent the mean percentage stimulation of hypoxia-induced EPO production more than that produced by hypoxia alone ± 1 SD. (Courtesy of Faquin WC, Schneider TJ, Goldberg MA: *Blood* 79:1987–1994, 1992.)

was obscure but not likely a consequence of an enhanced clearance of EPO, because with sufficient hypoxia, patients with cancer, for example, can make substantial quantities of EPO. Now, using an oxygen-sensitive, EPO-producing hepatocyte cell line, Faquin and his colleagues have demonstrated that certain inflammatory cytokines selectively depress EPO production by inhibiting expression of EPO messenger RNA. Interestingly, IL-6, an acute-phase reactant, enhanced EPO production and could antagonize the inhibitory effects of IL-1 and TNF-α. Similar data have been obtained by Jelkman et al. (1), implicating TNF-α but not gamma-interferon. Importantly, the concentrations of the cytokines active in vitro were similar to those achieved in vivo. The overlapping and antagonistic effects of the inflammatory cytokines suggest that the network of signals involved in influencing EPO production is complex because, in vivo, these cytokines also influence the production of other inflammatory mediators.—J.L. Spivak, M.D.

Reference

1. Jelkman W, et al: *Contrib Nephrol* 87:68, 1990.

Impaired Erythropoietin Response to Anemia After Bone Marrow Transplantation

Miller CB, Jones RJ, Zahurak ML, Piantadosi S, Burns WH, Santos GW, Spivak JL (Johns Hopkins Univ, Baltimore, Md)
Blood 80:2677–2682, 1992   1–5

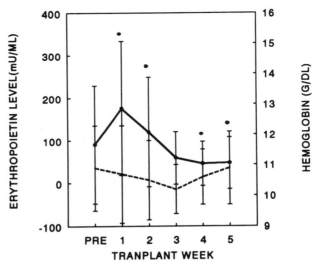

Fig 1–4.—Summary of mean ± SD EPO (*solid line*) and hemoglobin (*dashed line*) levels in the patients with BMT over time. *Asterisk* indicates EPO-hemoglobin ratios that were significantly different from pretransplant ratios. (Courtesy of Miller CB, Jones RJ, Zahurak ML, et al: *Blood* 80:2677–2682, 1992.)

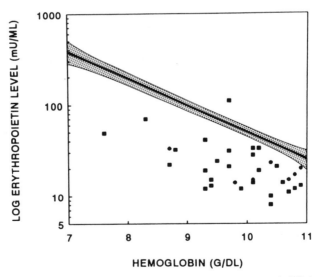

Fig 1–5.—Relationship of EPO/hemoglobin in anemic patients at 6-month (*filled circles*) and 12-month (*filled squares*) follow-up visits compared with EPO/hemoglobin relationship in iron-deficient patients represented by the *shaded area*. (Courtesy of Miller CB, Jones RJ, Zahurak ML, et al: *Blood* 80:2677–2682, 1992.)

Background.—All bone marrow transplant (BMT) patients require blood transfusion for anemia. Persistent anemia, lasting for as long as a year, is common among these patients. This anemia may be caused by depressed EPO levels. However, previous studies have reported conflicting findings regarding EPO levels after BMT. The EPO response in patients receiving a BMT was compared with the response of those with iron deficiency anemia.

Patients and Methods.—Seventy patients who had undergone autologous or allogenic BMT and 28 patients with uncomplicated iron deficiency anemia were examined. Blood samples were obtained from the BMT patients before transplant, weekly post-transplant until discharge, and at 6- and 12-month follow-ups. The EPO levels were monitored by radioimmunoassay. Renal function was assessed by measuring serum bilirubin and creatine levels.

Results.—Elevated EPO levels correlated with the degree of anemia 1 to 2 weeks after BMT, but by the estimated time of marrow recovery (weeks 4 and 5), they had become significantly suppressed (Fig 1–4). No differences in EPO response were found among those patients receiving an autologous or allogenic BMT, although those who had graft-vs.-host disease (GVHD) experienced a more severe depression in serum EPO. However, 6-month examinations showed that autologous BMT patients were less likely to be anemic. None of the patients with autologous BMT who were examined at the 12-month follow-up were anemic. All patients with BMT who were anemic at the 6- or 12- month follow-ups displayed a depressed EPO response (Fig 1–5). The EPO levels in these anemic patients were not related to the type of graft, GVHD, or renal function.

Conclusion.—The prolonged anemia found in autologous and allogenic patients with BMT may be caused by an inadequate EPO response. Because the delayed erythroid recovery after BMT is associated with inadequate EPO, exogenous EPO administration may prove to be as beneficial in these as in other anemic patients.

▶ Serum EPO levels before and after BMT have been examined by a number of investigators, and this large study confirms that the EPO response to anemia in patients undergoing allogeneic BMT is often inadequate and remains so for as long as 12 months. The mechanisms for this are unexplained, but obvious candidates include subclinical renal dysfunction, drugs (cyclosporine, amphotericin B), infection, and GVHD. In this study, acute GVHD but not chronic GVHD or cytomegalovirus infection could be implicated in reducing EPO production in allogeneic BMT; however, at least in autologous BMT, cyclosporine A could not. Importantly, when the bilirubin was greater than 2 mg/dL, an inappropriately high EPO level was observed. The association between anemia and impaired production of EPO post-BMT provides a correctable mechanism for the anemia, and recent studies (1) using recombinant human EPO indicate that the hormone can enhance the rate of red cell engraftment and reduce the transfusion requirement without perturbing the recovery of platelets or leukocytes (so much for the concept of stem cell competition). Recombinant EPO may also be useful in avoiding allogeneic transfusion in marrow donors, particularly children (2). —J.L. Spivak, M.D.

References

1. Steegmann JL, et al: *Bone Marrow Transplant* 10:541, 1992.
2. York A, et al: *Bone Marrow Transplant* 10:415, 1992.

Increased Plasma Viscosity as a Reason for Inappropriate Erythropoietin Formation

Singh A, Eckardt KU, Zimmermann A, Götz KH, Hamann M, Ratcliffe PJ, Kurtz A, Reinhart WH (Univ of Bern, Switzerland; Univ of Regensburg, Germany; John Radcliff Hosp, Oxford, England)

J Clin Invest 91:251–256, 1992   1–6

Introduction.—Patients with multiple myeloma and Waldenström's disease often have concurrent anemia. Recent studies have demonstrated that these patients have low EPO levels, which improve with administration of recombinant human EPO. The relationship between production of EPO and plasma viscosity or renal function in anemic individuals with hypergammaglobulinemias was determined. The effect of plasma viscosity on EPO formation was also assessed in rats.

Patients and Methods.—Patients with verified cases of monoclonal paraproteinemia without any major renal function impairment or chronic inflammatory disease participated in the study to determine

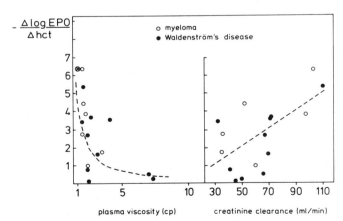

Fig 1–6.—**Left,** relationship between plasma viscosity and EPO response in patients with multiple myelomas and Waldenström's disease. The *dashed line* represents regression line. The **symbol with a cross** represents a value for nonrenal anemias. **Right,** the relationship between creatinine clearance and EPO response in patients with multiple myelomas and Waldenström's disease. (Courtesy of Singh A, Eckardt KU, Zimmerman A, et al: *J Clin Invest* 91:251-256, 1992.)

whether a low EPO production rate could be related to the hyperviscosity associated with multiple myeloma or Waldenström's disease. Sixteen patients with anemia and monoclonal paraproteinemia were studied. Their EPO levels ranged from 15 to 246 mU/mL. Blood exchange experiments in rats also were conducted to further elucidate the relationship between plasma viscosity and EPO production.

Results.—Those patients with the highest EPO levels had the most bone marrow failure. Initially, the plasma EPO levels seemed relatively low. The EPO response correlated with the plasma viscosity and creatinine clearance value (Fig 1–6). In the rats, EPO production was stimulated by a sharp decrease of the hemoglobin levels through exchange transfusion. Increasing the gamma-globulin level to approximately 40 mg/mL of plasma in the animals blocked the increase in serum EPO levels, although the hematocrit decreased by 20%. The reductions in serum EPO levels at higher plasma viscosities were associated with a reduction in the renal EPO messenger RNA levels.

Conclusion.—Plasma viscosity may significantly inhibit the production of EPO. The raised plama viscosity of patients with hypergammaglobulinemia appears to decrease the EPO response to anemia. Clinically, administering EPO to patients with low EPO levels could be dangerous unless the hyperviscosity that produced the low EPO level is corrected.

▶ This important study documents that hyperviscosity can blunt hypoxia-induced EPO production. This is a key observation from a clinical perspective because raising the hematocrit in the presence of plasma hyperviscosity would be dangerous. Anemia is actually beneficial in this instance. Of course, this would also be more true of blood transfusions than therapy with recombinant EPO because the effect on blood viscosity would be more immediate.

The reported observations have a wider significance because they corroborate important early work by Kilbridge et al. (1) showing that erythrocytosis, whether absolute or relative, also blunts EPO production. This is true even when the blood is incapable of carrying oxygen. Indeed, this type of behavior could be considered a paradigm for EPO production. That is to say, the body assiduously attempts to down-regulate production of this hormone even in the presence of hypoxia. The important corollary is that serum EPO is usually within the range of normal in patients with secondary erythrocytosis because erythrocytosis, in addition to the other complementary mechanisms for alleviating tissue hypoxia, suppresses EPO synthesis. For example, patients with polycythemia vera have very low EPO levels because of feedback inhibition by the high red cell mass. Because the normal range for serum EPO is wide (4–26 mU/mL), it is possible for the EPO level to be within the normal range but still be high for that individual. Without a premorbid baseline level, this, of course, cannot be known. It is known, however, that most patients with compensated hypoxia, whether secondary to cyanotic heart disease or pulmonary disease, have a "normal" serum EPO level caused by the nonspecific suppression by a high blood viscosity. Thus, the serum EPO level is often not a helpful guide to the cause of erythrocytosis. Of interest in this regard is that patients with compensated hypoxia, if phlebotomized, will elevate their serum EPO level to a greater degree for a given hematocrit than will a normal individual. Therefore, in these individuals, the capacity to produce EPO is apparently increased while the threshold for the initiation of its synthesis has also increased.—J.L. Spivak, M.D.

Reference

1. Kilbridge TM, et al: *Blood* 33:104–113, 1969.

Recombinant Human Erythropoietin in the Treatment of Anemia Associated With Human Immunodeficiency Virus (HIV) Infection and Zidovudine Therapy: Overview of Four Clinical Trials

Henry DH, Beall GN, Benson CA, Carey J, Cone LA, Eron LJ, Fiala M, Fischl MA, Gabin SJ, Gottlieb MS, Galpin JE, Groopman JE, Hooton TM, Jemsek JG, Levine RL, Miles SA, Rinehart JJ, Rios A, Robbins WJ, Ruckdeschel JC, Smith JA, Spruance SL, Starrett B, Toney J, Zalusky R, Abels RI, Bryant, EC, Larholt KM, Sampson AR, Rudnick SA (Tuttleman Ctr, Philadelphia; Harbor-Univ of California, Los Angeles Med Ctr, Torrance; Chicago; et al)
Ann Intern Med 117:739–748, 1992   1–7

Background.—Patients with AIDS frequently have anemia, a complication that can be further aggravated by zidovudine therapy. Although transfusions may temporarily alleviate the symptoms, additional infections, transfusion reactions, or depression of the immune system may result. The use of recombinant human (r-Hu) EPO in the treatment of patients with anemia and AIDS was evaluated.

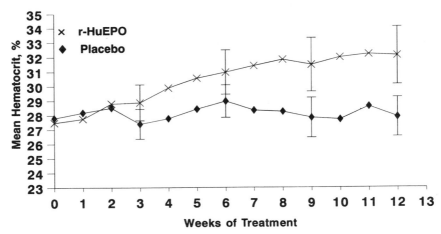

Fig 1–7.—*Abbreviation: r-HuEPO,* recombinant human EPO. Mean weekly hematocrit for patients with EPO levels less than or equal to 500 IU/L. *Bars* represent 95% confidence intervals. (Courtesy of Henry DH, Beall GN, Benson CA, et al: *Ann Intern Med* 117:739–748, 1992.)

Methods.—A total of 255 patients with stable anemia and AIDS receiving zidovudine completed this 12-week study. Patients received either a placebo or 100–200 units/kg body weight of r-HuEPO 3 times a week for as long as 12 weeks.

Results.—One hundred seventy-seven patients (69%) entering the study had low EPO levels ($\leq$ 500 IU/L). The administration of r-HuEPO increased their mean hematocrit level by 3.9%, compared with a .5% increase seen in those receiving the placebo (Fig 1–7). This resulted in a decreased number of blood units transfused to those patients given r-HuEPO (3.2 units per patient compared with 5.3 units per patient for those receiving placebo). Additionally, 21 (43%) of the patients receiving r-HuEPO no longer needed transfusions, compared with 8 (18%) of the patients treated with the placebo. In contrast, treatment with r-HuEPO did not alter any of these variables in patients who entered the study with higher endogenous EPO levels.

Conclusion.—Treatment with r-HuEPO is safe and may increase the mean hematocrit level in those patients with anemia, AIDS, and low endogenous EPO levels. An initial administration of 100 units/kg body weight, intravenously or subcutaneously, 3 times a week, is recommended.

▶ This study nicely summarizes 4 clinical trials of r-HuEPO in patients with HIV infection taking zidovudine. For unknown reasons, zidovudine increases EPO production in patients with HIV infection and also causes macrocytosis. Although some studies suggest only a subset of patients have this develop, in our studies, the mean corpuscular volume increased approximately 10 fL in every patient taking zidovudine. Obviously, the development of absolute macrocytosis will depend entirely on the initial mean corpuscular volume. More important, in a subset of patients, zidovudine increased serum EPO above 500 mU/mL, and these patients failed to respond to exogenous EPO. Thus, the serum EPO level can serve as a marker in this population for patients with anemia most likely to respond to the hormone. The role of EPO therapy here is not to restore the hematocrit to normal but rather to reduce or abolish the need for blood transfusions, which can be deleterious in these patients. I would, however, part with the authors on their proposed starting dose of 100 units/kg because their data suggest 150–200 units/kg is more effective.—J.L. Spivak, M.D.

Enhancement of Erythropoiesis by Recombinant Human Erythropoietin in Low Birth Weight Infants: A Pilot Study
Shannon KM, Mentzer WC, Abels RI, Wertz M, Thayer-Moriyama J, Li WY, Thompson D, Decelle S, Phibbs RH (Univ of California, San Francisco; US Naval Hosp, Oakland, Calif; RW Johnson Pharmaceutical Research Inst, Raritan, NJ)
J Pediatr 120:586–592, 1992   1–8

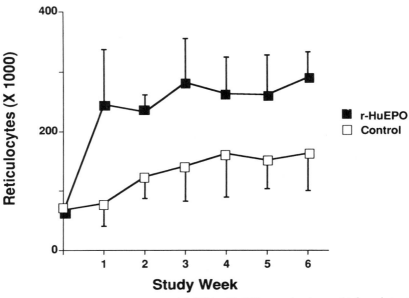

Fig 1–8.—Absolute reticulocyte counts (± SD) in r-HuEPO–treated and control infants during trial. (Courtesy of Shannon KM, Mentzer WC, Abels RI, et al: *J Pediatr* 120:586–592, 1992.)

Background.—The inadequate production of EPO is an important contributing factor to the anemia of prematurity. Some evidence suggests that treatment with recombinant human EPO (r-HuEPO) may prevent this anemia. The use of r-HuEPO in anemic premature infants was examined.

Patients and Methods.—Four of 8 symptom-free premature infants with birth weights of 1,250 g or less who were at high risk of requiring erythrocyte transfusions for anemia were randomly allocated to 6 weeks of intensive treatment with subcutaneous r-HuEPO, and 4 received placebo. The initial dosage of r-HuEPO was 100 units/kg/day, 5 days a week. If the target reticulocyte count was not achieved after 2 or 3 weeks, the r-HuEPO dosage was increased to 200 units/kg/day. All infants were given supplemental oral iron therapy starting at 3 mg/kg/day given in 3 divided doses. The iron dosage was increased to 6 mg/kg/day, as tolerated.

Results.—The 4 infants assigned to r-HuEPO therapy had higher reticulocyte counts during treatment and higher hematocrit values at the end of therapy than the 4 infants assigned to placebo (Fig 1–8). The treatment was well tolerated and there were no adverse events. One of 4 r-HuEPO–treated infants, and 3 of 4 placebo-treated infants required blood transfusions. The total volume of blood given was 17 mL for r-HuEPO–treated infants and 101 mL for placebo-treated infants.

Conclusion.—Recombinant human EPO stimulated endogenous erythropoiesis in premature infants who received supplemental oral iron therapy in this small study. The enhanced rate of erythropoiesis in r-HuEPO–treated infants lowered the need for blood transfusion.

▶ Anemic, premature infants have the lowest serum EPO levels of any group we have studied. Because these infants have a full complement of EPO-responsive erythroid progenitor cells, they seemed to be an ideal group to receive recombinant EPO to prevent the need for red cell transfusions with their attendant risks. However, this intuitively obvious proposition has been difficult to prove. This report by Shannon et al., as well as a recent study by Carnielli et al. (1), provides an additional impetus for a large-scale, blinded clinical trial in which factors such as birth weight, phlebotomy requirements, iron stores, and caloric intake can be controlled. Such a study might also confirm or refute the concept of stem cell competition with respect to erythropoiesis and granulopoiesis in this patient population.—J.L. Spivak, M.D.

Reference

1. Carnielli V, et al: *J Pediatr* 121:98, 1992.

Hemolytic Anemia

Molecular Basis for Membrane Rigidity of Hereditary Ovalocytosis: A Novel Mechanism Involving the Cytoplasmic Domain of Band 3

Mohandas N, Winardi R, Knowles D, Leung A, Parra M, George E, Conboy J, Chasis J (Univ of California, Berkeley; Univ of British Columbia, Vancouver; Universiti Kebangsaan Malaysia, Kuala Lumpur)

J Clin Invest 89:686–692, 1992   1–9

Background.—Hereditary ovalocytosis is an erythrocytic disorder in which cell membrane rigidity is markedly increased and the cells resist invasion by malarial parasites. The disorder is prevalent in several ethnic groups in Southeast Asia. The linkage between the ovalocytic phenotype and a structural polymorphism in the band 3 protein, the red cell anion transporter, has been described.

Objective.—An attempt was made to define the mutation in the band 3 gene in several Malayan subjects and to establish its biophysical effects.

Findings.—All 6 Malayans studied who had the ovalocytic phenotype were heterozygous for a band 3 deletional mutation. Amino acids 400–408 are deleted in the boundary between the cytoplasmic and the first transmembrane domains of band 3 (Fig 1–9). A reduction in the lateral mobility of band 3 resulted and, in turn, increased the extensional rigidity of the red cell membrane. A much higher membrane tension was required to aspirate an equivalent cell length of ovalocyte, compared

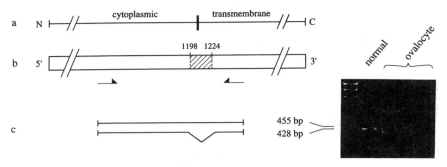

Fig 1–9.—Scheme for band 3 messenger RNA analysis by PCR. **A,** schematic model of band 3 protein indicating the location of cytoplasmic and first transmembrane domain. **B,** model of band 3 complementary DNA (cDNA). *Arrow* indicates the location of primer set (p5-p6) used in PCR to define the deletion in mutant cDNA. *Hatched area* represents the location of the deletion identified in mutant cDNA from ovalocytes. **C,** polyacrylamide gel electrophoresis of amplified DNA products. The larger 455-bp band represents the normal allele and the smaller 428-bp band represents the mutant allele. Two higher molecular weight bands seen in ovalocytes represent heteroduplexes. The molecular weight marker is HaeIII-digested ϕX174 DNA. (Courtesy of Mohandas N, Winardi R, Knowles D, et al: *J Clin Invest* 89:686–692, 1992.)

with normal red cell, into a pipette. The ability of the ovalocytic red cell membrane to undergo truly elastic deformation was compromised.

An Explanation.—The deletion of 9 amino acids from the boundary between the cytoplasm and transmembrane domains of band 3 produces a conformational change in the cytoplasmic domain, which markedly increases its association with the skeletal protein network. As a result, spectrin tetramers are less well able to uncoil and extend during induced deformation (Fig 1–10).

▶ This article defines the molecular basis for red cell membrane rigidity in hereditary ovalocytosis and establishes the principle that interactions between intergral membrane proteins and the cytoskeleton can have important implications for red cell membrane behavior. In this instance, a loss of 9 amino acids in a highly conserved region between the cytoplasmic and transmembrane domains of the red cell anion transporter, band 3, produced a change in the conformation of its cytoplasmic domain that interfered with the normal movement of spectrin tetramers and also inhibited the lateral mobility of band 3. In addition, the abnormal band 3 protein also lacks anion transport acitivty (1). In one sense, this has proved to be a "useful" mutation because the increase in membrane rigidity and impaired anion transport result in resistance to invasion by malaria parasites.—J.L. Spivak, M.D.

Reference

1. Schofield AE, et al: *Nature* 355:836, 1992.

A

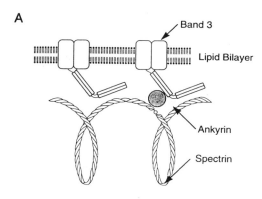

B

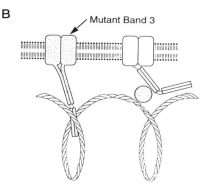

Fig 1–10.—Model for role of cytoplasmic domain of band 3 in regulating membrane extensional rigidity. Conformation of the cytoplasmic domain of normal band 3 (**A**) offers little resistance to the extension of spectrin tetramers during membrane deformation. In contrast, the conformationally altered cytoplasmic domain of mutant band 3 (**B**), by getting entangled in the spectrin network, sterically hinders the extension of spectrin tetramers. For reasons of clarity, all the individual components of the skeletal network have not been delineated. (Courtesy of Mohandas N, Winardi R, Knowles D, et al: *J Clin Invest* 89:686–692, 1992.)

Sideroblastic Anemia

Enzymatic Defect in "X-Linked" Sideroblastic Anemia: Molecular Evidence for Erythroid δ-Aminolevulinate Synthase Deficiency

Cotter PD, Baumann M, Bishop DF (Mount Sinai School of Medicine, New York; Frankenhaus Spaudau, Berlin)

Proc Natl Acad Sci USA 89:4028–4032, 1992   1–10

Introduction.—The human gene encoding erythroid-specific δ-aminolevulinate synthase (ALAS) was localized to the chromosomal region Xp21–Xq21. This assignment suggested that the gene might express the enzymatic defect responsible for "X-linked" sideroblastic anemia (XLSA). The erythroid (ALAS2) coding regions were amplified and se-

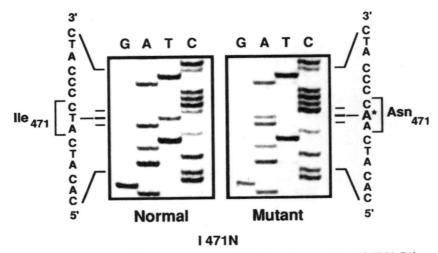

I 471N

Fig 1–11.—Exon 9 nucleotide sequence in region of 1471N mutation in patient with XLSA. Dideoxy-nucleotide sequencing was conducted with ^{35}S-labeled dATP and exon 9 DNA was amplified and sub-cloned from a normal person and from the proband. Normal and mutant reaction products were electrophoresed on .4-mm thick 8% polyacrylamide/7 M urea sequencing gels and autoradiographed by using Kodak X-Omat AR film. (Courtesy of Cotter PD, Baumann M, Bishop DF: *Proc Natl Acad Sci USA* 89:4028–4032, 1992.)

quenced from a man with pyroxidine-responsive XLSA to examine this association.

Observations.—The patient was a Chinese man aged 30 years with the classic phenotype of XLSA, including microcytic, hypochromic anemia with abundant ringed sideroblasts in the marrow; marked anisocytosis and poikilocytosis; broadened and flattened osmotic curve; iron overload with beginning hemosiderosis; and moderate hypersplenism. Treatment with pyroxidine, 300 mg/day subcutaneously, resulted in complete disappearance of pathologic marrow cells. The 11 exonic coding regions of the ALAS gene in this patient were amplified and sequenced. There was a single T→A transition in codon 471 in a highly conserved region of exon 9, which resulted in an isoleucine→ asparagine substitution, designated as I471N (Fig 1–11). Contiguous hydrophobic residues were interrupted by this mutation, which was predicted to transform a region of β-sheet structure to a random-coil structure. The mutant construct expressed low levels of enzymatic activity on prokaryotic expression of normal and mutant complement DNAs, with the latter requiring a higher concentration of pyridoxal 5'-phosphate to achieve maximal activation. The amino acid substitution was in the exon containing the putative pyridoxal 5'-phosphate binding site and may account for the reduced ability of the cofactor to catalyze the formation of δ-aminolevulinic acid.

Conclusion.—An exonic point mutation in the ALAS2 gene that predicts the substitution of asparagine for a highly conserved isoleucine has been reported. This mutation, designated as I471N, occurs as the 3' end of exon 9 in this gene and is in the highly conserved SHIP box region that is present in all reported eukaryotic ALAS sequences. Therefore, the defect in XLSA may be deficient activity of the erythroid form of ALAS.

▶ This article defines a molecular defect responsible for XLSA: an isoleucine for asparagine substitution that disrupts the secondary structure of δ-ALAS in such a fashion that its affinity for its cofactor, pyridoxal 5'-phosphate, is reduced. As the authors note, this may not be the only erythroid-specific abnormality in ALAS that is associated with XLSA, but it is certainly the first. This article was interesting to me for several other reasons as well. First, the authors actually entertained a diagnosis of myelodysplasia in this patient but failed to obtain marrow cytogenetics, although a large number of irrelevant hematologic studies were performed. Second, although the patient's anemia corrected with pyridoxine as did his thrombocytosis, microcytic erythrocytosis persisted. Therefore, even in the presence of a normal hemoglobin electrophoresis, I wonder whether this Chinese patient also had a hemoglobinopathy. Finally, it is noteworthy that with hematologic remission, the serum ferritin was 1210 μg/L and the spleen was still enlarged, which raises the possibility of continuing tissue iron overload and portal hypertension. This situation calls for an esophogram, an echocardiogram, and a liver biopsy because phlebotomy therapy and study of other family members might be indicated. The only patient whom I have seen with this disorder had severe tissue iron overload.—J.L. Spivak, M.D.

Aplastic Anemia

Multicenter Randomized Study Comparing Cyclosporine-A Alone and Antithymocyte Globulin With Prednisone for Treatment of Severe Aplastic Anemia
Gluckman E, Esperou-Bourdeau H, Baruchel A, Boogaerts M, Briere J, Donadio D, Leverger G, Leporrier M, Reiffers J, Janvier M, Michallet M, Stryckmans P, and the Cooperative Group on the Treatment of Aplastic Anemia (Hôpital Saint Louis, Paris; U Z Gasthuisberg, Leuven, Belgium; Hôpital Beaujon, Paris; et al)
Blood 79:2540–2546, 1992   1–11

Objective.—The best curative treatment for severe aplastic anemia (SAA) is bone marrow transplantation from an HLA-matched sibling donor, which provides up to 80% long-term survival in young patients. When no compatible donor is found, long-term survival of up to 70% can be achieved with antithymocyte globulin (ATG), with or without androgens. The response rate to ATG is only 20%, however, in young patients and those with less than .2 × 10⁹/L granulocytes. The efficacy of ATG and prednisone was compared with cyclosporin A (CsA) as first-line therapy for SAA.

Methods.—The analysis included 94 patients with SAA seen at 37 European centers who were randomized to receive either ATG and prednisone or CsA. Antithymocyte globulin was given as a 6-hour infusion at a dosage of 12 mg/kg for 5 consecutive days, with methylprednisolone beginning at 5 mg/kg intravenously. Cyclosporin A was given at a dosage of 6 mg/kg/day orally, which was subsequently modified according to weekly blood or serum levels to achieve a level of 100–200 ng/mL in serum or 400–800 ng/L in blood. Patients who failed to respond or who had only a minimal response at 3 months were given the alternative therapy.

Results.—Overall actuarial survival was 67% at a median follow-up of 19 months. At 1 year, there was no significant difference between groups in survival (70% with CsA and 64% with ATG), and there was little difference in the percentage of complete and partial response (32% and 30%, respectively). The absolute neutrophil count at entry was the main prognostic factor; survival was significantly lower in patients with an absolute neutrophil count of less than .2 $\times$ 10^9/L. At 1 year, 62 evaluable patients were still alive; 36 had had a complete or partial response. Bone marrow recovery was better in patients who responded to their first treatment, compared with those who had sequential immunosuppression. Infection was the most important complication, and it occurred with greater frequency and lethality in patients receiving ATG.

Conclusion.—This randomized study showed comparable response and survival rates for patients with SAA treated with either CsA or ATG and prednisone, followed by crossover therapy for nonresponders. Treatment with CsA appears to result in less infection, toxicity, and mortality, and it may possibly be used on an outpatient basis.

▶ This article, which documents the superiority of CsA alone over ATG plus methylprednisolone for the treatment of SAA not amenable to marrow transplantation, comes on the heels of a large study (1) that documented the superiority of ATG, methylprednisolone, and CsA rather than ATG and methylprednisolone alone and also the limitations on therapy imposed by severe neutropenia. Although there was no difference in survival between the ATG plus methylprednisolone and CsA treatment groups, the ATG group before or after CsA had a higher incidence of lethal infections. As might be expected, these appeared to cluster in the patients with the lowest neutrophil counts, suggesting that although CsA might be the initial treatment of choice for SAA not amenable to transplantation, additional studies on the usefulness of therapy with hematopoietic growth factors are indicated in the patients with very low neutrophil counts. There are 2 other recent reports on ATG therapy. Doney et al. (2) did not find a difference in the response rate for individual receiving low-dose methylprednisolone (.5 mg/kg) with ATG as compared with those receiving ATG with a dose of methylprednisolone 40-fold higher. In Gluckman and co-workers' article (Abstract 1–11), the methylprednisolone dosage was 5 mg/kg daily initially, suggesting that a lower dosage might be associated with fewer infections. Crump et al. (3) used ATG and methylprednisolone as first-line therapy before bone marrow transplantation with good results. Given Gluckman's results, a similar trial with CsA might be in order.—J.L. Spivak, M.D.

References

1. Frickhofen N, et al: *N Engl J Med* 324:1297, 1991.
2. Doney K, et al: *Blood* 79:2566, 1992.
3. Crump M, et al: *Am J Med* 92:596, 1992.

Effect of Interleukin-3 on Responsiveness to Granulocyte-Colony-Stimulating Factor in Severe Aplastic Anemia
Geissler K, Forstinger C, Kalhs P, Knöbl P, Kier P, Kyrle P, Lechner K (Univ of Vienna)
Ann Intern Med 117:223–225, 1992   1–12

Background.—Patients with severe aplastic anemia rarely respond to monotherapy with hematopoietic growth factors, probably because they have a profound deficiency of hematopoietic progenitors. In primates, IL-3 expands the hematopoietic progenitor pool, which raises the possibility that it could be used therapeutically to make hematopoiesis more

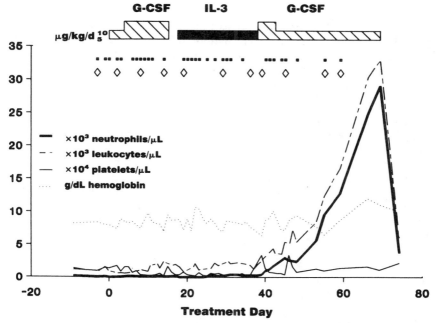

Fig 1–12.—Blood cell counts during treatment with cytokine in patient with severely neutropenic aplastic anemia. Days at which patient received RBC (*diamonds*) or platelet (*squares*) transfusions are indicated. (Courtesy of Geissler K, Forstinger C, Kalhs P, et al: *Ann Intern Med* 117:223-225, 1992.)

responsive to late-acting cytokines. Pretreatment IL-3 followed by G-CSF in 1 patient with refractory aplastic anemia was reported.

Case Report.—Woman, 35, with severe aplastic anemia and no suitable bone marrow donor was treated with antithymocyte globulin and high-dose methylprednisolone. Her granulocyte count was normalized and the erythropoiesis and thrombopoiesis improved temporarily, but the patient eventually became severely pancytopenic and required weekly erythrocyte and platelet transfusions. The patient had fever, blood cultures positive for staphylococci, and recurrent oropharyngeal infections. The treatment with G-CSF, beginning at 5 μg/kg/day subcutaneously, had no effect on the neutrophil count or any other hematologic measure (Fig 1–12). The patient then received recombinant human IL-3, 5 μg/kg/day subcutaneously for 20 days, which resulted in only a minor increase in neutrophils but a few circulating hematopoietic progenitor cells, whereas none had been detected before. Under the assumption that IL-3 may have primed residual hematopoiesis, G-CSF was then readministered. The neutrophil count reached 1,000/mm^3 within 2 days, and fever and recurrent infections resolved rapidly. Reconstitution of myelopoiesis was associated with a shift toward less mature neutorphil precursors and a further increase in the number of circulating progenitors. Bone marrow aspiration showed prominent granulopoiesis with no evidence of erythropoiesis or thrombopoietic reconstitution. Neutrophil counts decreased rapidly after G-CSF was withdrawn, but another course 6 weeks later was able to re-stimulate neutropoiesis.

Conclusion.—Patients with aplastic anemia who do not respond to growth factor monotherapy may benefit from IL-3 followed by repeat treatment with the same cytokines. Combinations of hematopoietins other than those used in this case may be as effective or more so. Clinical trials are warranted in patients with severe aplastic anemia.

▶ This article records an interesting but anecdotal observation: IL-3 apparently induced responsiveness to G-CSF in a patient with severe aplastic anemia when neither agent alone had any effect. Growth factor synergy has been well studied in vitro, and studies in humans are in progress. Such studies are logical because, with the exception of EPO, none of the other growth factors behaves like a hormone, and their production appears to be initiated or upregulated in a coordinated fashion. Furthermore, given the hierarchy of hematopoietic progenitor cells as well as the differential sensitivity of these progenitor cells to specific growth factors, it is logical to employ together or in tandem growth factors that target primitive progenitor cells and those that target committed progenitor cells. It must be remembered, however, that growth factor specificity has largely been defined in the culture dish, which may not reflect the in vivo situation. For example, G-CSF, which was once thought to stimulate neutrophil along formation, enhances erythroid burst-forming unit proliferation in vivo (1) and appears to not only stimulate CFU-S proliferation (2) but also to synergize with IL-3 in inducing blast cells to proliferate (3).

With these observations, it is possible to consider other explanations for the observations of Geissler et al. First, given either a low number of progenitor cells or defective progenitors in this patient with aplastic anemia, perhaps either a higher dose of G-CSF alone would have been effective or a trial longer than 16 days was needed. Alternatively, the G-CSF could have potentiated the IL-3, as seen in in vitro studies. It is, of course, impossible in a single case to determine which explanation is correct, a problem made more difficult because the in vivo production of these growth factors cannot be measured yet. However, given the expense of recombinant hematopoietic growth factors, it will be important to substantiate anecdotal claims such as those described by our Austrian colleagues.—J.L. Spivak, M.D.

References

1. Miles SA, et al: *Blood* 75:2137, 1990.
2. Spivak JL, et al: *J Clin Invest* 83:100, 1989.
3. Ikebuchi K, et al: *Proc Natl Acad Sci USA* 85:3445, 1988.

Very Low Doses of GM-CSF Administered Alone or With Erythropoietin in Aplastic Anemia
Kurzrock R, Talpaz M, Gutterman JU (Univ of Texas MD Anderson Cancer Ctr, Houston)
Am J Med 93:41–48, 1992   1–13

Objective.—In none of the previous reports of the use of GM-CSF in aplastic anemia have dosages of less than $15\mu g/m^2/day$ been used. However, the use of much lower dosages, if effective, would supply significant economic and side effect benefits. The use of very-low-dose GM-CSF in patients with aplastic anemia, including some who received EPO concomitantly, was examined.

Methods.—Twelve patients with aplastic anemia were treated with recombinant human GM-CSF, 5–20 $\mu g/m^2/day$ subcutaneously. A 13th patient also received EPO 4,000 unit/day subcutaneously from the start of treatment. Three of 12 patients who had an adequate neutrophil response but remained dependent on the RBC transfusions received EPO later. In each patient, aplastic anemia was confirmed by bone marrow examination and manifested by peripheral blood pancytopenia and bone marrow hypocellularity.

Results.—Five of the patients had at least a doubling of their neutrophil count, and 1 achieved a bilineage response. The median time to response was 2.5 weeks. A sixth patient had an increase in platelet count with no concomitant increase in neutrophil count. Minimal constitutional side effects were noted. The patient who received GM-CSF and EPO together from the start of treatment had a bilineage response, and 1 of the patients who began EPO later demonstrated a neutrophil re-

Response to Very-Low-Dose GM-CSF Treatment

Patient	Neutrophils (×10⁹/L) Before	After	Platelets (×10⁹/L) Before	After	Therapy Duration* (mo)	Comment
1	**0.3†**	**1.75**	**8**	**169**	18	Response occurred slowly over a period of several months (see Results)
2	0.03	0.2	**19**	**80**	4+	Platelet response was accompanied by an increase in eosinophils (0.03 → 0.3 × 10⁹/L) but not neutrophils
3	**0.8**	**1.6**	10	10	11+	Neutrophils increased from 0.8 → 1.6 × 10⁹/L with GM-CSF alone. Further neutrophil increase to 3.75 × 10⁹/L, increase in platelets (10 → 34 × 10⁹/L), and elimination of RBC transfusion requirement occurred after EPO added
4	**0.7**	**1.5**	79	80	2+	
5	**0.6**	**4.1**	12	12	1.5	
6	**1.4**	**2.8**	7	8	4	
7	0.4	1.0	5	3	0.5	Patient developed bleeding diathesis (severe bruising, gum bleeding, epistaxis) that reversed when GM-CSF was stopped
8	0.9	1.1	10	10	4	
9	0.8	1.4	13	5	2.5	
10	0.4	0.4	9	8	2.5	
11	0.2	0.2	5	11	1	
12	0.1	0.02	6	6	3	

*Total time that patients were treated with very-low-dose GM-CSF. Patients 3, 6, and 12 were treated with EPO in addition to GM-CSF during the latter 6+, 3, and 2 months, respectively, of this period. Responses are those achieved during the interval with GM-CSF alone.
†Boldface numbers reflect pretherapy and post-therapy values for patients who showed hematologic response to very-low-dose GM-CSF treatment.
(Courtesy of Kurzrock R, Talpaz M, Gutterman JU: Am J Med 93:41–48, 1992.)

sponse to GM-CSF alone and a trilineage response to the combination (table). The addition of EPO appeared to add no toxicity.

Conclusion.—Patients with aplastic anemia may begin GM-CSF treatment at very low doses, which are increased only for patients who do not respond. Adding EPO can have additive and sometimes synergistic effects in some patients. This combination therapy is being used in larger numbers of patients with a variety of bone marrow failure states.

▶ The title of this article caught my attention because of the suggestion that low-dose GM-CSF might be efficacious in aplastic anemia. Given the expense of growth factor therapy in general and the toxicity of GM-CSF in particular, the concept that, in this situation, less could be more intrigued me. Unfortunately, the data presented are not convincing. Foremost, one must ask whether the patients described are really representative of the aplastic anemia patient population because they are from a major referral center. In this regard, it is noteworthy that 8 patients had their disease for more than a year, whereas only 3 had been ill for less than 4 months. Thus, most of the patients had already survived the greatest risk period. Next, the time required to achieve a response was slow, raising the question of whether improvement was spontaneous as opposed to drug induced. Finally, the group treated with the EPO and GM-CSF was too small to base any conclusions on. Overall, more data will be required to support the authors' contentions about low-dose therapy with GM-CSF.—J.L. Spivak, M.D.

Aplastic Anemia and Viral Hepatitis: Non-A, Non-B, Non-C?
Hibbs JR, Frickhofen N, Rosenfeld SJ, Feinstone SM, Kojima S, Bacigalupo A, Locasciulli A, Tzakis AG, Alter HJ, Young NS (Natl Heart, Lung and Blood Inst, Bethesda, Md; Univ of Ulm, Germany; US Food and Drug Adminstration, Kensington, Md; et al)
JAMA 267:2051–2054, 1992   1–14

Introduction.—Aplastic anemia is a rare and often fatal disease of unknown cause. Hepatitis-associated aplasia (HAA) is a variant in which clinical hepatitis precedes aplastic anemia by weeks to months. A viral infection may precipitate aplastic anemia, the most common of which is non-A, non-B hepatitis. The recently identified hepatitis C virus (HCV) could be responsible for both HAA and aplastic anemia. To understand the association between aplastic anemia and HCV, 31 patients wtih aplastic anemia were examined for the presence of HCV.

Study Design.—The subjects were 28 patients with an onset of aplastic anemia within 90 days of seeking medical attention for jaundice or with serum transaminase levels 150% or more of normal plus 3 patients who had aplastic anemia after liver transplantation for non-A, non-B hepatitis. Three newly diagnosed HAA patients were evaluated at the NIH between July 1, 1990 and June 30, 1991. The 3 patients were typical of HAA in that all were between the ages 5 and 24 years, 2 of 3 were male, and aplasia followed hepatitis by 40–50 days (table). Hepatitis C virus was assessed in serum, bone marrow, and liver samples by an antibody test and PCR. The amount of activated peripheral cytotoxic T lymphocytes was determined by immunophenotyping.

Onset, Transfusions, and Virologic Testing, Hepatitis-Associated Aplasia Patients Evaluated at the NIH, Bethesda, Md, 7/1/90 to 6/30/91

Patient No.	Age, y/Sex	Date of Hepatitis Onset	Aplasia Onset (d After Hepatitis Onset)	Blood Products Received at First HCV Sampling, U	Anti-HCV	HCV In Bone Marrow†	HCV Viremia† (1/2/3 mo After Aplasia Onset)	CD8+, DR+ lymphocytes‡
1	17/M	8/1/90	48	11	No	No	No/No/No	2.9
2	11/M	12/1/90	40	19	No	No	No/No/No	11.6
3	8/F	2/10/91	49	0	No	No	No/NR/NR	22.0

† Hepatitis C virus RNA detected by PCR. NR indicates specimen not received for HCV testing.
‡ Percentage of total lymphocytes; CD8+ and DR+ lymphocytes normally represent .4% to .9% of total lymphocytes.
(Courtesy of Hibbs JR, Frickhofen N, Rosenfeld SJ, et al: *JAMA* 267:2051–2054, 1992.)

Findings.—The RNA from HCV was detected in the serum of 10 patients. However, HCV viremia was associated with transfusions received after the onset of aplasia. Of the 12 patients with HAA who had received 21 or more units of blood, 58% were viremic, whereas among the 16 patients with HAA who received 20 or less units of blood, only 19% were viremic. No HCV was detected in the blood or bone marrow of 3 NIH case patients who were tested at diagnosis. None of the livers from the 3 patients who had aplastic anemia after transplantation contained HCV. Activated CD8+ T lymphocytes were increased 3- to 20-fold early in the course of HAA.

Discussion.—Although the presence of HCV is associated with transfusions used to treat anemia, it is not often seen in the serum or bone marrow of patients with HAA at diagnosis. Therefore, HCV does not appear to be the cause of the hepatitis that precedes HAA. A non-A, non-B, non-C hepatitis virus may be responsible for the hepatitis and aplastic anemia of HAA.

▶ The agent responsible for acute hepatitis-associated aplastic anemia is unknown, but until a reliable diagnostic test for hepatitis C was developed, this virus remained a candidate. Now, using reverse transcriptase PCR, Hibbs et al. appear to have excluded this virus as a candidate as well. They suggest that an as-yet unrecognized virus may be involved, but given the paucity of such cases, the issue will not be easily resolved. However, given the high mortality rate of hepatitis-associated aplastic anemia, a registry of such cases may be initiated (1). It is equally tempting to wonder whether these patients might have an unrecognized genetic disorder, such as Fanconi's anemia, that makes them susceptible to a viral agent.—J.L. Spivak, M.D.

Reference

1. Schlitt HJ, et al: *Transplantation* 54:936, 1992.

Clonal Remission in Aplastic Anemia After Treatment With Antithymocyte Globulin

Wun T, Lewis JP (Univ of California, Sacramento)
Am J Hematol 40:229–231, 1992   1–15

Introduction.—A patient with otherwise typical aplastic anemia was found to be a constitutional mosaic, and she exhibited clonal evolution. The clone carrying a translocation disappeared after treatment with antithymocyte globulin, and the patient remitted completely.

Case Report.—Woman, 69, with chest pain was found to be pancytopenic with a WBC of 3,500 μL (33% neutrophils), hemoglobin 5 g/dL, platelets 24,000/μL, and an absolute reticulocyte of 3,200/μL . An iliac crest bone marrow aspiration and biopsy showed less than 5% cellularity with only 1 small area of granulocyte activity and lymphoid aggregates. She responded well to 4 units of red cells and to 15 units of donor platelets. A vague history of rheumatoid arthritis and gout was reported. Drugs included enalapril, propoxyphene, allopurinol, and conjugated estrogens. Large ecchymoses were noted at phlebotomy sites, and there were mild signs of rheumatoid arthritis. The rheumatoid factor titer was positive at 1:80. Reticulocytes remained absent, and an iliac crest marrow biopsy showed fewer than 5% cellularity. A mosaic sex chromosome distribution was demonstrated cytogenetically. Antithymocyte globulin was given for 8 days, causing fever, hypertension, rash, and ulceration. These effects lessened when prednisone was given. Marrow cellularity was 30% to 40% after 70 days, with normal maturation of all cell lines. Only XXX cells were present in post-treatment bone marrow.

Discussion.—The presence of a cytogenetic abnormality in a patient with aplastic anemia does not preclude a response to antithymocyte globulin. More frequent cytogenetic studies using new techniques may reveal additional cases in which a clonal disorder is present and evolution takes place.

▶ Patients with aplastic anemia have a small but real risk of having a clonal disorder—usually myelodysplastic syndrome or acute leukemia (1–3). Appelbaum et al. (3) reported 176 patients with aplastic anemia, 7 of whom had clonal cytogenetic abnormalities. Two of 7 progressed into myelodysplastic syndrome. Five were transplanted and 4 are alive and disease free. The present study indicates that a clonal disorder, in the setting of aplastic anemia, can respond to antithymocyte globulin. Although antithymocyte globulin was initially used on the assumption that it would be reversing an immunologic attack on bone marrow, this issue has become quite cloudy because it has a number of effects beyond its potential immunosuppressive action. Perhaps one of the most intriguing effects is its ability to induce potent cytokines that could then impact on a diseased marrow by stimulating differentiation or a normal coexistent clone of cells. The isolated clonality described in this case is unfortunately unclear. The authors state that "in contrast to the mosaicism of her peripheral T lymphocytes and skin biopsy," her marrow was predominantly 47,XXX. However, the skin biopsy showed 93.2% XXX with 6.8% XX. This is an unusual type of "mosaicism"! Nevertheless, this article is a reasonable vehicle to highlight the existence of clonal disorders in the setting of aplastic anemia and their potential response to therapy.—P.J. Quesenberry, M.D.

References

1. DePlanque MM, et al: *Br J Haematol* 70:55–62, 1988.
2. Tichelli A, et al: *Br J Haematol* 69:413–418, 1988.
3. Appelbaum FR, et al: *Exp Hematol* 15:1134–1139, 1987.

Sickle Cell Anemia

Prevalence and Pathologic Features of Sickle Cell Nephropathy and Response to Inhibition of Angiotensin-Converting Enzyme
Falk RJ, Scheinman J, Phillips G, Orringer E, Johnson A, Jennette JC (Univ of North Carolina, Chapel Hill; Duke Univ, Durham, NC)
N Engl J Med 326:910–915, 1992   1–16

Introduction.—Renal failure may occur in as many as 18% of patients with sickle cell disease, but the pathogenesis of sickle cell nephropathy remains poorly understood. The renal pathologic changes in patients with sickle cell disease were investigated prospectively, and the effects of enalapril, an angiotensin-converting enzyme inhibitor, on protein excretion were evaluated.

Patients and Methods.—Serum creatinine and urinary protein excretion were measured in 310 adults and 71 children with sickle cell disease. Twenty-six adults (7%) but none of the children had levels of serum creatinine above the normal range, and 101 patients (26%) had proteinuria at least 1+. Ten patients with homozygous sickle cell disease and proteinuria and minimal renal dysfunction had a renal biopsy. The glomeru-

Characteristics of 10 Patients With Sickle Cell Disease, Proteinuria, and Minimal Renal Dysfunction

PATIENT No.	AGE AT BIOPSY	SERUM CREATI- NINE	PROTEIN EXCRE- TION	GFR	RENAL PLASMA FLOW	FOCAL AND SEGMENTAL GLOMERULO- SCLEROSIS	GLOMERULUS	
							MEAN AREA *	MEAN DIAM. †
	yr	μmol/liter	g/day		ml/sec		μm^2 $(\times 10^{-3})$	μm
1	38	88	1.4	2.3	NA	0 ‡	22.6	163
2	49	133	1.6	0.9	5.4	+	28.8	186
3	54	71	10.8	0.9	11.9	+	22.8	166
4	24	71	2.1	1.4	14.4	+	26.3	176
5	48	71	1.0	1.6	8.1	+	31.4	198
6	27	53	0.8	1.7	18.6	0 ‡	28.2	187
7	39	88	1.5	1.3	10.5	+	30.2	191
8	40	88	0.9	1.4	10.3	+	34.8	204
9	35	159	2.2	0.7	8.1	+	27.9	184
10	38	150	1.4	0.8	22.1	+	34.0	205

Abbreviations: GFR, glomerular filtration rate; NA, not available.
° Mean value (± SD) for control patients was 15.8 ± 4.3 × 10^3 μm^2.
† Mean value (± SD) for control patients was 137.9 ± 19.3 μm.
‡ Focal global but not segmental sclerosis was present.
(Courtesy of Falk RJ, Scheinman J, Phillips G, et al: N Engl J Med 326:910–915, 1992.)

lar filtration rate, effective renal plasma flow, and urinary excretion of protein were measured at baseline, after 2 weeks of enalapril therapy, and again 2–3 weeks after enalapril had been discontinued. Enalapril was given orally in dosages of 5–10 mg/day for 2 weeks.

Results.—Renal biopsy showed perihilar focal and segmental glomerulosclerosis in 8 of 10 patients with sickle cell disease (table). Some had global sclerosis. Administration of enalapril decreased the mean 24-hour urinary excretion of protein to 57% below baseline levels, but 2–3 weeks after enalapril had been discontinued, proteinuria had increased to 25% below baseline levels. Enalapril had no significant effect on the glomerular filtration rate or on the effective renal plasma flow.

Conclusion.—Approximately 25% of patients with sickle cell disease have proteinuria. Enalapril reduces the degree of proteinuria, suggesting that glomerular capillary hypertension may have a role in the pathogenicity of sickle cell nephropathy.

▶ Sickle cell disease, the first molecular disease, continues to be well studied, and because patients are living longer, the effects of red cell sickling on various organs are becoming more apparent. We have previously featured articles on the natural history of pulmonary disease, leg ulcers, and osteonecrosis in sickle cell anemia and, more to the point of the current article, a large prospective series on chronic renal failure by Powars et al. (1), which, amazingly, Falk et al. neglected to cite. This could not have been "citation ignorance," so it must have been "citation amnesia"; neither, of course, is academically acceptable. This is not a trivial consideration because Powars's data suggest that the highest mortality rate occurs before age 30, whereas most of Falk's patients who had a renal biopsy were much older. Nevertheless, Falk et al. prospectively screened patients with sickle cell disease for evidence of intrinsic renal disease. Proteinuria was common, and glomerular enlargement and focal glomerular sclerosis were seen on renal biopsy, but immune complex nephropathy was not. This observation is important because the angiotensin-converting enzyme inhibitor, enalapril, reduced proteinuria in these patients. Whether enalapril will prevent progressive renal failure, whether it would benefit patients younger than 30 years of age, who undoubtably need it the most, and why only a portion of patients with sickle cell disease have progressive renal failure are all unknown. That the impact of age was not raised by the authors indicates that neither they nor their reviewers have done their readers a service.—J.L. Spivak, M.D.

Reference

1. Powars DR, et al: *Ann Intern Med* 115:614, 1991.

Hip Arthroplasty in Patients With Sickle-Cell Haemoglobinopathy

Acurio MT, Friedman RJ (Med Univ of South Carolina, Charleston)
J Bone Joint Surg [Br] 74-B:367–371, 1992   1–17

Introduction.—Sickle cell hemoglobinopathy is associated with the development of osteonecrosis of the femoral head. The small blood vessels of the femoral head are particularly liable to occlusion by sickled cells, leading to collapse of the bone and joint destruction. Twenty-five patients with osteonecrosis secondary to sickle cell hemoglobinopathy were examined to assess long-term results of hip arthroplasty.

Patients and Methods.—Twenty-five patients were treated with 35 primary hip arthroplasties between 1970 and 1986. The mean age of the group was 25 years at onset of symptoms and 30 years at the initial hip arthroplasty. Eleven had sickle cell disease, 6 had sickle thalassemia, 5 had sickle cell trait, and 3 had sickle C disease. Two patients died of unrelated causes; the remaining 23 patients had physical and radiographic examinations and they completed a detailed questionnaire.

Results.—Two thirds of the patients had results judged unacceptable at the latest evaluation. At a mean follow-up of 8.6 years, 14 of 35 primary operations had required revision surgery. Nine resection arthroplasties were performed, 5 for infection, 1 for suspected infection, and 3 for severe bone loss. Infection was more common in cemented arthroplasties (5 of 17) than in uncemented arthroplasties (2 of 18). Sixteen cemented hips, but only 7 uncemented hips, were either loose or had undergone revision.

Conclusion.—In patients with sickle cell hemoglobinopathies, hip arthroplasty for osteonecrosis is associated with an excessively high rate of failure, infection, and complications. The use of methylmethacrylate cement appeared to contribute to high infection and revision rates. The risk-to-benefit ratio of hip arthroplasty is high.

▶ This pessimistic, but important, report about the long-term results of hip arthroplasty in patients with sickle cell disease details a disappointingly high rate of failure and infection. Although the high failure rate in this series may reflect the experience of the particular center, the results are sobering. The results of the Cooperative Study discussed in these pages last year (1) suggest that early detection of osteonecrosis of the femoral head may make it possible to prevent progression and thus obviate the need for arthroplasty.—J.L. Spivak, M.D.

Reference

1. 1992 Year Book of Hematology, p 46.

Stroke in a Cohort of Patients With Homozygous Sickle Cell Disease

Balkaran B, Char G, Morris JS, Thomas PW, Serjeant BE, Serjeant GR (Univ of the West Indies, Kingston, Jamaica)
J Pediatr 120:360–366, 1992   1–18

Introduction.—The risk factors for stroke among patients with homozygous sickle cell disease are largely unknown. To identify factors predictive of stroke, 310 children with sickle cell disease from birth were followed.

Methods.—The incidence of stroke was determined by survival analysis. Hematologic risk factors were assessed by comparing steady-state indexes immediately preceding the stroke with steady-state values in cohort children who did not have strokes.

Results.—Seventeen children had a stroke, for an overall incidence of 7.8% by age 14 years. The median age for stroke was 6 years, 3 months; 82% occurred between 3 and 10 years of age. Fourteen children had hemiplegia, 10 had impaired speech, and 8 had cranial nerve lesions. Convulsions preceded the stroke in 3 patients. Two patients had subarachnoid hemorrhages and 15 were presumed to have cerebral infarction, although evidence was available in only 8 patients. One child with subarachnoid hemorrhage had complete resolution of symptoms after aneurysm surgery; 5 of 9 survivors of cerebral infarction have recovered completely. Patients with stroke had higher hemoglobin A_2 and leukocyte levels than those without stroke (table). Patients with stroke also had a significantly higher mean leukocyte count during both the steady-state phase preceding the stroke and at age 1 year. No hematologic dif-

Preceding Steady-State Hematologic Data in 15 Patients With Presumed Cerebral Infarction Compared With Cohort Patients With Sickle Cell Disease But Without Stroke

Variable	n	z score (mean ± SD)	Significance t	p
HbA$_2$ (%)	11	0.47 ± 0.61	2.53	0.030
$\sqrt{HbF}$	15	−0.30 ± 0.71	−1.64	0.123
Hb (gm/dl)	15	−0.32 ± 0.63	−2.00	0.066
MCHC (gm/dl)	15	0.0073 ± 0.901	0.03	0.975
$\log_e (RBC + 1) \times 10^{12}$	15	−0.33 ± 0.77	−1.68	0.115
MCV (fl)	15	0.17 ± 0.80	0.82	0.425
$\sqrt{Reticulocytes}$	15	0.43 ± 0.85	1.99	0.066
Platelets ($\times 10^9$/L)	13	−0.33 ± 0.98	−1.21	0.251
$\log_e (WBC + 1) \times 10^9$	15	0.83 ± 0.93	3.49	0.004

Abbreviations: N, number of patients; *Hb,* hemoglobin; *MCHC,* mean corpuscular hemoglobin concentration; *MCV,* mean corpuscular volume.
(Courtesy of Balkaran B, Char G, Morris JS, et al: *J Pediatr* 120:360–366, 1992.)

ferences were seen between patients who had stroke with and without recurrence. In 5 patients, acute anemia was associated with the initial stroke. In 7 patients with presumed infarction, painful crisis preceded the initial stroke.

Conclusion.—The identification of risk factors for stroke could allow therapy to be directed against these factors. A high leukocyte count and an acute decrease of hemoglobin may identify patients with sickle cell disease at risk for stroke.

The Use of Transcranial Ultrasonography to Predict Stroke in Sickle Cell Disease

Adams R, McKie V, Nichols F, Carl E, Zhang D-L, McKie K, Figueroa R, Litaker M, Thompson W, Hess D (Med College of Georgia, Augusta)
N Engl J Med 326:605–610, 1992   1–19

Background.—A major cause of morbidity and mortality in children with sickle cell anemia is stroke, especially cerebral infarction. Primary prevention by tranfusion therapy may be possible if the patients at greatest risk can be identified. The use of transcranial ultrasonography to predict stroke in children with sickle cell disease was investigated.

Methods.—The velocity of cerebral blood flow in children and young adults with sickle cell disease was measured prospectively by transcranial Doppler ultrasonography. Findings were categorized as normal or abnormal on the basis of the highest velocity of flow in the middle cerebral artery. Abnormal velocity was defined as a flow of 170 cm/sec or more. In 190 patients (aged 3–18 years), 283 transcranial ultrasound assessments were done.

Findings.—After an average 29-month follow-up, 7 patients had had a cerebral infarction. Ultrasound examination results were abnormal in 23 patients and normal in 167. The 2 groups were comparable clinically and hematologically. Six of 7 strokes occurred among the 23 patients with abnormal ultrasound findings. The relative risk of stroke in this group was 44.

Conclusion.—Children with sickle cell disease who are at greatest risk for cerebral infarction can apparently be identified with transcranial ultrasonography. Through periodic ultrasound assessment and selective transfusion therapy, the primary prevention of stroke may become an attainable goal.

▶ Stroke is a complication of sickle cell disease most often seen by our pediatric colleagues. Long-term transfusion therapy is effective in reducing recurrences, but the factors identifying patients at risk of cerebral infarction are not fully understood. Abstract 1–18 represents an analysis of stroke in 310 children with sickle cell disease followed from birth. A higher leukocyte count and an acute decrease in hemoglobin were the 2 predictive factors, but the former appears to lack the sensitivity needed to be a clinical predictor. Abstract 1–19 presents another approach to the problem: transcranial ultrasonography. This is an attractive, noninvasive screening option, but it appears to be operator-dependent, and there is currently no proof that long-term transfusion therapy will prevent cerebral infarction in patients with abnormalities detected by ultrasonography. Furthermore, only 30% of the patients with an abnormal ultrasound sustained a clinical stroke during 29 months of follow-up. Nevertheless, a coupling of transcranial ultrasonography with known risk factors may improve the predictability of this test (see also the comments after Abstrct 1-20). Ultrasonography may also be useful in predicting which patients are at risk of stroke after discontinuation of transfusions (1).—J.L. Spivak, M.D.

Reference

1.   1992 YEAR BOOK OF HEMATOLOGY, p 61.

A Modified Transfusion Program for Prevention of Stroke in Sickle Cell Disease
Cohen AR, Martin MB, Silber JH, Kim HC, Ohene-Frempong K, Schwartz E (The Children's Hosp, Philadelphia; Univ of Pennsylvania, Philadelphia)
Blood 79:1657–1661, 1992   1–20

Introduction.—Approximately 6% to 10% of children with sickle cell disease will have a stroke, and two thirds of those who have had a stroke will have a recurrence. Regular RBC transfusions dramatically reduce the risk of recurrent stroke, but they also lead to iron overload. The efficacy

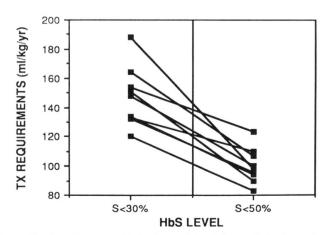

Fig 1–13.—Blood requirements with simple transfusion before and after increasing the pretransfusion HbS level from 30% to 50%. (Courtesy of Cohen AR, Martin MB, Silber JH, et al: *Blood* 79:1657-1661, 1992.)

of a modified transfusion program, which still affords protection against recurrent stroke while reducing the rate of iron loading was examined.

Patients and Methods.—Fifteen patients with homozygous sickle cell disease who were free of recurrent stroke for at least 4 years and whose hemoglobin S (HbS) level had been maintained below 30% during those 4 years were enrolled in the study. The target pretransfusion HbS level was increased from 30% to 50%. The transfusion regimens included simple transfusion (Fig 1–13) and manual or automated partial exchange transfusion. The duration of follow-up ranged from 14 to 130 months; the median follow-up was 84 months.

Results.—Before the transfusion protocol was modified, the target HbS level was maintained below 30% during a total of 1,184 patient-months. None of the patients had a recurrent cerebral infarction during the 1,023 patient-months when the target HbS level was maintained below 50%. Two patients had neurologic complications other than stroke during the modified transfusion program. A man had a fatal intraventricular hemorrhage at age 23 years when the HbS was 30%, and a woman had a fatal subarachnoid hemorrhage in the 40th week of pregnancy at age 21 years when the HbS was 29%. When the target pretransfusion HbS level was increased from 30% to 50%, mean blood requirements decreased by 31% for simple transfusion and by 67% for manual or automated partial exchange transfusion. The differences were statistically significant.

Conclusion.—Increasing the target HbS level from 30% to 50% provides a major reduction in blood requirements and lowers the rate of iron accumulation while providing continuing protection against recurrent stroke.

▶ Chronic transfusion programs have been very successful in preventing recurrent strokes in patients with sickle cell disease. The problems of alloimmunization to red cell antigens, iron overload, and disease transmission are real, so that assessments of how long these transfusion programs must be maintained and how intensive they must be are critical. Wang et al. (1) showed an unacceptably high rate of recurrence when transfusions were stopped 5 years after the last occurrence, leading to a reluctance to curtail transfusions for these patients. This important study by Cohen and co-workers suggests that transfusions are equally effective if the HbS level is allowed to increase from 30% to 50% before the next transfusion episode; this modification results in a 31% reduction of transfusion requirements with the likely, but as yet undocumented, reduction of transfusion complications.—P.M. Ness, M.D.

▶ With respect to transfusion therapy in sickle cell anemia, the observations of Rackoff et al. (2) are worth noting. These authors observed serious neurologic events in 6 patients having sickle cell with priapism treated with partial-exchange transfusion. Admittedly, the postexchange hemoglobin appeared to be too high, but at the same time, on arteriography, these patients demonstrated vascular anatomical abnormalities. If others have had a similar experience, perhaps transcranial ultrasonography (Abstract 1-19) might be gainfully used to assess the risk for a neurologic event with transfusion therapy in patients with no previous history of neurologic disease.—J.L. Spivak, M.D.

References

1. Wang WC, et al: *J Pediatr* 118:377, 1991.
2. Rackoff WR, et al: *J Pediatr* 120:882, 1992.

Treating Sickle Cell Pain Like Cancer Pain
Brookoff D, Polomano R (Hosp of the Univ of Pennsylvania, Philadelphia)
Ann Intern Med 116:364–368, 1992   1–21

Introduction.—To avoid the phenomenon of cycles of pain and sedation with pain relief, continuous opioid infusions and long-acting oral opioids have been used for patients with cancer. This strategy provides satisfactory pain relief with lower doses of narcotics and fewer side effects. In patients without cancer, however, physicians have been overly concerned about the possibility of addiction. Whether the protocols used for cancer pain can benefit patients with sickle cell pain was examined.

Methods.—In the last half of 1988, the Hospital of the University of Pennsylvania replaced its protocol of intermittent doses of short-acting opiods with one of intravenous morphine infusions and oral controlled-release morphine for patients seen in the emergency department with sickle cell pain. Dosage was adjusted to patient need and supplemented when necessary. Patients received a 2-week supply of controlled-release morphine at discharge. Researchers examined records for the periods before and after initiation of the protocol.

Results.—All patients with sickle cell crisis who were treated remained stable, but the total number of emergency department visits for sickle cell pain decreased by 67%, the number of admissions was reduced 44%, the number of inpatient days decreased by 57%, and the hospital stay was shortened by 23%. Patients with high levels of hospital use decreased their number of admissions and hospital days after the morphine protocol (table). No evidence of addiction was found in any patient, and the morphine regimen appeared to be as safe as the previous regimen.

Conclusion.—The combination of continuous intravenously and orally administered morphine and patient education reduced hospital use by these adult patients with sickle cell pain. Undertreatment of the pain of sickle cell disease has led to repeated and unsatisfactory hospitalizations and conflict between patient and physician.

Hospital Admissions and Inpatient Days Before and After the Institution of the Morphine Protocol for 15 Patients With Sickle Cell Disease and High Levels of Hospital Use

Patient	Before Morphine Protocol		During Morphine Protocol	
	Admissions	Inpatient Days	Admissions	Inpatient Days
	←————————		n	————————→
1†	6	38	9	57
2	6	42	5	20
3	3	14	0	0
4	5	15	0	0
5	4	20	0	0
6	5	48	1	7
7	7	61	3	12
8	13	83	2	9
9	7	35	3	10
10	3	15	7	39
11	4	13	0	0
12	3	12	5	19
13	3	10	0	0
14	5	31	0	0
15	3	25	0	0
Total	77	462	35	173

Note: Data were collected from January 1 to June 30 in both 1988 (before institution of the morphine protocol) and 1989 (after institution of the morphine protocol).
† Treated with hydromorphone during the protocol period.
(Courtesy of Brookoff D, Polomano R: Ann Intern Med 116:364–368, 1992.)

▶ This article, which aroused both criticism and compliments, will be an important contribution if it helps change the way many physicians approach the management of pain in patients with sickle cell anemia and promotes further studies of the problem. Perhaps in the future, agents, such as hydroxyurea and butyrate, that promote hemoglobin F synthesis will alleviate the frequency and severity of sickle cell crises and the need for narcotic analgesia. However, presently, painful crises are a reality for patients with sickle cell disease, and failure to obtain adequate pain relief is unfortunately all too often a reality. In today's "drug culture," it is easily forgotten that analgesia adequate to relieve pain, even if received on multiple occasions, does not routinely lead to addiction. Of course, as discussed in these pages last year (1), the data from the Cooperative Study indicated that the number of pain episodes per year is a measure of clinical severity and, in patients older than age 20 years, correlates with early death. Thus, simply alleviating pain is not a sufficient end.—J.L. Spivak, M.D.

Reference

1. 1992 YEAR BOOK OF HEMATOLOGY, p 48.

Thalassemia

A Short-Term Trial of Butyrate to Stimulate Fetal-Globin-Gene Expression in the β-Globin Disorders

Perrine SP, Ginder GD, Faller DV, Dover GH, Ikuta T, Witkowska HE, Cai S-p, Vichinsky EP, Olivieri NF (Children's Hosp, Oakland, Calif; Hosp for Sick Children, Toronto; Univ of Minnesota, Minneapolis; et al)
N Engl J Med 328:81–86, 1993   1–22

Background.—Sickle cell anemia and the β-thalassemia syndromes are caused by mutations of the adult globin (β-globin) chain of hemoglobin A. Fetal (γ)-globin chains inhibit the polymerization of sickle hemoglobin and can substitute functionally for defective or absent β-globin chains in patient with β-thalassemia. There is evidence that butyrate selectively stimulates the promoter of the human γ-globin gene and enhances expression of the gene in cultured cells and in the developing fetus.

Patients and Methods.—Because butyrate is not very toxic, a phase I trial of arginine butyrate was undertaken in 3 patients, aged 3–13 years, with sickle cell anemia and 3 others, aged 7–27 years, with β-thalassemia syndromes. The drug was infused continuously for 2 or 3 weeks in an initial dose of 500 mg/kg daily. If no side effects occurred, the dose was increased to a maximum of 2 g/kg daily.

Results.—The γ-globin synthesis increased by 6% to 45% in all 6 patients. The proportion of fetal reticulocytes increased by about twofold, and the level of γ-globin messenger RNA increased twofold to sixfold. Globin chain ratios improved in the patients with thalassemia. In 1 patient with hemoglobin Lepore who was treated for 7 weeks, the hemoglobin increased from 4.7 to 10.2 g/dL. Side effects were minimal. One patient had a transient rise in serum aminotransferase at the time of a viral infection.

Conclusion.—Butyrate, a natural fatty acid that does not produce significant side effects, may prove to be an effective means of enhancing fetal hemoglobin production to ameliorate β-globin disorders. Dramatic increases in expression of the γ-globin gene occurred in the present patients with β-hemoglobinopathies when they were given arginine butyrate.

▶ The most direct method for reversing the organ damage associated with hemoglobinopathies is to encourage the synthesis of normal globin chains. The obvious strategy is to turn on the production of γ-globin chains that can inhibit the polymerization of sickle globin chains and substitute functionally for defective or absent β-globin chains. Consequently, a large and productive industry devoted to the study of hemoglobin switching and the expression of γ-globin chains has evolved that can serve as a model for how basic research can be translated into clinical benefits. In this instance, the observations that infants of diabetic mothers who have high plasma α-amino-*n*-butyric acid levels do not switch from γ-globin to β-globin synthesis at birth and that butyrate stimulates γ-globin expression in vitro led to clinical trials of arginine butyrate in patients with sickle cell anemia and β-thalassemia. These studies were bolstered by the knowledge that butyrate therapy proved to be nontoxic in patients with inborn metabolic errors of the urea cycle (1). The preliminary results detailed by Perrine et al. are impressive with respect to the rapid stimulation of γ-globin synthesis in vivo, particularly when measured against other agents, such as hydroxyurea, that are being used for the same purpose or such alternative experimental therapies as bone marrow transplantation or gene replacement.—J.L. Spivak, M.D.

Reference

1. Blau CA, et al: *Blood* 81:529, 1993.

Bone Marrow Transplantation in Adult Thalassemia
Lucarelli G, Galimberti M, Polchi P, Angelucci E, Baronciani D, Durazzi SMT, Giardini C, Albertini F, Clift RA (Ospedale di Pesaro, Italy; Fred Hutchinson Cancer Research Ctr, Seattle)
Blood 80:1603–1607, 1992   1–23

Introduction.—Treatment of young adults with homozygous thalassemia by allogenic bone marrow transplants (BMTs) has previously been unsuccessful because of complications from acute graft-vs.-host disease. However, from recent transplant successes in younger patients, 3 important diagnostic factors—degree of hepatomegaly, presence of portal fibrosis, and history of inadequate chelation therapy—have been identified that are used to classify patient risk. Class 1 patients have none of these risk factors, class 2 patients have 1 or 2 adverse risk factors, and class 3 patients have all 3. The results of new treatment regimes in patients with class 2 and 3 thalassemia receiving BMTs were examined.

Treatment.—Five class 2 patients and 15 class 3 patients between ages 17 and 26 years received BMTs (Table 1). All patients had a history of inadequate chelation. Class 2 patients were prepared for transplantation for 4 consecutive days with daily oral administration of 3.5 mg of busulfan per kg followed by an intravenous administration of 50 mg of cyclophosphamide (CY) per kg. Treatments for acute graft-vs.-host disease were begun 2 days preoperatively and consisted of 5 mg of cyclosporine per kg intravenously administered until day 5, followed by a daily intravenous administration of 3 mg/kg until day 21, and finally oral administra-

TABLE 1.—Patients of Group B: Pretransplant Characteristics

UPN	Age/Sex	No. Tx	Ferritin †	Liver ‡	Spleen†	SD	FS	CAH	CPH	Protocol
								Liver Biopsy		
Class 2 disease										
504	17/M	205	1,561	2	Out	MO	SE	SE	NO	6
595	17/M	274	3,063	2	2	MO	MO	MI	NO	6
624	19/M	450	1,971	2	Out	MO	NO	NO	NO	6
662	17/M	480	1,546	2	Out	MO	SE	MO	NO	6
704	21/F	428	1,478	1	1	MI	MI	MO	NO	6
Class 3 disease										
626	17/M	188	805	4	Out	MO	MO	MI	NO	12
636	21/F	250	5,206	3	2	SE	SE	NO	NO	12
643	17/M	260	6,338	3	2	SE	SE	NO	NO	12
675	23/F	300	7,818	6	Out	SE	SE	NO	MI	12
679	21/F	600	4,680	3	Out	SE	SE	MI	NO	12
683	19/M	570	2,231	3	1	SE	MI	NO	NO	12
684	26/M	162	1,913	3	Out	MI	MI	NO	MI	12
686	19/M	252	2,078	6	Out	SE	SE	SE	NO	12
687	21/M	310	6,805	4	Out	SE	SE	NO	MI	12
688	19/M	456	9,071	5	4	SE	MI	MO	NO	12
690	24/M	314	930	4	Out	NO	MO	NO	NO	12
709	18/M	230	1,857	3	Out	SE	SE	MO	MI	12
712	17/M	230	6,738	3	1	SE	SE	NO	MI	12
716	18/M	263	1,177	3	4	MO	MO	NO	MI	12
719	18/M	265	1,741	4	Out	MO	MI	NO	MI	12

Abbreviations: UPN, unique patient number; No. Tx, number of RBC units received before transplant; Out, splenectomized; SD, hemosiderosis; FS, portal fibrosis; CAH, chronic aggressive hepatitis; CPH, chronic persistent hepatitis; NO, absent; MI, mild; MO, moderate; SE, severe.
† Serum ferritin levels (μg/L).
‡ Centimeters below costal margin.
(Courtesy of Lucarelli G, Galimberti M, Polchi P, et al: *Blood* 80:1603-1607, 1992.)

tion of 12.5 mg/kg for 1 year. Class 3 patients received the same busulfan regime, followed by intravenous administration of 60 mg of CY per kg for 2 consecutive days. These patients also received a continuous infusion of equine antilymphocyte globulin at 10 mg/kg during 12 hours from 5 days preoperatively to 5 days postoperatively. In addition to the

TABLE 2.—Patients of Group B: Outcome of Transplantation

| UPN | Days to Donor's Type † | | Rejection | Grade | | Outcome | KS |
---	α/β	Karyotype		AGVHD	CGVHD		
504	14	14	No	2	0	Alive with graft d 1,083	80
595	39	13	No	3	0	Alive with graft d 726	100
624	13	13	No	0	1	Alive with graft d 635	90
626	13	—	No	0	0	Alive with graft d 628	100
636	13	—	No	2	0	Alive with graft d 600	100
643	13	—	No	0	0	Alive with graft d 579	100
662	21	13	No	0	0	Alive with graft d 509	100
675	18	—	No	0	0	Alive with graft d 467	100
679	13	13	No	0	1	Alive with graft d 461	90
683	21	13	No	4	0	Died d 76 (AGVHD, pneumonia)	—
684	39	26	No	0	0	Alive with graft d 446	100
686	13	13	No	0	2	Alive with graft d 397	80
687	13	—	No	4	0	Died d 70 (AGVHD, aspergillosis)	—
688	20	32	No	0	0	Alive with graft d 390	100
690	21	—	No	0	0	Alive with graft d 390	100
704	13	13	No	0	0	Alive with graft d 341	100
709	NE	NE	NE	0	—	Died d 15 (septic shock)	—
712	13	—	No	0	0	Alive with graft d 313	100
716	13	—	Yes (d 42)	0	0	Alive with thalassemia d 299	90
719	45	—	No	0	0	Alive with graft d 264	100

Abbreviations: UPN, unique patient number; NE, not evaluable; AGVHD, acute grave vs. host disease; CGVHD, chronic grave vs. host disease.
† Days from transplant to first appearance of donor α/β globin synthesis ratio or karyotype.
(Courtesy of Lucarelli G, Galimberti M, Polchi P, et al: *Blood* 80:1603-1607, 1992.)

cyclosporine treatment prescribed for class 2 patients, class 3 patients received 7.5 mg of CY per kg 1 day postoperatively and 10 mg/m^2 of methotrexate by intravenous administration 3 and 6 days after transplantation.

Results.—After a minimum follow-up of 9 months, there have been 3 deaths, and 1 patient has recurrent thalassemia (Table 2). The Kaplan-Meier projections for rejection, survival, and rejection-free survival are 5%, 85%, and 80%, respectively.

Conclusion.—All patients had extramedullary organ damage and a poor prognosis when treated with conventional therapy. Bone marrow transplantation provides a reasonable option for adult patients with thalassemia who have HLA-identical donors.

▶ I chose this article because we have previously discussed BMT in thalassemia (1) and sickle cell anemia. Hepatomegaly, portal fibrosis, and inadequate chelation therapy were found to be adverse risk factors for transplantation, but by modifying the conditioning regimen with respect to these factors as well as age, the authors obtained a reasonable success rate for disease-free survival and chronic graft-vs.-host disease. Of course, follow-up is still relatively short with respect to whether liver damage will either stabilize or improve. Nevertheless, marrow transplantation for hemoglobinopathies may become moot, if Perrine et al. (Abstract 1–22) prove correct.—J.L. Spivak, M.D.

References

1. 1989 YEAR BOOK OF HEMATOLOGY, p 20.
2. 1990 YEAR BOOK OF HEMATOLOGY, p 29.

Erythrocytosis and Polycythemia

Familial Erythrocytosis Genetically Linked to Erythropoietin Receptor Gene
de la Chapelle A, Sistonen P, Lehväslaiho H, Ikkala E, Juvonen E (Univ of Helsinki)
Lancet 341:82–84, 1993   1–24

Introduction.—A heterogenous group of disorders, familial erythrocytosis, results from abnormal hemoglobins, aberrations in 2,3-diphosphoglycerate metabolism, and increased EPO production. Both recessive and dominant types have been reported. The results of testing the sequence repeat polymorphism of the EPO receptor (EPOR) gene to determine whether a mutation in the gene causes the erythrocytosis were assessed in a large kindred with familial erythrocytosis.

Patients and Methods.—A family of at least 33 affected living members, in many of whom the erythrocystosis caused no symptoms, had a hemoglobin level of 18.1 g/dL or greater for males and 16.1 g/dL for females. Family members underwent linkage analysis of genomic DNA from the blood using simple, sequence repeat polymorphism in the 5′ region of the EPOR gene.

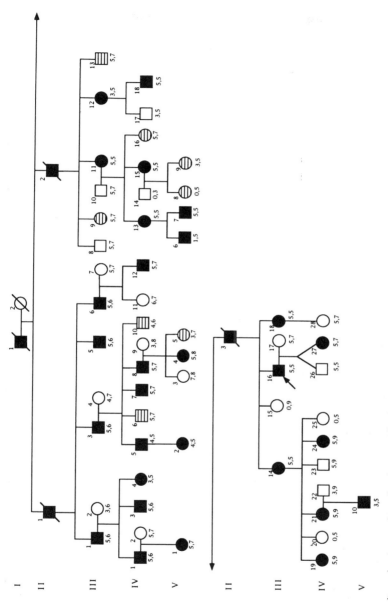

Fig 1-14.—Pedigree showing members of erythrocytosis family studied by linkage. Dead key members of generations I and II are shown for clarity; their status has been deduced from pedigree analysis and historical data. Alleles of EPOR gene polymorphism are shown under symbol for each individual. *Filled* = affected; *open* = unaffected; *hatched* = unknown status. (Courtesy of de la Chapelle A, Sistonen P, Lehväslaiho H, et al: *Lancet* 341:82–84, 1993.)

Results.—Based on the computer gene linkage program results, the disease phenotype co-segregated with allele 5 in all cases, whereas allele 5 did not occur in unaffected members at genetic risk (Fig 1–14). No recombinations occurred between the disease phenotype and the polymorphism, which was supported by the logarithm of odds score of 6.37 for the gene linkage at zero recombination, a highly significant result suggesting an EPOR gene mutation. Of the 8 family members with an unknown disease status, allele 5 appeared in 1 person but not in 2 others.

Conclusion.—Other studies have not shown mutational changes in EPOR, but the results of this report indicate that a mutation in EPOR probably causes familial erythrocytosis in the family described. Because EPOR mutations promote decreased erythropoietic activity, disease phenotypes producing anemia or other erythropoietic malfunction also may be associated with an EPOR mutation.

▶ We abstracted an article last year on familial autosomal dominant erythrocytosis that the authors attributed to increased sensitivity to EPO. The possibility of a mutation of the EPOR gene in this kindred has now been examined using the PCR to amplify a region 5′ to the transcription initiation site of the gene that contains a simple-sequence repeat polymorphism. Linkage analysis indicated that the disease phenotype co-segregated with a specific allele in all instances, whereas this allele was not present in unaffected family members. The data suggest that, in this family, a mutation in the EPOR gene may be responsible for the erythrocytosis. This is a fascinating observation, and I suspect that even as I am writing this, someone in Finland is sequencing the EPOR gene in this kindred and we will have more to comment on next year.—J.L.Spivak, M.D.

Familial and Congenital Polycythemia in Three Unrelated Families
Emanuel PD, Eaves CJ, Broudy VC, Papayannopoulou T, Moore MR, D'Andrea AD, Prchal JF, Eaves AC, Prchal JT (Univ of Alabama, Birmingham; British Columbia Cancer Agency, Vancouver, Canada; Univ of British Columbia, Vancouver, Canada; et al)
Blood 79:3019–3030, 1992   1–25

Purpose.—There have been a few reports of families having familial polycythemia with no evidence of excessive production of EPO. Clinical and laboratory findings, including results of EPO receptor studies, were presented for 3 unrelated white families with familial and congenital forms of "primary" polycythemia.

Patients.—In family 1 (Fig 1–15), the index case is a boy, now aged 9 years who has a slightly ruddy complexion but has never required any treatment for erythrocytosis. In family 2, a number of members have been affected in addition to the female index case, now aged 18 years, including her father, a paternal aunt and her children, and 8 others. The propositus has had hemoglobin concentration of 17–20 g/dL, and mini-

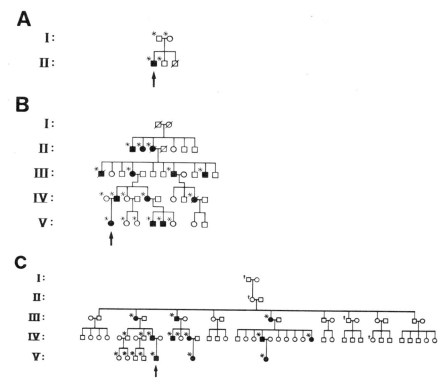

Fig 1–15.—Pedigrees of family 1 (**A**), family 2 (**B**), and family 3 (**C**). *Arrow* indicates the index case in each family; *filled circles* indicate family members with polycythemia; *asterisks* indicate subjects examined; *single daggers* indicate other family members with suggestive history; *slashes through squares or circles* indicate subject is deceased. (Courtesy of Emanuel PD, Eaves CJ, Broudy VC, et al: *Blood* 79:3019–3030, 1992.)

mal symptoms of headache, lack of energy, and irritability, and a somewhat ruddy complexion. Family 3, includes the index case and his father, both of whom have ruddy complexions, headaches, and lethargy, as well as 9 other relatives.

Findings.—Clinical and laboratory findings on members of the 3 families are summarized in (Table 1). Patients were found to have normal or low levels of EPO even after phlebotomy. In vitro erythroid colony growth in standard assay cultures containing EPO was normal. Without EPO, however, a few progenitors from most affected persons generated recognizable colonies of mature erythroblasts. These colonies tended to be smaller and proportionately less numerous than in polycythemia vera (PV). Southern blot analysis using 2 different probes derived from the human EPO receptor showed no evidence of chromosomal rearrangements or gene amplification in patients with hereditary polycythemia or PV. Neither were any nucleotide sequences homologous to the Friend

TABLE 1.—Clinical and Laboratory Data From Representative Polycythemic Patients and Normal Family Members

	Age	Sex	Hb (g/dL)	Hct (%)	WBC (10⁹/L)	Platelets (10⁹/L)	P₅₀	O₂ Saturation (%)	RBC Volume	Plasma Volume	Bone Marrow	Epo Level (mU/mL)	2,3-DPG* (nmol/gHb)
Family 1:													
Affected individual	9	M	20.5	59.3	6.2	315	30.5	94.5	37.7†	47.9‡	Iron deficient	16§	13,051
Normal family member	34	F	13.7	40.3	6.0	293	ND	ND	ND	ND	Normal	22¶	13,932
Family 2:													
Affected individual	18	F	20.3	62.7	6.7	218	27.4	97	30.8†	34.1‖	Relative erythroid hyperplasia	6	13,686
Normal family member	9	F	13.3	37.2	6.9	383	ND	ND	ND	ND	ND	5	ND
Family 3:													
Affected individual	13	M	18.4	66.7	5.3	260	28.4	99.1	2,136**	2188††	Normal	7	12,461

Abbreviation: ND, not done.
Note: Because plasma volumes and RBC were calculated in different laboritories, there are different normal ranges.
* Normal range 8,530–16,030 nmol/g of hemoglobin.
† Normal range 20–30 mL/kg.
‡ Normal mean 52.1 mL/kg.
§ Confirmed normal level by radioimmunoassay and bioassay (2 independent laboratories).
¶ Normal range 10–26 mU/mL.
‖ Normal range 30–45 mL/kg.
** Calculated upper limit of normal for size and gender, 1,718 mL.
†† Calculated upper limit of normal for size and gender, 2,477 mL.
(Courtesy of Emanuel PD, Eaves CJ, Broudy VC, et al: *Blood* 79:3019-3030, 1992.)

TABLE 2.—Idiopathic Polycythemia Syndromes

Type	Erythroid Progenitor Response In Vitro		Serum EPO Levels	
	EPO Sensitiviy	Endogenous Colonies	Baseline	Response to Phlebotomy
I (PV)	Increased	Present	Normal to low†	Normal
Ia (PV variant)	Increased	Present	Not increased† (by bioassay only)	Normal
II (this report)	Normal to slightly increased	None to trace	Normal to low†	Depressed
III	Increased	Present	Increased	Normal
IV	Normal	None	Increased	Depressed
V	Normal	None	Increased	Normal

†Because these types do not appear to be driven by increased levels of EPO, they may represent true or "primary" polycythemias.
(Courtesy of Emanuel PD, Eaves CJ, Broudy VC, et al: *Blood* 79:3019–3030, 1992.)

spleen focus-forming virus glycoprotein gp55, which binds to and activates the murine EPO receptor. No abnormalities were seen on functional studies of the number and binding affinity of the EPO receptor on erythroid progenitors from patients with hereditary polycythemia.

Conclusion.—These patients may have a new type or class of polycythemia (Table 2). In familial and congenital polycythemia, as well as in PV, the mechanisms of erythrocytosis may not involve the EPO receptor. In these cases, alterations in postreceptor responses may be involved.

▶ The development of sensitive techniques for the assay of EPO and erythroid progenitor cells and for the analysis of the EPO receptor has generated new interest in the mechanisms for inherited erythrocytosis and PV. This is a careful study of 3 unrelated families with erythrocytosis. Unfortunately, the authors, reviewers, and editor succumbed to the use of the term polycythemia when only erythrocytosis was present; their lapse into medical jargon contrasts so sharply with their science. In the families studied, no evidence for EPO receptor gene rearrangement or amplification was observed nor was any observed in 3 patients with PV, but more subtle changes would have been missed, as indicated by Abstract 1–24. No abnormalities in the regulation of EPO production were detected either. Thus, the mechanisms for familial erythrocytosis, like PV, remain obscure. The authors ruined good science with improper clinical judgment when they added a note in proof to the effect that familial erythrocytosis may require no treatment because their patients were asymptomatic. I won't repeat my comments on this subject from last year. Instead, I'll ask you first to inspect Figure 1–14 from Abstract 1-24 for the number of deceased, affected individuals with familial erythrocytosis and then to read the brief report (1) about a patient with hypoxic erythrocytosis who had angina (hemoglobin 18.2 g/dL; hematocrit 52%) secondary to high-altitude exposure with normal coronary arteries but decreased coronary flow. The red cell mass was elevated, but the plasma volume was normal. Phlebotomy to an hematocrit of less than 45% relieved the angina.—J.L. Spivak, M.D.

Reference

1. Kershenovich S, et al: *Am Heart J* 123:521, 1992.

Increased Thromboxane Biosynthesis in Patients With Polycythemia Vera: Evidence for Aspirin-Suppressible Platelet Activation In Vivo
Landolfi R, Ciabattoni G, Patrignani P, Castellana MAL, Pogliani E, Bizzi B, Patrono C (Catholic Univ, Rome; Univ of Milan, Monza, Italy; Univ of Chieti, Italy)
Blood 80:1965–1971, 1992   1–26

Whole Blood TXB_2 Production in Relation to Platelet Count in Patients With Polycythemia Vera and Healthy Controls

Group	Serum TXB_2 (nmol/L)	Blood Platelets (10^9/L)	Serum TXB_2 (nmol/10^9 Platelets)
Healthy controls (n = 177)	811 ± 292	212 ± 42	3.8 ± 2.4
Polycythemia vera patients (n = 13)	1,678 ± 1,899	434 ± 294	3.8 ± 1.4

Note: Values are mean ± SD. Normal values are from a previous study.
(Courtesy of Landolfi R, Ciabattoni G, Patrignani P, et al: *Blood* 80:1965–1971, 1992.)

Background.—Thrombohemorrhagic diathesis, a major complication of myeloproliferative disorders, is characterized by chronic episodes of cutaneomucosal bleeding and venous and arterial thrombosis. In vitro platelet isolation from patients with polycythemia vera has demonstrated increased thromboxane (TX) A_2 production and modified aspirin sensitivity. The urinary excretion of TXB_2 major enzymatic metabolites was examined to correlate these capacity-related measurements to the actual rate of TXA_2 biosynthesis in vivo, and its suppression via oral aspirin.

Patients and Methods.—Seventeen patients with polycythemia vera and 23 healthy participants were studied. Radioimmunoassays were used to measure urinary 11-dehydro-TXB_2 and 2, 3-dinor-TXB_2, and 5-lipoxygenase arachidonate metabolism was examined via urinary immunoreactive leukotriene (LT) E_4 measurements.

Results.—A significantly higher excretion rate of 11-dehydro-TXB_2 was found in the polycythemia vera patients vs. controls. Urinary excretion of 2,3-dinor-TXB_2 was also significantly higher in patients than in controls. Excretion of both enzymes was significantly correlated, implying an underlying increase in TXA_2 production. The TXB_2 production during blood clotting was twofold higher in patients with polycythemia vera than in 177 previously measured healthy controls (table). When these levels where corrected for platelet count, identical values were obtained. However, no correlation was found between urinary 11-dehydro-TXB_2 or 2,3-dinor-TXB_2 excretion and platelet levels, indicating that there was no direct relationship between enhanced metabolite excretion and platelet count. Moreover, no relation between current treatment or clinical history of thrombotic complications and metabolite excretion was noted. The TXA_2 receptor binding to a receptor agonist and antagonist was similar between patient and control groups. Interestingly, urinary LTE_4 levels did not differ significantly between patients and controls, implying a modified arachidonate metabolism in the polycythemia vera patients. A greater than 80% metabolite excretion suppression was found in 9 patients during platelet-selective aspirin therapy (50 mg/day for 7–14 days).

Conclusion.—Each patient exhibited selective alterations involving the cyclo-oxygenase/TX-synthase pathway. Platelets provided the major source of enhanced TXA_2 biosynthesis. However, increased platelet count is not related to this aspirin-suppressible abnormality, and it may reflect in vivo platelet activation.

▶ This YEAR BOOK is primarily devoted to new developments in hematology and information worth knowing, but occasionally it is necessary to deal with dubious information, particularly when it is published in a well-respected journal. This article is an example of the latter. My initial thought when I read it was that I must be missing something. My next thought was that my favorite parable for life, "The Emperor's New Clothes," was still operative. My third thought was to ignore it (the article), but since we all swore an oath "to first do no harm," I could not. The authors' premise for this study was that because both thrombotic events and platelet abnormalities are prevalent in polycythemia vera, they must be related and, therefore, might be correctable by aspirin therapy. They studied TX synthesis in patients with polycythemia vera and its suppression by aspirin and observed that, indeed, TX synthesis was increased and was suppressible with aspirin.

I have no problem with their experimental observations; however, the authors, reviewers, editor, and I part company with their conclusions. First, it is noteworthy that TX metabolite excretion did not correlate with either the platelet count or the history of the thrombotic events. Second, TX concentrations on a per platelet basis were identical for patients with polycythemia vera and controls, and their platelet TX receptors also behaved similarly. Third, the use of aspirin to suppress TX synthesis does not prove a platelet origin for this compound. Whether I am correct about all of this is only relevant because the authors conclude that because of enhanced TX synthesis in polycythemia vera and its suppression by aspirin, these patients should be treated with a "platelet-selective dose" of aspirin. The data of the polycythemia vera study demonstrated unequivocally that aspirin was toxic to patients with polycythemia vera. It has also been demonstrated that patients with thrombocytosis are at risk of bleeding, not thrombosis. Indeed, no controlled study has ever been published that definitively links the platelet count to thrombosis. When thromboses do occur, they usually do so in the setting of migraine or erythromelalgia. The authors' contention that low-dose aspirin will have less toxicity is unsupported. More to the point, based on their hematocrit values, 15 of the authors' 17 patients had not received adequate phlebotomy therapy. I do not believe that this problem is peculiar to the authors; it seems rather to be a consistent error on the part of many hematologists. The bottom line here is that if patients with polycythemia vera are phlebotomized to achieve a hemoglobin level of 15 g/dL or less for men and 12 g/dL or less for women, thrombotic events are not an issue. The role of aspirin in patients with polycythemia vera, aside from the treatment of erythromelalgia, is not established. I am convinced that thrombocytosis is bad for you if it reflects an underlying malignancy, chronic myeloid leukemia, or myelodysplasia (5q-syndrome), or if your physician thinks it is bad for you. But don't trust me. For a good review of this problem, see Andrew Schafer's review in *Blood* (1).—J.L. Spivak, M.D.

Reference

1. Schafer AI: *Blood* 64:1, 1984.

Gaucher's Disease

Gaucher Disease: Clinical, Laboratory, Radiologic, and Genetic Features of 53 Patients
Zimran A, Kay A, Gelbart T, Garver P, Thurston D, Saven A, Beutler E (Shaare Zedek Med Ctr, Jerusalem; The Scripps Research Inst; Scripps Clinic and Re-

search Found, La Jolla, Calif)
Medicine 71:337–353, 1992

Background. —Gaucher's disease, a prevalent lipid storage disorder, can occur in 3 forms. Of these, type 1 is the most common, especially

TABLE 1.—Follow-Up Data

Patient ID No.	Age At First Evaluation	Year	Number of Evaluations	Longest Time Interval (yrs)	SSI (initial)	SSI (final)	Disease Progression
1	72	1987	2	3	1	1	None
3	62	1986	4	6	2	2	Minimal changes in x-ray of rt. femur head
4	54	1988	3	3	2	2	None
5	61	1987	5	5	2	2	None (platelet counts stable over 26 y)
7	34	1982	2	3	3	3	None
9	65	1985	2	4	3	3	None
11	70	1986	5	6	3	3	None
13	32	1984	3	7	4	4	None
16	31	1988	2	3	8	8	None
18	25	1984	3	7	10	10	None
19	37	1978	5	4	14	14	Steady deterioration in joints and rt. femoral head
21	6	1985	6	6	8	8	Minimal skeletal x-ray changes*
23	29	1987	3	5	14	15	Slight increase in liver size axial transverse dimension; increase in spleen size; Hb (g/dl) $11.1 \rightarrow 9.1$, WBC ($10^3/\mu l$) $5400 \rightarrow 2900$
24	33	1988	2	3	15	15	None/improved mobility following bilateral total hip replacement
25	43	1981	3	9	17	17	None
28	41	1981	4	9	6	6	None
30	49	1986	4	4	12	12	None

(continued)

among Ashkenazi Jews. The assumption that Gaucher's disease is a relentless, progressive ailment was examined in 53 patients with the disease.

Patients.—Among the patients, 39 were Ashkenazi Jews, 1 had 1 Jewish parent, and 13 were non-Jewish. The mean age of diagnosis was 21

Table 1 *(continued)*

31	38	1984	5	7	8	12	Slight increase in liver size in the transverse dimension 227 mm → 264 mm; in 1990 development of pulmonary manifestations → shortness of breath
32	29	1978	4	13	14	14	New AVN of rt. humoral head
34	47	1988	3	3	14	14	New rt. humeral head AVN; slight increase in antero-posterior dimension of liver
35	22	1980	6	12	16	16	None
36	23	1984	5	5	20	24	Significant deterioration in pulmonary functions
41	34	1984	2	4	6	6	None
43	6	1987	2	4	7	9	Progressive bone disease
44	32	1989	2	2	19	19	None
46	12	1972	4	10	12	12	None/slight improvement in liver size
48	1	1989	3	2	8	8	Progressive pancytopenia
51	65	1987	4	5	9	9	None (bleeding from varices; relation to Gaucher unclear)
53	6	1984	8	7	8	9	Progression of bone disease

Abbreviation: AVN, avascular necrosis.
* Interval growth in liver or spleen size consistent with growth in patient size.
(Courtesy of Zimran A, Kay A, Gelbart T, et al: *Medicine* 71:337–353, 1992.)

TABLE 2.—Mutations in Gaucher's Disease Analyzed in the Present Study

Position		Base Pair Substitution	Exon	Amino-acid Change	Restriction Site Created (+) or Removed (−) by the Mutation	Frequency in Patients		Reference
cDNA	Genomic					Jewish (12)	Non-Jewish (Unpublished)	
Common Mutations								
1226	5841	A→G	9	$370^{Asn \to Ser}$	+CviJI*	77%	24	51
84GG	1035	G→GG	2	Stop		13	1	8, 11
1448	6433	T→C	10	$444^{Leu \to Pro}$	+NciI	3	39	50
Uncommon Mutations								
XOVR†								57
476	3060	G→A	5	$120^{Arg \to Gln}$	+BstNI, EcoRII			26
535†	3119	G→C	5	$140^{Asp \to His}$	+BspHI, NlaIII			21
586	3170	A→C	5	$157^{Lys \to Gln}$	+EcoRII, +ScrFI			35
764	4113	T→A	7	$216^{Phe \to Tyr}$	+KpnI			10
1043	5259	C→T	8	$309^{Ala \to Val}$	−BanI, +MaeIII			35
1053	5269	G→T	8	$312^{Trp \to Cys}$	−KpnI, −BanI, −NlaIV			35
1090	5306	G→A	8	$325^{Gly \to Arg}$	−HaeI + Bsu361			22
1093‡	5309	G→A	8	$326^{Glu \to Lys}$	+BbvII, MboII, −BsmAI			21
1141	5357	T→G	8	$342^{Cys \to Gly}$	−StuI			22
1208	5424	G→C	8	$364^{Ser \to Thr}$	−CviJI, +TaqII-2			35
1297	5912	G→C	9	$394^{Val \to Leu}$	−HgiEII			49
1342	5957	G→C	9	$409^{Asp \to His}$	−StyI			49
1343	5958	A→T	9	$409^{Asp \to Val}$	−AflIII, +MaeIII			49
1361	5976	C→G	9	$415^{Pro \to Arg}$	+HhaI			52
1504	6489	C→T	10	$463^{Arg \to Cys}$	+BsrI, −MspI			30
1604	6683	G→A	11	$496^{Arg \to His}$	+HphI			13

* Commercially unavailable at present.
† XOVR, crossover mutation. Similar, but not identical, recombinant mutations have recently been described.
‡ Both mutations found on the same allele.
(Courtesy of Zimran A, Kay A, Gelbart T, et al: *Medicine* 71:337–353, 1992.)

years, and the first evaluation in the present study occurred approximately 20 years after initial diagnosis.

Findings.—Common disease symptoms, including nose bleeds, a predisposition to bruising, or prolonged bleeding after superficial injury, were found in 23 patients. Another common symptom, thrombocytopenia, was noted in 28 patients. Twenty-two patients had anemia, and 3 had pancytopenia. Chest x-ray studies were usually normal. A widening of the distal femur was noted in 32 patients, and 9 had avascular necrosis in the femur head. Five patients had undergone hip replacements and 2 had kneecap replacements. In the skeletal-involved cases, the bony disease usually developed before age 30 years, and then stabilized (Table 1). Spleen and liver enlargement were another common finding. Of the 53 patients, only 5 had normal-size spleens and 12 had normal-size livers. The glucocerebrosidase gene was examined for 20 previously reported mutation occurrences; 7 were found in this patient group (Table 2). A 1226G-point mutation was noted in 61% of the examined genes, followed by a 1448C-point mutation and an 84GG nonsense mutation in 10%. The long-term follow-up studies indicated that an earlier onset of symptoms was associated with increased disease severity. Milder disease forms were noted in 1226G mutations, whereas 1448C mutations (associated with neuronopathic manifestations) were clinically more severe. The 84GG nonsense gene was also correlated with severe symptoms because of a lack of enzyme production.

Conclusion.—Contrary to popular belief, it is suggested that Gaucher's disease progresses from childhood until early adulthood but is stable thereafter.

▶ Gaucher's disease was first described 100 years ago, but probably more has been learned about it in the past decade than in the preceding century. The article by Zimran et al. is extremely important for a variety of reasons. It represents a model for clinical studies of other chronic disorders for which new and as-yet unproved therapies are becoming available. As the authors note, unless the natural history of a disease is understood, it is very difficult to judge the indications for particular forms of therapy and also their positive or negative impact. This is greatly important when the therapy is expensive (e.g., enzyme replacement) or involves high risk (e.g., bone marrow transplantation or gene transfer). Another noteworthy aspect is the observation that this inherited metabolic disorder is not necessarily a progressive disorder in adults, and this appears to be predictable by genotype. Furthermore, splenectomy, which is frequently necessary because of thrombocytopenia or mechanical reasons, is not necessarily associated with increasing skeletal disease. Most important, however, this study emphasizes that treatment for Gaucher's disease must be individualized and that the risks of some forms of therapy, such as allogeneic marrow transplantation, may outweigh the adverse consequences of the disease itself.

There is, of course, a certain irony here. Until 2 decades ago, the bulk of the papers in better internal medicine journals dealt with the natural history of various diseases. As new drugs and other forms of therapy became available, these scholarly, comprehensive treatises were superseded by articles devoted to treatment and its complications. Furthermore, almost in tandem with the development of "sound bite" journalism came the minimal publishable unit, and, as a consequence, today some journals are mere shadows of their previous forms. The pendulum now seems to have come full circle, as this article and such endeavors as the Cooperative Study of Sickle Cell Disease suggest. Although they are sometimes difficult to abstract, I always try to feature excellent clinical reviews in these pages.—J.L. Spivak, M.D.

2 White Bood Cells

Introduction

This year, there has been continuing emphasis on gene therapy and its application clinically. A relatively large number of protocols has now been approved, and the first marking studies have been carried out. Work from St. Jude's appears to indicate that, in some patients, relapse of acute lymphocytic leukemia is coming from the infused autologous cells. This is an important first step in defining the autologous marrow as the source of relapse in at least some instances. These type of data will provide guidance as to how much effort should be invested in pursuing various marrow-purging techniques. Relatively intense interest is being focused on the potential for inserting the multiple drug resistance gene into marrow to induce a chemotherapy refractory state. As shown in Abstract 2–25, these approaches are clearly feasible in animals and should work when applied in a clinical setting. Perhaps the major concern here is the insertion of the multiple drug resistance gene into contaminating tumor cells. This is being approached both by purifying marrow stem cells and by trying to engineer vectors with a self-destruct mechanism such that exposure to gancyclovir would abort an engrafted tumor population.

A number of other gene therapy proposals are being activated, but one of the more promising targets is that of HIV infection. The transferring of genetic resistance in HIV infection to hematopoietic stem cells appears to be feasisble and is intriguing. As pointed out in previous editions of the YEAR BOOK, the first reports of infection of CD34+ cells by HIV appear to have been erroneous. Most of the data are consistent with the idea that marrow suppression occurs via the release of inhibitors by accessory cell populations impacted by HIV and is not caused by a direct infection of stem cells. These data indicate that it may be feasible to purify CD34+ stem cells, transduce them with retroviral vectors encoding antisense to various critical HIV proteins, and, thus, induce a population of hematopoietic stem cells resistant to HIV infection. These could then be used in various transplantation approaches to attempt to repopulate HIV-positive individuals with HIV-resistant marrow cells. In the best of all worlds, this could lead to a resistant population of T lymphocytes and reverse the developing immunodeficiency in these patients. Obvious problems will relate to whether infection of monocyte/macrophage tissue populations or other nonhematopoietic cell types might eventually lead to a neurologic or other debilitating consequence, negating the positive effects of this approach. However, presently given the virtual lack of effective therapeutic approaches to AIDS, this seems to be the most promising avenue of new therapy. In this vein, it is appropriate to point out that recent studies on azidothymidine (AZT) appear to indicate that this drug is virtually without clinical benefit to patients infected with HIV. This is not too surprising, considering the first reports showed relatively marginal effects in HIV-infected individuals. That this drug has become a mainstay in the clinical therapy of AIDS indicates how desperate the situation is with these patients. Given the toxicity of AZT and its lack of survival and even palliative advantage, perhaps clinicians should relegate it back to an investigational status and stop routinely administering it to HIV-positive patients.

Stem cells continue to be highlighted this year, with an especially exciting presentation at the American Society of Hematology meetings in Anaheim, California on the existence of a stem cell common to stromal and hematopoietic elements. Many have suspected that such a cell might exist, but this is the first apparent demonstration that it does exist, at least in fetal marrow. Anytime an observation of this importance is reported, critics demand a high level of convincing before accepting. Thus, many wait to see studies on single-cell transfer that absolutely establish that 1 cell gave rise to these stromal and hematopoietic lineages. Even this may not be enough because some have suggested that 1 cell may be carrying passenger cells inside its cytoplasm. Several important questions remain to be answered in this area. The data appear to be fairly convincing, i.e., that these are single cells, but could this be basically a fetal characteristic, i.e., do these cells exist in adult hematopoietic tissues? Given the existence of these cells, they provide very interesting potential targets for gene insertion and for reconstitution to both hematopoietic and stromal cells in a transplant setting. Work from this laboratory will be followed with intense interest, and evolving data should continue to enliven various stem cell meetings.

The whole arena of short-term and long-term repopulating cells continues to generate a good deal of interest. Two of the contributions, Abstract 2–4 and Abstract 2–5, indicate that lymphoid and myeloid cells share a common stem cell. One of these presentations, surprisingly, indicates that very short-term repopulation may be caused by a stem cell that gives rise to both lineages. The uncertainty surrounding long- and short-term repopulation in human marrow transplantation may be clarified by some of the gene-cell marking studies that have been approved for clinical use. A few questions are, What is the full capacity of peripheral blood stem cells to repopulate? Do they represent simply an early intermediate scaffold transplant on which the final repopulation of donor cell occurs, or do they mediate long-term repopulation? Differential neo marking of both marrow and peripheral blood cells with evaluation of their ability to engraft and persist at varying time intervals posttransplantation should provide answers to these important, basic questions in stem cell transplantation biology.

Relatively few of this year's contributions address inhibitors, although a lot of progress and action have been made in this area, as reflected by presentations at various meetings. The macrophage inhibitory protein-1α (MIP-1α) is a stem cell inhibitor that appears to be able to reversibly move early stem cells out of the cell cycle, and it has interesting potential for ameliorating myelotoxicity associated with various chemotherapeutic approaches. Transforming growth factor-β is another inhibitor acting on relatively early stem cells. The MIP-1α appears to work in hours, whereas transforming growth factor-β may take days to exert its maximum effect. Both agents appear to have potential for protecting marrow cells from cytotoxic agents. Both agents also appear to be able to stimulate more differentiated progenitor cells, while inhibiting more primitive stem cells. Some of the more interesting developments in the inhibitor area relate to ongoing studies on the tetrapeptide of Frindel and Guigon and the pentapeptide inhibitors described by Paukovitz and Laerum. The pentapeptide pGlu-Glu-Asp-Cys-Lys and the tetrapeptide N-acetyl-Ser-Asp-Lys-Pro are rapidly acting inhibitors of the cell cycle in early hematopoietic stem cells. An important aspect of the action of the tetrapeptide is that is appears to have no affect on leukemic cells, but it blocks normal hematopoietic stem cells from entering the S phase. Phase 1 clinical studies addressing the ability of these agents to protect marrow against the cytotoxic affects of chemotherapy have been initiated.

One area not covered in this YEAR BOOK, but in which progress continues is that of the definition of the hematopoietic receptor families. Some of the more intriguing data relate to the formation of receptors for IL-6, leukemic inhibitor factor (LIF), oncostatin-M, and ciliary neurotrophic factor. One receptor chain, GP-130, appears to form a high-infinity receptor with the IL-6–specific chain or LIF-specific chain. Oncostatin-M appears to be able to bind to the GP-130/LIF receptor with high infinity, whereas ciliary neurotrophic factor can bind with low infinity. A tri-part chain, including a GPI-linked ciliary neurotrophic factor receptor, GP-130, and the LIF chain, constitutes the high-infinity receptor for the ciliary neurotrophic factor but also binds LIF and oncostatin-M with high affinity. The complexity of the receptor systems continues to unfold, with the possibility of even additional chains modulating both their signal transmitting activity and the affinity of their binding to various ligands. Investigators continue to try to unravel the second messenger pathways upstream of the receptors mediating the proliferative and differentiated effects of various growth factors. Abstract 2–31 is a step in that direction, but at the present time, it must be acknowledged that we have little understanding of how messages are transmitted to the nucleus or how many second messenger pathways may mediate various cytokine signals.

The clinical use of cytokines is expanding, at the least in the United States. We have covered this area in rather exhaustive detail in previous YEAR BOOKS, but it warrants some more comment. There is little question that in the United States the growth factors G-CSF and GM-CSF are being overused in the clinical setting. It is worth emphasizing that there is still no information indicating that the use of these growth factors has prolonged survival or increased cure rates. In addition, although I believe that they are probably beneficial in some patients with cancer treated with chemotherapy, it is unclear whether an equivalent result might be obtained by a dose reduction of the chemotherapeutic agent. The critical issue here remains the effect of the growth factors on the natural history of tumor progression. In other words, could we be harming some of our patients by using these potent biologicals? Cost-effectiveness has been cited as a reason to use the growth factors. I feel that these are false arguments. In fact, in the structured manner in which they have been studied, they may have some cost-effectiveness, although the studies have not included the appropriate controls, i.e., patients discharged at the same time intervals not on growth factors regardless of the level of their count. This is a relatively minor point, however. The manner in which G-CSF and GM-CSF are currently being used is not by the rigid protocols reported in the literature. Cytokines are frequently administered to patients who have little hope of tumor response or ultimate recovery. They have become a major cost item in the marrow transplant setting. Used in this fashion, they are extraordinarily cost-ineffective and promise to become one of the major expenses in most hospital pharmacies. These fascinating biologicals undoubtedly have a role to play in specific clinical settings. My recommendation now would be to use them only under defined protocol conditions in which specific experimental questions are being asked.

The feasibility of in vitro transplantation, as outlined in Abstracts 2–2 and 2–3, suggests important potential applications to various human genetic diseases. In fact, in vitro transplantation has been carried out in patients with severe combined immunodeficiency, β-thalassemia, Hurler syndrome, and bare lymphocyte syndrome with a least some evidence of engraftment in some patients. The information suggesting a period of tolerance in early gestation for unrelated or histoimcompatible cells is particularly compelling. The data from a sheep model suggest that one can transplant human cells at this point and get engraftment. Major questions relate to the degree of engraftment, its longevity, and its potential long-term side effects.

Peter J. Quesenberry, M.D.

Hematopoietic Stem Cells

Formation of Haematopoietic Microenvironment and Haematopoietic Stem Cells From Single Human Bone Marrow Stem Cells

Huang S, Terstappen LWMM (Becton Dickinson Immunocytometry Systems, San Jose, Calif)

Nature 360:745–749, 1992

2–1

Background.—Methods of enriching human hematopoietic stem cells have relied on the expression of CD34, which is present on progenitor cells in the bone marrow. Most of these cells, however, are committed to their lineage. Recently, attempts have been made to characterize a pluripotent subset of CD34+ cells.

Objective.—The expression of CD38 and HLA-DR on CD34+cells was investigated in samples of human fetal bone marrow of gestational age 16–22 weeks. The presence of primitive mesenchymal elements among HLA-DR−, CD38− cells prompted a search for stem cells not dependent on hematopoietic growth factors.

Findings.—Cells from fetal bone marrow that were CD34+ and HLA-DR+ but CD38− were found capable of differentiating into all hematopoietic lineages. The subset of CD34+, HLA-DR−, CD38− cells was capable of differentiating into both hematopoietic precursors and stromal cells that supported the differentiation of these precursors. The cells demonstrated self-renewal by repeated reconstruction after disruption and supplementation with cytokines.

Conclusion.—This is the first demonstration that a single cell is able to reconstitute both hematopoietic cells and their associated supportive stromal cells from the marrow microenvironment. Presumably, common stem cells first generate stromal stem cells in utero, and these produce a microenvironment where common stem cells are induced to form hematopoietic stem cells. Purified common stem cells would conceivably be an ideal target for gene therapy. In addition, the role of these cells in hematopoietic malignancies deserves investigation.

▶ This was one of the hot presentations at the American Society of Hematology meeting last December. The observation that a single CD34+ HLA-DR− CD38− cell can differentiate into both hematopoietic and stromal cells with extensive replication capacity is fascinating. The data presented are quite convincing, but many investigators still would like to see single-cell transfer for demonstration of these common stem cells. These investigators are experts in the area of fluorescent-activated cell sorting, but there is still concern for whether doublets may have accounted for some of these results. Another possibility is that 1 cell was carried intracytoplasmically in another cell. Although these criteria may appear to be overly rigorous, they seem appropriate given the basic importance of the observations reported. The demonstration of a common stromal-hematopoietic stem cell clearly changes our thinking with regard to control of hematopoiesis. Another possibility, of course, is that this is a fetal characteristic and will not hold for adult cells. This will be an exciting experimental tract to follow during the next several years.—P.J. Quesenberry, M.D.

Sustained Human Hematopoiesis in Sheep Transplanted In Utero During Early Gestation With Fractionated Adult Human Bone Marrow Cells

Srour EF, Zanjani ED, Brandt JE, Leemhuis T, Briddell RA, Heerema NA, Hoffman R (Indiana Univ, Indianapolis; VA Med Ctr, Reno, Nev)

Blood 79:1404–1412, 1992   2-2

Introduction.—A small fraction of adult human bone marrow cells express CD34 and low or undetectable levels of HLA-DR and are capable of sustaining long-term hematopoiesis in vitro. The human hematopoietic stem cell or a cell having many of its functional features is probably present among CD34+HLA-DR⁻ marrow cells.

Methods.—If these cells are present and they are used as marrow grafts, immunologic tolerance to sheep self-antigens might be inducible in progeny cells after the human cells differentiate and mature in a "nonself" environment. Fractionated adult human marrow cells enriched for hematopoietic progenitor and stem cells were transplanted into immunologically immature sheep fetuses.

Results.—Chimerism was documented in 3 of 7 sheep fetuses, by either monoclonal antibodies against human-specific hematopoietic cell lines or cytogenetic analysis of recipient marrow and blood cells. Only chimeric sheep marrow cells expressing CD45, which formed 6% of all marrow cells, formed human hematopoietic colonies in response to recombinant human cytokines. Human T-cell colonies containing CD3+, CD4+, and CD8+ cells developed from CD45+ marrow cells. The DNA taken from chimeric marrow cells 3 months after birth had a fingerprinting pattern identical to that of DNA from the human donor of the hematopoietic stem cell graft.

Applications.—This model may prove helpful in determining the ability of human marrow subpopulations to sustain hematopoiesis in vivo over the long term. It may prove feasible to use cell populations from adult human marrow across HLA barriers to correct congenital metabolic or hematologic abnormalities in utero.

▶ These authors have demonstrated that human marrow stem cells can be successfully transplanted to sheep fetuses at gestational ages between 42 and 48 days, when the animals are immunologically tolerant. Three of 7 animals showed chimerism, and the documentation in 1 animal that human cells were present 3 months after birth suggests that low-level stable engraftment occurred. These data do not tell us what level the stem or progenitor cell may have engrafted but suggest the feasibility of current attempts at in utero engraftment for various human genetic diseases.—P.J. Quesenberry, M.D.

Liver-Derived Fetal Hematopoietic Stem Cells Selectively and Preferentially Home to the Fetal Bone Marrow

Zanjani ED, Ascensao JL, Tavassoli M (Univ of Nevada, Reno; Univ of Mississippi, Jackson)
Blood 81:399–404, 1993

2–3

Background.—During fetal development, the homing site for hematopoietic stem cells (HSC) shifts from the yolk sac to the liver and spleen and then to the bone marrow. Thus far, this pattern has been established mostly on a morphologic basis.

Objective.—The pattern of migration of the HSCs was examined by the in utero transplantation of allogeneic or xenogeneic cells into preimmune sheep fetuses. The path of the transplanted cells was followed using the sex chromosome, type of hemoglobin, and species-specific surface markers as indicators.

Findings.—Initially both liver- and marrow-derived HSC homed only to the liver and spleen. As bone marrow developed at about 60 days' gestation, homing occurred also in the nascent marrow. By day 80, the marrow was the exclusive site of homing and remained so until term at 145 days. The liver remained the major source of HSCs during most of the prenatal period, without participation by the marrow itself. Only perinatally did the bone marrow assume hematopoietic function.

Conclusion.—The stroma of immature fetal bone marrow apparently is not adequate to support the differentiation and maturation of hematopoietic progenitors. After day 80, marrow sites preferentially accept HSC from fetal liver until the perinatal period. Measures allowing the bone marrow to support the differentiation and egress of mature donor cells early in gestation could make in utero stem cell transplantation more effective, especially when the disease is active even before birth (as in Hurler syndrome).

▶ The ultimate origin of hematopoiesis during embryonic development remains controversial. The classic work of Moore et al. (1) indicating that there was stem cell migration from the yolk sac to the fetal liver to the marrow has been challenged by Duane and colleagues, who have proposed a mesenchymal origin for hematopoiesis. The contribution by Huang and Terstappen (Abstract 2–1) suggests that early cells may have the potential to form both stroma and hematopoiesis locally. This article by Zanjani and colleagues holds the promise of further defining the issue of developmental migratory streams from 1 organ to another. They have shown that marrow becomes the exclusive site of stem cell homing after day 80 of gestation in sheep, but this, of course does not yet speak to the origin of hematopoiesis during normal development. The observation that the marrow site did not support differentiation in maturation is quite intriguing and suggests that there may be developmental processes that need to occur in microenvironmental tissues to allow the full hematopoietic differentiation program to proceed. —P.J. Quesenberry, M.D.

Reference

1. Moore MAS, Metcalf D: *Br J Haematol* 18:279, 1970.

The Same Exhaustible Multilineage Precursor Produces Both Myeloid and Lymphoid Cells as Early as 3–4 Weeks After Marrow Transplantation
Harrison DE, Zhong R-k (Jackson Lab, Bar Harbor, Me)
Proc Natl Acad Sci USA 89:10134–10138, 1992   2–4

Introduction.—Throughout life, a wide range of myeloid and lymphoid cells develop from common precursors. An important issue in immunology is the role of the lymphoid-specific precursor in repopulation. The myeloid-specific precursor is the common precursor of myeloid but not lymphoid cells. Mice were used as marrow donors to assess the populations of marrow precursors from which both myeloid and lymphoid lineages descend shortly after transplantation.

Observations.—Few or none of the marrow precursors exhibited long-term repopulating ability. When a mixture of marrow cells from different strains of mice was transplanted, significant correlations between proportions of B6-type T cells, B cells, granulocytes, and platelets were noted 3 weeks later, indicating that many lymphoid and myeloid cells are descended from common precursors. More differentiated myeloid-specific precursors did not contribute significantly to myeloid cell populations. The variance in cell types increased substantially 3 to 12 weeks after transplantation, indicating that most or all of the initially active multilineage precursors were exhausted at this time.

Conclusion.—The ability of a hematopoietic stem cell to differentiate into desparate lineages does not correlate necessarily with its long-term repopulating ability. It is possible that 2 or more types of stem cells exist that can produce both myeloid and lymphoid descendents but have vastly different long-term repopulating ability.

Bipotential Precursors of B Cells and Macrophages in Murine Fetal Liver
Cumano A, Paige CJ, Iscove NN, Brady G (Ontario Cancer Inst, Toronto)
Nature 356:612–615, 1992   2–5

Background.—Lymphocytes are derived from the same multipotential stem cells that produce myeloid cells, including granulocytes, macrophages, and erythrocytes. Clonal studies have demonstrated tripotential and bipotential myeloid intermediates between the early multipotential stem cells and the later unipotential cells. Committed pre-B cells also have been detected in murine fetal liver, but earlier progenitors that possess non-B lineage options have not been found in normal tissues.

Objective.—An attempt was made to characterize murine fetal liver cells that generate clones containing both macrophages and B cells. Precursors were extensively purified to assess the clonal progeny of single isolated cells.

Results.—Cultures of single precursor cells confirmed a common origin for macrophages and B cells. Their unrearranged immunoglobulin loci placed the precursor cells before exclusive B-lineage commitment in hematopoietic development.

Conclusion.—This study established the ability of normal murine hematopoietic precursors to generate clones containing both lymphoid and myeloid cells. About half the B-cell precursors in fetal liver have dual potential on day 12. Both B cells and macrophage-like cells derive from untransformed cells that have not rearranged their immunoglobulin loci.

▶ These 2 contributions (Abstracts 2–4 and 2–5) are discussed together because they address the "stemness" of cells that give rise to both lymphocytes and myeloid cells. These studies relate to the issue of whether there is a common stem cell for lymphopoiesis, i.e., B and T cells per se, or whether all lymphopoiesis originates from myeloid-lymphopoietic stem cell. The Harrison and Zhong data indicate that a surprisingly early, albeit short-term, repopulation is derived from a cell that gives rise to both the lymphocyte populations and myeloid cells. They further define these early cells as separate from long-term repopulating cells. Harrison and Zhong use a different approach from many investigators, studing competing marrow mixtures and determining correlations between cell types to then ascertain the origin of these cells. Their approach appears valid, albeit unique, and these data are a convincing demonstration that early repopulation is carried out by a somewhat differentiated stem cell with the potential to make both lymphoid and myeloid populations. The contribution by Cumano et al. further emphasizes this point, showing that macrophages and B cells are derived from a common progenitor in mouse fetal liver. Ogawa, Weissman, and colleagues (1, 2) have also presented evidence indicating the presence of short-lived clones giving rise to lymphoid and myeloid populations.—P.J. Quesenberry, M.D.

References

1. Hirayama R, et al: *Proc Natl Acad Sci USA* 89:5907–5911, 1992.
2. Smith LG, et al: *Proc Natl Acad Sci USA* 88:2788–2792, 1991.

"Stem Cell" Origin of the Hematopoietic Defect in Dyskeratosis Congenita

Marsh JCW, Will AJ, Hows JM, Sartori P, Darbyshire PJ, Williamson PJ, Oscier DG, Dexter TM, Testa NG (Christie Hosp, Manchester, England; Hammersmith Hosp, London; Children's Hosp, Birmingham, England; et al)
Blood 79:3138–3144, 1992   2–6

Purpose.—Dyskeratosis congenita (DC), is the rare congenital and familial disorder, characterized by abnormal skin pigmentation, nail dystrophy, and leukoplakia of mucosal membranes, with about half of patients having bone marrow (BM) failure. The pathogenesis of BM failure in patients with DC has been assessed using only clonogenic assays, which showed markedly reduced or absent multilineage colonies and granulocyte-macrophage colonies. In-depth analysis of hematopoiesis was undertaken in 3 patients using long-term BM culture (LTBMC), as well as a modification of this system to assess hematopoietic and stromal cell function.

Methods and Results.—The study included 3 patients with classic signs of DC. Two of them also had aplastic anemia, whereas the third had a normal blood count, other than mild macrocytosis, and normal BM cellularity. Compared with normal LTBMC, the number of hematopoietic foci was reduced to less than 10% for the first 2 patients and 25% for the third. The first 2 patients also showed severe functional hematopoietic defects, more marked for granulocyte-macrophage colony-forming cells than for total cell numbers. In all cases, the marrow stroma was normal in its ability to support the growth of seeded hematopoietic progenitors from normal BM. However, when patient marrow cells were inoculated onto normal stromas, the generation of hematopoietic progenitors was reduced. The parents and unaffected brother of 1 patient showed normal hematopoietic and stromal cell function on LTBMC.

Conclusion.—This study documents normal stromal function but severe defects of stem cell function in patients with DC. Defects in stem cell function may relate to the pathogenesis and outcome of this disease. The LTBMC system used in this study appears to be sufficiently sensitive to detect a stem cell defect before BM failure develops.

▶ This is an interesting (albeit of necessity), somewhat anecdotal study of the nature of the defect present in the rare DC disorder. The marrow failure occurring in these patients is clearly separate from that seen in patients with Fanconi's anemia as discerned by normal diepoxybutane tests (1). The work of Marsh and colleagues suggests that the defect in patients with DC and marrow failure resides at the stem cell level. This would be consistent with the fact that of 5 patients with DC who have been transplanted for marrow failure with HLA-identical sibling donors, engraftment has occurred in all and 3 have shown long-term engraftment for 2, 4, and 7 years (2–5). These observations plus the data suggesting that stromal cells are not translatable point to a stem cell origin for the marrow problems in DC. In addition, the authors cite 2 instances of acute myelocytic leukemia (unpublished data) in patients with DC. Thus, we can probably include DC as another stem cell disorder.—P.J. Quesenberry, M.D.

References

1. Auerbach AD, et al: *Blood* 73:391, 1989.
2. Berthou C, et al: *Br J Haematol* 70:335, 1991.
3. Ling NS, et al: *Arch Dermatol* 121:1424, 1985.
4. Mahmoud HK, et al: *Blut* 51:57, 1985.
5. Conter V, et al: *Am J Pediatr Hematol Oncol* 10:99, 1988.

CD4 Is Expressed on Murine Pluripotent Hematopoietic Stem Cells

Wineman JP, Gilmore GL, Gritzmacher C, Torbett BE, Müller-Sieburg CE (Med Biology Inst, La Jolla, Calif; Scripps Clinic and Research Found, La Jolla, Calif)
Blood 80:1717–1724, 1992   2–7

Introduction.—The expression of CD4 antigen on primitive stem cells was clarified. Previously, hematopoietic stem cells were found to lack this antigen, although some early hematopoietic precursors have recently been shown to express CD4.

Findings.—Pluripotent hematopoietic stem cells from mice expressed CD4 antigen. The CD4+cells from murine bone marrow repopulated all hematopoietic cell lineages in long-term repopulation assays and competitive repopulation assays. The CD4⁻ population exhibited significant life-sparing activity. A majority of cells responding to the stroma in cultures with B-cell differentiation were CD4⁻cells. The molecular weight and epitope makeup of CD4 molecules expressed on marrow cells resembled those of the CD4 found on thymocytes.

Conclusion.—This study and others suggest that CD4 is expressed throughout the course of early hematopoietic differentiation, except for B-lineage cells. Such a widely expressed antigen may well have functional significance. The presence of CD4 on mature T cells could have a role in cell-cell interactions through interacting with class II major histocompatibility antigens expressed on antigen-presenting cells. In this way, CD4 might enhance the interaction of hematopoietic cells with their microenvironment.

▶ A great deal of recent attention has focused on characterization of both murine and human hematopoietic stem cells. The claim to have isolated "the stem cell" (1) has generated an enthusiastic debate. Further work has indicated that the originally reported lineage-negative Sca+ Thy-1^{lo} cell is further subsetted by rhodamine staining into short-term and long-term repopulating cells. The work by Wineman et al. indicates that CD4 is expressed on murine pluripotent hematopoietic stem cells with extensive repopulation capacity. This is worrisome for those following the Spangrude (1) separation technique, as a depletion of CD4+cells is an early step. However, relatively low levels of CD4 are expressed, necessitating high concentrations of antibody for separation. Future work in this area needs to pay attention to this point, especially with steps designed to deplete populations of T cells.—P.J. Quesenberry, M.D.

Reference

1. Sprangrude GJ, et al: *Science* 241:58, 1988.

Demonstration of Stem Cell Inhibition and Myeloprotective Effects of SCI/rhMIP 1α In Vivo

Dunlop DJ, Wright EG, Lorimore S, Graham GJ, Holyoake T, Kerr DJ, Wolpe SD, Pragnell IB (CRC Beatson Lab, Bearsden, Glasgow, Scotland; MRC Radiobiology Unit, Chilton, Didcot, Oxom; Western Infirmary, Glasgow, Scotland; et al)
Blood 79:2221–2225, 1992   2–8

Background.—Both positive and negative regulating factors influence the proliferation of stem cells in the bone marrow, and these factors have potential clinical value for manipulating the proliferation of stem cells in vivo in patients treated for neoplastic disease.

Methods.—The proliferation of primitive murine progenitor cells was evaluated both in vitro and in vivo after exposure to a stem cell inhibitor (SCI), the human recombinant homologue of murine macrophage inflammatory protein-1α (rhMIP-1α). The recombinant protein is similar to LD78, the human homologue of MIP-1α.

Results.—In vitro studies of stem cell CFU(-S) showed rhMIP-1α to be active in a dose-dependent manner at day 12, and to a slightly lesser degree at day 8. In vivo activity was demonstrated in 2 models of marrow regeneration where the initially high proliferative level of CFU-S was reduced to quiescence after a single inoculation of SCI/rhMIP-1α. Measurements of improvement in the kinetics of neutrophil recovery confirmed the inhibitory action of SCI/rhMIP-1α.

Conclusion.—Because myelosuppression may limit the dose of chemotherapy, myeloprotective cytokines may permit dose intensification and thereby help eliminate chemosensitive malignancies. The present findings indicate the feasibility of testing SCI/rhMIP-1α in conjunction with various chemotherapeutic regimens.

▶ MIP-1α appears to have the capacity to inhibit CFU-S cycle entry in normal bone marrow in a reversible fashion (1, 2). This article shows that in 2 models of marrow regeneration, MIP-1α improved the kinetics of neutrophil recovery. A number of other inhibitors of early hematopoietic stem cells have also been described, including transforming growth factor-β, which suppresses CFU-S progenitor proliferation in a dose-dependent manner (3). The regulatory pentapeptide, pEEDCK, has also been described as effective in protecting the CFU-S compartment. In a similar vein, a tetrapeptide, AcSKDP, results in some decrease in lethal toxicity induced by a combination of Aac and cytoxin (4). At a recent meeting in Paris, preliminary data on the initial clinical trials with both the pentapeptide and tetrapeptide were presented, both showing that they could be tolerated in vivo and suggesting, in a tantalizing fashion, the possibility of better chemotherapy tolerance and/or clinical results. Using these various inhibitors to protect early marrow stem cells in the setting of chemotherapy is the current direction being taken, and hopefully it could result in therapeutic agents that might lessen the toxicity of chemotherapy to the normal marrow stem cells but not to the malignant tumor.—P.J. Quesenberry, M.D.

Reference

1. Lord BI, et al: *Br J Haematol* 34:441, 1976.
2. Broxmeyer JE, et al: *Blood* 76:1110, 1990.
3. Migdalska A, et al: *Growth Factors* 4:239, 1991.
4. Bogden AE, et al: *Ann NY Acad Sci* 628:126, 1991.

Hematopoietic Stroma

Binding of Primitive Hematopoietic Progenitor Cells to Marrow Stromal Cells Involves Heparan Sulfate

Siczkowski M, Clarke D, Gordon MY (Inst of Cancer Research, London)
Blood 80:912–919, 1992   2–9

Introduction.—Both blast colony-forming cells (Bl-CFCs) and pre–CFU-granulocyte, monocyte (Pre-CFU-GM) cells in human bone marrow bind to marrow-derived stromal layers grown in the presence of methylprednisolone (MP). The binding of these progenitor cells to stroma depends on the presence of heparan sulfate proteoglycan (HS-PG) in the extracellular matrix secreted by stromal cells. An attempt was made to distinguish the functional and biochemical characteristics of HS-PG isolated from MP-positive and MP-negative stromal cultures. Marrow cells were obtained from adult donors of marrow for allogeneic transplantation.

Results.—Both HS-PG and isolated HS glycosaminoglycan (GAG) side chains partly blocked progenitor cell binding when added to the 2-hour binding phase of a Bl-CFC or the pre–CFU-GM assay. Gel electrophoresis of HS-PG yielded more bands in matrix preparations from MP-positive than from MP-negative cultures. The blocking activity of eluted MP-positive HS-PG bands depended partly on the amount of GAG attached to the protein core. The HS-dependent phase of the interaction was limited to the first 30 to 60 minutes of the 2-hour binding phase.

Conclusion.—These findings are consistent with an initial phase of adhesion in which HS-GAG is specifically recognized by an anchored cell adhesion component, followed by further adhesion events that remain to be identified. The HS-GAG in MP-positive stroma has a higher degree of sulfation and higher negative charge-to-mass ratio than does that in MP-negative stroma.

▶ This is one possible explanation for the importance of corticosteroids in the establishment of Dexter long-term cultures, the binding of critical early progenitor cells. Deficiencies in progenitor surface ligand binding to specific HS-GAG may explain the failure of chronic mylogous leukemic blasts to bind to stroma, and this, in turn, may explain why long-term Dexter cultures appear to select against the malignant chronic mylogous leukemic clone and why they can be used effectively, at least short term, for autologous transplantation in this disease.—P.J. Quesenberry, M.D.

Biologic Significance of Constitutive and Subliminal Growth Factor Production by Bone Marrow Stroma
Kittler ELW, McGrath H, Temeles D, Crittenden RB, Kister VK, Quesenberry PJ (Univ of Virginia, Charlottesville)
Blood 79:3168–3178, 1992   2–10

Background.—The murine bone marrow culture system described by Dexter et al. (1) provides a useful in vitro model of the microenvironment of the bone marrow. The adherent stromal cells of these cultures produce CSF-1 constitutively, but the constitutive production of other hemolymphopoietic cytokines had not been confirmed. We have previously described the detection and evaluation of GM-CSF.

Methods.—The production of stromal cytokine messenger RNA was examined by Northern blot analysis in normal or irradiated Dexter-type explant bone marrow cultures established with marrow from female BALB/c mice (6 to 8 weeks of age).

Results.—Messanger RNAs for CSF-1, GM-CSF, G-CSF, c-*kit* ligand (KL), and IL-6 were constitutively produced by the Dexter stromal cells at 4 weeks. Messenger RNAs for IL-3, IL-4, and IL-5 were not detected. The exposure of stromal cells to pokeweed mitogen or IL-1 induced messages for GM-CSF, G-CSF, KL, and IL-6. The use of the PCR method to amplify complementary DNA demonstrated IL-3 message in irradiated stromal cells. Factor-dependent cell lines (FDC-P1 or 32D) were supported by stromal cells without the need for exogenous growth factors, and their growth was inhibited by exposure to an IL-3 monoclonal antibody, indicating the production of biologically active IL-3 in this hemesystem.

Conclusion.—Dexter stromal cells produce a number of cytokines constitutively. Stromal IL-3 messenger RNA is only detectable by PCR techniques but is biologically active. "Subliminal" levels of IL-3 and possibly other cytokines may be important in stromal in vitro hematopoiesis regulation.

Reference

1. Dexter TM, et al: Conditions controlling the proliferation of haemopoietic stem cells in vitro. *J Cell Physiol* 91:335, 1977.

▶ This article needs to be considered in the context of Abstract 2–29 where it is demonstrated that very low concentration ("subliminal") of cytokines can act in a synergistic fashion when certain critical "anchor" factors (Steel) are present at optimum concentrations. This contribution states that very low amounts of IL-3 messenger RNA, only detectable by reverse transcriptase PCR methodology, produce biologically active protein. These data suggest that primitive hematopoietic stem cells adhere directly to stromal cell membranes, presumably through a variety of adhesion proteins, and then are exposed and respond to a relatively large number of membrane-based or soluble cytokines, some of which may be biologically active at very low concentrations. Recent data from our laboratory (1) indicate the possibility that growth on stroma of target cells may also turn on autocrine loops, which introduces even more complexity into this fascinating model.—P.J. Quesenberry M.D.

Reference

1. Kittler EW, Quesenberry PJ: Unpublished.

The Generation of Human Natural Killer Cells From CD34⁺/DR⁻ Primitive Progenitors in Long-Term Bone Marrow Culture

The Generation of Human Natural Killer Cells From CD34$^+$/DR$^-$ Primitive Progenitors in Long-Term Bone Marrow Culture

Miller JS, Verfaillie C, McGlave P (Univ of Minnesota, Minneapolis)
Blood 80:2182–2187, 1992
2–11

Background.—It has been proposed that primitive progenitors of both myeloid and lymphoid lineage may be found among bone marrow mononuclear cells that express CD34. Cells with phenotypic and cytotoxic characteristics of natural killer (NK) cells have been cultured from primitive lymphoid progenitors.

Objective and Methods.—The stroma-dependent long-term bone marrow culture system was used to examine the development of human NK cells from the population of CD34+/HLA-DR⁻ bone marrow mononuclear cells. Such cells, obtained from 20 healthy adults by fluorescence-activated cell sorting, were plated on irradiated allogeneic bone marrow stromal layers.

Results.—Marked expansion of cells resembling large granular lymphocytes was noted after 5 weeks of culture in the presence of recombinant IL-2 and human serum. The cultured cells expressed the CD56+/CD3− phenotype characteristic of NK cells. Some cells also expressed markers of lymphoid lineage associated with mature NK cells, such as CD2, CD7, CD8, and CD16. The cultured cells were cytotoxic against K562 and Raji target cell lines.

Conclusion.—Cells of the human CD34+/DR− population that do not express lineage-specific antigens are able to differentiate into NK cells.

▶ A number of studies have now established the importance of stromal support of myelopoiesis and B lymphopoiesis in different culture systems. Presumptively, stroma provides both soluble cytokines and membrane-based cytokines along with critical adhesion factors for appropriate proliferation and differentiation of hematopoietic cell populations. Previous data have shown that a population of rat NK cells can be generated from bone marrow cells only in the presence of stroma (1), and this article extends this to the generation of human NK cells from isolated CD34+/DR− cells plated on allogeneic, irradiated human stromal layers. This occurred in the presence of recombinant IL-2 and human serum.—P.J. Quesenberry M.D.

Reference

1. van der Brink MRM, et al: *J Exp Med* 172:303, 1990.

Characterization of Endothelial Cells in Murine Long-Term Marrow Culture. Implication for Hemopoietic Regulation
Hasthorpe S, Bogdanovski M, Rogerson J, Radley JM (Peter MacCallum Cancer Inst, Melbourne, Australia)
Exp Hematol 20:476–481, 1992   2–12

Introduction.—The interaction between hematopoietic cells and stroma in the bone marrow appears critical in the regulation of hematopoiesis. A thorough understanding of stromal cell–related hematopoiesis requires a knowledge of the various cell types present in long-term marrow culture (LTMC). In particular, the identity of very large cells or "blanket cells" remains uncertain.

Methods.—Dual immunogold labeling with monoclonal antibody, H513E3, and antihuman factor VIII antibodies was used in attempt to locate endothelial cells in mouse LTMC. This monoclonal antibody reacts specifically with vascular endothelium.

Findings.—The LTMC endothelial cells had exactly the location and ultrastructural features as previously described blanket cells. They were relatively large, had thinly spread cytoplasm, and also overlay macrophages, granulocytes, and other less differentiated hematopoietic cells. Micrographs of LTMC-adherent stroma showed the upper endothelial

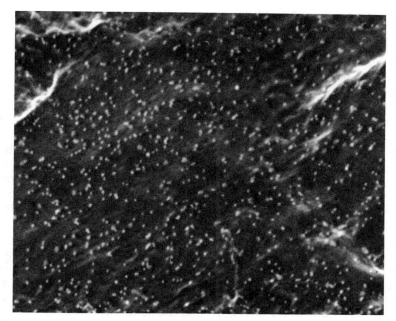

Fig 2–1.—Scanning electron microscope micrograph of mouse LTMC-adherent stroma labeled with H513E3 monoclonal antibody-protein A-10-nm gold with silver enhancement of gold grains. The upper endothelial cell layer is heavily labeled with the H513E3 monoclonal antibody, with numerous silver grains apparent. (Courtesy of Hasthorpe S, Bogdanovski M, Rogerson J, et al: *Exp Hematol* 20:476–481, 1992.)

cell layer to be heavily labeled with H513E3 monoclonal antibody (Fig 2-1).

Discussion.—Appellations such as blanket cells may now be dropped and these cells accepted as endothelium. Their functional role remains to be established, but morphologic studies suggest that they actively synthesize proteins and take up molecules from their milieu.

▶ This carefully done study documents the existence of endothelial cells in murine Dexter cultures and their probable identify with blanket cells. One note of caution is that these cultures were supplemented with 20% fetal calf serum, whereas standard murine Dexter cultures have ordinarily used horse serum. This could explain some of the different results in the literature with regard to the presence of endothelial cells in Dexter cultures. Even different lots of horse serum can markedly alter cytokine messenger RNA production, and correlation of this with growth in the system is poor. Thus, Dexter cultures may vary from laboratory to laboratory, depending on the serum supplementation.—P.J. Quesenberry, M.D.

Interleukins and Growth Factors

In Vivo Effect of Interleukin-1α on Hematopoiesis: Role of Colony-Stimulating Factor Receptor Modulation

Hestdal K, Jacobsen SEW, Ruscetti FW, Dubois CM, Longo DL, Chizzonite R, Oppenheim JJ, Keller JR (Natl Cancer Inst, Frederick, Md; Hoffman-LaRoche, Nutley, NJ)
Blood 80:2486–2494, 1992   2–13

Introduction.—A potent potentiator of hematopoietic cell growth in vitro and in vivo is IL-1. It enhances granulopoiesis and also hastens the recovery of myeloid cells treated with sublethal doses of chemotherapeutic drugs. Because IL-1 rapidly induces the production of hematopoietic growth factors, its hematopoietic effects in vivo may be indirectly mediated through various cytokines.

Objective.—The mechanisms by which IL-1 promotes granulopoiesis in vivo were studied to determine the effects of administering IL-1α to mice on the expression of CSF receptors on murine bone marrow cells.

Results.—Administration of IL-1α upregulated both GM-CSF and IL-3 receptors. These effects were more evident in a progenitor-enriched cell population. Enhanced expression of GM-CSF and IL-3 receptors correlated with increased stimulation by the factors of CFU culture or CFU-mixture. The number of colony-forming cells having high proliferative potential increased fivefold. Binding of G-CSF was reduced after IL-1α administration. The effects of IL-1α on GM-CSF and IL-3 receptors were blocked by pretreating mice with anti-type I IL-1 receptor antibody.

Interpretation.—Interleukin-1α may stimulate the expression of functional GM-CSF and IL-3 receptors on bone marrow cells. Along with induction of CSFs, this may explain the ability of IL-1α to stimulate hematopoiesis.

▶ This nice study indicates the IL-1α may induce expression of GM-CSF and IL-3 receptors. This may well explain some of the synergistic effects of IL-1α in different systems and provides a general model for further fine-tuning cytokine modulation of early marrow stem cells.—P.J. Quesenberry, M.D.

Elevated Serum Levels of Interleukin-5 in Patients With the Syndrome of Episodic Angioedema and Eosinophilia

Butterfield JH, Leiferman KM, Abrams J, Silver JE, Bower J, Gonchoroff N, Gleich GJ (Mayo Clinic and Mayo Found, Rochester, Minn; DNAX Research Inst, Palo Alto, Calif and Lykens, Pa)
Blood 79:688–692, 1992   2–14

Introduction.—In 1984, Gleich et al. described 4 patients with recurrent angioedema, urticaria, fever, marked episodic weight gain, and eosinophilia. The levels of IgM were increased, and eosinophilic infiltration and degranulation were seen in the dermis. The risk of cardiovascular morbidity is not increased, in contrast to idiopathic hypereosinophilic syndrome.

Patient Studies.—Because IL-5 specifically stimulates human eosinophil differentiation and activates eosinophils, serum IL-5 levels were assayed in 4 patients with episodic angioedema and eosinophilia. The 3 previously reported patients all had increased serum IL-5 levels during attacks. In the 1 new patient, IL-5 levels peaked several days before maximum eosinophilia and then decreased. The lymphocytes included 28% activated T cells staining for both CD3 and HLA-DR, 10 days before peak eosinophilia, but no increase at the time of the peak. No IL-5 was detected after glucocorticoid treatment in 3 of 4 patients.

Conclusion.—Increased production of IL-5 may explain many aspects of the syndrome of episodic angioedema and eosinophilia.

▶ Another growth factor disease! Well, at least it appears that IL-5 plays a role here. Apparently, IL-5 is the primary eosinophil regulator stimulating human eosinophil differentiation (1), prolonging in vitro survival (2), and converting normodense to hypodense eosinophils (3), while acting as an eosinophil chemoattractant (2, 4). The GM-CSF and IL-3 also act on the eosinophil lineage, and these 3 cytokines have dimeric receptors on eosinophils that consist of a unique alpha-chain and a beta-chain that are common to all 3 receptors. The basis for this unusual syndrome remains unknown, and although activated T cells may be the source of IL-5, we still have little clue to basic pathophysiology or inciting events. This is a good one for syndromologists.—P.J. Quesenberry, M.D.

References

1. Clutterbuck EJ, et al: *Blood* 71:646, 1988.
2. Yamagucki Y, et al: *J Exp Med* 167:1737, 1988.
3. Rothenberg ME, et al: *J Immunol* 143:2311, 1989.
4. Wang JM, et al: *Eur J Immunol* 19:701, 1989.

Interleukin-5 Is an Autocrine Growth Factor for Epstein-Barr Virus-Transformed B Lymphocytes
Baumann MA, Paul CC (Wright State Univ, Dayton, Ohio)
Blood 79:1763–1767, 1992   2–15

Background.—Normal B cells transformed by the Epstein-Barr virus (EBV) were recently shown to constitutively produce IL-5. Whether EBV-transformed B lymphocytes (EBV-B cells) might use IL-5 by an autocrine mechanism was investigated.

Observations.—The proliferation of EBV-B cells known to produce IL-5 was augmented in a dose-related fashion by the addition of exogenous IL-5. These effects were decreased by the addition of a neutralizing anti–IL-5 antibody, which also inhibited the proliferation and decreased the viability of unsupplemented EBV-B cells in a dose-dependent manner. The effect of the antibody peaked at about 120 hours. Burkitt's lymphoma cell lines had no stimulatory effect from IL-5 and no inhibitory effect from anti–IL-5 antibody. Binding of IL-5 to EBV-B cells cultured in fresh medium was demonstrated with biotinylated IL-5, second labeling with streptavidin–fluorescein isothiocyanate, and flow cytometry. Excess unlabeled IL-5 competed for this binding, suggesting that binding sites specific for IL-5 were present. In cells cultured for longer periods, IL-5 binding was decreased; however, binding was restored by extensive washing of cells before labeling with biotinylated IL-5. This suggested that surface binding sites had become occupied by endogenously produced IL-5.

Conclusion.—Epstein-Barr–altered B cells producing IL-5 were shown to bind IL-5 specifically, to have their growth inhibited by anti–IL-5 antibody, and to respond to IL-5 by augmented proliferation. This suggests that EBV-B cells produce and use IL-5 in an autocrine fashion.

▶ Not surprisingly, IL-5 has proliferative effects on human B lymphocytes, and although this may be confined to EBV-infected cells, it seems more likely that normal human B cells will also be responsive to IL-5. The possibility of autocrine IL-5 production is exciting. Evolving studies suggest that autocrine loops may be an important mechanism in normal cell regulation. The observation that IL-5 shares receptor chains with IL-3 and GM-CSF raises the possibility that these 3 factors may show unique actions and/or synergies on both eosinophils and B-cell growth.—P.J. Quesenberry, M.D.

Cytokine Serum Level During Severe Sepsis in Human IL-6 as a Marker of Severity

Damas P, Ledoux D, Nys M, Vrindts Y, De Groote D, Franchimont P, Lamy M (Univ of Liège, Belgium; Medgenix, Fleurus, Belgium)
Ann Surg 215:356–362, 1992   2–16

Background.—Cytokines IL-β and tumor necrosis factor (TNF-α) are produced mainly by activated macrophages in response to injury. Many consequences of bacterial sepsis are currently believed to be caused by the release of these polypeptides. Another cytokine, IL-6, appears to be the most efficient stimulator of liver production of acute-phase proteins. The role of IL-1β, TNF-α, and IL-6 in human infection, particularly septic shock, was investigated.

Methods.—Forty critically ill surgical patients with documented infections were studied while in the intensive care unit. Nineteen developed septic shock and 16 died, 9 from septic shock. Interleukin-1β, TNF-α,

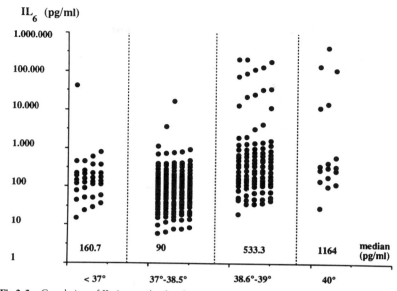

Fig 2–2.—Correlation of IL-6 serum level with maximum recorded temperature on the same day for the entire group of 40 patients. Median is the mean of the log of IL-6 serum level. The differences between these mean values are highly significant ($P < .001$). (Courtesy of Damas P, Ledoux D, Nys M, et al: *Ann Surg* 215:356–362, 1992.)

and IL-6 were measured every day. When septic shock occurred, they were measured every 1 or 2 hours.

Findings.—Interleukin-1β was never found, and TNF-α was observed most often in serum at a level under 100 pg/mL, except during septic shock. During these acute episodes, TNF-α levels reached several hundred pg/mL for a few hours; however, IL-6 was always elevated in the serum of acutely ill patients, peaking at 500,000 pg/mL (Fig 2–2). Interleukin-6 peak serum levels were directly correlated with TNF-α peak serum levels during septic shock. Also correlated were IL-6 serum levels and temperature or C-reactive protein serum levels. Interleukin-6 was also ssociated with Acute Physiology and Chronic Health Evaluation II scores. The death rate was increased significantly in patients with IL-6 serum levels exceeding 1,000 pg/mL.

Conclusion.—In contrast to IL-1β and TNF-α, IL-6 was often found at a serum level correlating with severity of illness in these critically ill patients. Interleukin-6 was also correlated with acute-phase response. It may, therefore, be a good marker of illness severity during bacterial infection.

▶ Although the title of this contribution does not make sense, the data are fairly straightforward. Measuring an IL-6 serum level, and to some extent TNF, gives a gauge of severity of illness presumably relating to the impact of various bacterial products, especially endotoxin, on cellular sources of these cytokines.

We have carried out studies evaluating IL-6, G-CSF, and GM-CSF in a marrow transplant setting and found an impressive correlation of elevations of G-CSF and IL-6, but not GM-CSF, when patients became severly cytopenic. The common denominator here is presumptively the infectious element associated either with severe neutropenia or as a complication of surgery. The present observations are clearly of pathophysiologic interest, although I have a sneaking suspicion that determining the sedimentation rate might provide equally discriminative information.—P.J. Quesenberry, M.D.

Increased Osteoclast Development After Estrogen Loss: Mediation by Interleukin-6

Jilka RL, Hangoc G, Girasole G, Passeri G, Williams DC, Abrams JS, Boyce B, Broxmeyer H, Manolagas SC (Indiana Univ, Indianapolis; Lilly Research Labs, Indianapolis, Ind; DNAX Research Inst for Cellular and Molecular Biology, Palo Alto, Calif; et al)
Science 257:88–91, 1992   2–17

Background.—Loss of ovarian function is followed by a marked loss of bone that can be prevented by replacing estrogen. It is now believed that osteoclasts arise from hematopoietic progenitors (probably CFUs for granulocytes and macrophages) and that development of osteoclasts is controlled by cytokines such as IL-6. The production of IL-6 by bone marrow stromal cells and osteoblasts is inhibited by 17β-estradiol.

Objective.—Whether estrogen loss leads to up-regulation of osteoclast formation through increased production of IL-6 was studied in ovariectomized mice. Some mice were treated with 17β-estradiol in a dosage that prevented loss of trabecular bone in pilot studies.

Results.—An ovariectomy increased the number of CFUs for granulocytes and macrophages and increased osteoclast formation in ex vivo cultures of bone marrow. In addition, the number of osteoclasts in trabecular bone increased. All these changes were prevented by administering either 17β-estradiol or antibody to IL-6.

Conclusion.—These findings are consistent with a loss of inhibitory effects of estrogen on cytokine production or action when estrogen is deficient, leading to increased osteoclast development in the bone marrow. This may explain the increased bone resorption associated with the estrogen-deficient state.

▶ Interleukin-6 seems to play a role in the development of increased osteoclast activity postovariectomy. Presumably, IL-6 also plays a role in the development of osteoporosis in postmenopausal women. Interleukin-6 appears to be involved in bone resorption seen with Paget's disease and multiple myeloma (1). The idea that estrogen inhibits IL-6 release in the marrow, and that the loss of this inhibitory effect relates to bone resorption, is an intriguing one. This issue is not settled yet, of course, because there is also evidence that in IL-1, tumor necrosis factor and GM-CSF production by monocytes increase after ovariectomy in humans (2).—P.J. Quesenberry, M.D.

References

1. Roodman GD, et al: *Blood* 78:1198, 1991.
2. Pacifici R, et al: *Proc Natl Acad Sci USA* 88:5134, 1991.

Recombinant Glycosylated Human Interleukin-6 Accelerates Peripheral Blood Platelet Count Recovery in Radiation-Induced Bone Marrow Depression in Baboons
Herodin F, Mestries J-C, Janodet D, Martin S, Mathieu J, Gascon M-P, Pernin M-O, Ythier A (Ctr de Recherches du Service de Santé des Armées, La Tronche, France; Ares Serono, Geneva)
Blood 80:688–695, 1992   2–18

Introduction.—Interleukin-6 is a key cytokine in immune function as well as in stimulating hematopoiesis. Maturation of murine and human megakaryocytes exposed to recombinant human IL-6 (rhIL-6) alone has been demonstrated in vitro.

Study Design.—The ability of rhIL-6 to restore functional platelet production was examined in baboons exposed to a dose of neutron radiation producing reversible bone marrow depression. A dose-finding study demonstrated a dose-dependent response of peripheral platelets. The highest doses of rhIL-6 produce an elevated white cell count and a reversible normochromic normocytic anemia.

Findings.—Treatment with rhIL-6 was clinically well tolerated. A dosage of 10 µg/kg/day for 13 days significantly lessened the degree of induced thrombocytopenia and also led to earlier recovery than in control animals. The mean time to return to a baseline platelet count was 8 days less in rhIL-6–treated animals. There was no apparent effect on the recovery of white blood cells, and IL-6 did not worsen radiation-induced anemia.

Conclusion.—The finding that rhIL-6 is a potent thrombopoietic factor in clinically tolerated doses suggests its usefulness for treating induced thrombocytopenia.

▶ Interleukin-6 is a major candidate for a clinical platelet-elevating agent, along with IL-11. Interleukin-3 was showing promise, but it appears to induce unacceptable side effects reminiscent of systemic mastocytosis. Interleukin-6 may also have a problem with toxicity. One major concern is whether significant anemia may be induced in the setting of IL-6 administration. In this report, IL-6 hastened platelet recovery in irradiated baboons without worsening the anemia. Apparently, the clinical platelet agent will either be IL-6, IL-11, or some synergistic combination of growth factors.—P.J. Quesenberry, M.D.

Castleman's Disease in POEMS Syndrome With Elevated Interleukin-6

Mandler RN, Kerrigan DP, Smart J, Kuis W, Villiger P, Lotz M (Univ of New Mexico, Albuquerque; Univ of California at San Diego)
Cancer 69:2697–2703, 1992   2–19

Introduction.—The POEMS syndrome—so called for its signs of peripheral neuropathy, organomegaly, endocrinopathy, monoclonal protein, and skin lesions—is a rare multisystem disease with a poor prognosis. The pathogenesis is unknown, but immune dysfunction may play a role. The clinical and laboratory findings in a patient with POEMS syndrome and Castleman's disease were reported.

Case Report.—Woman, 26, had a number of classic features of POEMS syndrome, including chronic progressive polyradiculoneuropathy, modestly elevated paraprotein levels with lambda-chain preponderance; phrenic nerve involvement; anasarca; intercostal chest pains; hepatomegaly; increased intracranial pressure; diffuse, patchy skin hyperpigmentation; and endocrinopathy. She had a combination of POEMS and the plasma cell variant of Castleman's disease associated with systemic symptoms and a poor prognosis. The biopsy of a right axillary lymph node showed some plasma cells in the interfollicular area with a mixture of kappa- and lambda-immunoreactivity; this abnormal lymph node was the probable site of abnormal plasma cell differentiation. The biopsy was followed by a temporary improvement in some of the symptoms.

A second biopsy, done during a worsening of patient's symptoms, showed the mixed variant of Castleman's disease with features of hyalinized-vascular and plasma cell types. Focal monoclonality in the plasma cell component correlated with the M spike noted in the patient's cerebrospinal fluid and serum. The cerebrospinal fluid and serum contained elevated levels of IL-6. These levels decreased transiently after the start of immunosuppressive therapies, but the trend was toward elevation that paralleled the progressive course of the disease.

Discussion.—A case of Castleman's disease associated with POEMS syndrome was presented. Increased serum IL-6 levels previously noted in Castleman's syndrome, could play a pathogenetic role in POEMS syndrome, but further study is needed. The observation that lymph node biopsy improved the patient's symptoms suggests some relationship between hyperplastic lymph nodes and the multisystem manifestations of POEMS syndrome.

▶ This is a great one for clinical roundsmanship. The association of Castleman's disease and POEMS syndrome is apparently a real one and is likely to stump most of your colleagues on rounds. The best bet here is that IL-6 may be the link between the tissue abnormalities and the clinical symptoms.—P.J. Quesenberry, M.D.

Effects of Intravenous IL-8 Administration in Nonhuman Primates
Van Zee KJ, Fischer E, Hawes AS, Hébert CA, Terrell TG, Baker JB, Lowry SF, Moldawer LL (Cornell Univ, New York; Genentech, Inc, South San Francisco)
J Immunol 148:1746–1752, 1992   2–20

Introduction.—Interleukin-8, which has been observed in the circulation during septic shock and endotoxemia and after IL-1α administration, may augment host defenses. However, IL-8 may also contribute to the pathologic findings in endotoxemia and sepsis associated with neutrophilic infiltration and activation. Animals were used to evaluate the acute hemodynamic, hematologic, cytokine, and histologic responses to both brief and prolonged physiologic quantities of intravenous recombinant human IL-8.

Methods.—Recombinant human IL-8 was administered to healthy anesthetized baboons as a single rapid intravenous bolus or as a primed continuous 8-hour intravenous infusion. Control animals received human serum albumin. At the end of a 24-hour observation period, the histopathology was studied along with tumor necrosis factor (TNF-α), IL-1β, IL-8, and IL-6 levels and leukocyte and platelet counts.

Findings.—There were no hemodynamic α changes or detectable changes in circulating TNF-α, IL-1β, or IL-6 response after either IL-8 administration regimen. The animals were clinically stable during the observation period. Interleukin-8 did elicit rapid and profound changes in circulating granulocytes, suggesting that IL-8 may contribute to the dynamics of circulating leukocytes seen in sepsis. On necropsy, there was mild to moderate neutrophilic margination in lung, liver, and spleen, which was greater in the baboons receiving the 8-hour infusion, but there was no associated neutrophilic infiltration or tissue injury.

Conclusion.—Interleukin-8 administered to healthy animals as either a bolus dose or as a continuous infusion for as much as 8 hours did not induce the hemodynamic and metabolic aberrations or the acute organ damage seen during sepsis. The IL-8 elicited profound and rapid changes in circulating granulocytes but did not induce hemodynamic changes or increases in TNF-α, IL-1β, or IL-6 levels. Further work is needed to define the role of IL-8 in sepsis and other disease states.

▶ A single injection of endotoxin results in an initial rapid decline in peripheral granulocytes caused by a sequestration in the reticuloendothelial system of the lung, liver, and spleen, with a subsequent release of marrow granulocytes and a granulocytosis within 6 to 8 hours followed then by an increase in the total production of granulocytes. Endotoxin is a potent inducer of cytokines, including IL-1, IL-6, G-CSF, and TNF. We can now add IL-8 to the list. The TNF and IL-1 also induce a neutropenia, but with a different and longer time course, and thus the mechanisms may be distinct. One possible mechanism for these neutropenias is cell stiffening with trapping in capillaries, but alternatively there may be an up-regulation of various adhesion proteins with increased adhesion of neutrophils to endothelium. An intriguing part of the IL-8 effect is that segmented neutrophils alone appear to be increased, suggesting that this is not caused by a release from the bone marrow, but rather probably by a demargination of circulating and splenic sequestered granulocytes. Along this line, IL-8 induces a loss of lectin adhesion molecule-1 from neutrophil surfaces, which presumably leads to a decrease in adhesion to vascular endothelium. As with virtually all other aspects of the cytokine network, the modulation of granulocyte release and margination becomes progressively more complex.—P.J. Quesenberry, M.D.

Synergistic Effects of Interleukin 3 and Interleukin 11 on Murine Megakaryopoiesis in Serum-Free Culture
Yonemura Y, Kawakita M, Masuda T, Fujimoto K, Kato K, Takatsuki K (Kumamoto Univ, Japan)
Exp Hematol 20:1011–1016, 1992   2–21

Introduction.—The cytokine IL-11, similarly to IL-6, acts synergistically with IL-3 to promote murine megakaryocyte colony formation in serum-containing culture. The ability of IL-11 to augment murine megakaryocyte colony formation in serum-free culture and the role of IL-11 in megakaryocyte maturation were assessed.

Methods.—Recombinant IL-11 was added to serum-free cultures of nonadherent, nonphagocytic, and T-cell–depleted bone marrow cells. Megakaryocyte size and DNA content were studied, along with acetylcholinesterase activity and the number of cells per megakaryocyte colony.

Findings.—By itself, IL-11 did not influence colony formation, but it did augment colony growth when supported by suboptimal (and optimal) levels of IL-3. The size of megakaryocyte colonies and cells also increased. The cytokine induced acetylcholinesterase in a dose-dependent manner, but its effect was much greater when combined with IL-3.

Conclusion.—The finding that IL-11 augments megakaryopoiesis in vitro suggests that stromal cells can have an important role in megakaryocyte development.

▶ The list of megakaryocyte colony-stimulating and differentiating factors continues to grow. At present and in various systems, the following cytokines have been observed to stimulate various aspects of megakaryocyte colony formation usually in association with evidence of effects on maturation: Steel factor, IL-3, GM-CSF, G-CSF, IL-6, IL-11, IL-4, EPO, leukemia inhibitory factor, and basic fibroblast growth factor. Most of these will show synergistic effects when tested with other cytokines. It is probably time to drop the hypothesis (nice in its time) that there is a megakaryocyte CSF and a megakaryocyte potentiator or thrombopoiesis-stimulating factor. Many megakaryocyte CSFs, either alone or more likely in synergistic combination, function as thrombopoiesis or thrombopoietin. Even more megakaryocyte-active factors will be elucidated. Count on it.—P.J. Quesenberry, M.D.

Effects of Recombinant Human Interleukin-11 on Hematopoietic Reconstitution in Transplant Mice: Acceleration of Recovery of Peripheral Blood Neutrophils and Platelets

Du XX, Neben T, Goldman S, Williams DA (Indiana Univ, Indianapolis; Howard Hughes Med Inst, Indianapolis, Ind; Genetics Inst, Cambridge, Mass)
Blood 81:27–34, 1993   2–22

Background.—Human IL-11 stimulates the proliferation of IL-6–dependent murine plasmacytoma cells, but little is known of its functional role in normal hematopoiesis. Recent observations have suggested that IL-11 may increase platelet production in normal and splenectomized mice when administered in vivo. A murine bone marrow and spleen cell transplantation model was examined to determine the effects of recombinant human IL-11 (rhIL-11) on the recovery of peripheral blood cell counts and on the proliferation of progenitors and hematopoietic stem cells.

Results.—Daily administration of rhIL-11 accelerated the recovery of leukocytes, particularly neutrophils. Neutropenia lasted about 2 weeks in control transplant recipients, but IL-treated animals regained normal neutrophil counts within 8–10 days. Treatment increased counts of granulocyte-macrophage progenitors derived from both spleen and bone marrow cells. Bone marrow and spleen cellularity was increased in treated mice, but the number of hematopoietic stem cells was not increased. Platelet counts in the peripheral blood increased threefold in IL-11–treated animals.

Conclusion.—The effects of IL-11 in accelerating the recovery of leukocytes (mainly neutrophils) and platelets in transplant mice suggest it may be clinically useful in bone marrow transplantation or in treating chemotherapy-related cytopenias or those associated with irradiation.

▶ Interleukin-11 is the other major candidate for a platelet-active agent in patients with chemotherapy suppression of bone marrow. This contribution indicates that IL-11 can accelerate recovery of platelets and also leukocytes after total body irradiation and marrow transplantation in mice. Interleukin-11 is a stromal cell cytokine first cloned from an immortalized IL-1–induced primate bone marrow stromal cell line PU35 (1, 2). This cytokine is induced in response to IL-1, tumor growth factor-β and platelet-derived growth factor (3, 4). It is a pleiotropic agent with many actions, including in-creasing I-secreting B cells in a murine assay and in a T-cell–dependent fash-ion (2, 5) and synergizing with IL-3 on stimulation of early progenitors (6) and megakaryocyte colonies (2, 7). It also acts to inhibit the differentiation of a preadipocytic cell line in vitro (8) and, in normal mice, increases the platelet count (9). Yin et al. (5) showed that IL-11 in vivo in normal and lymphopenic mice (after cytoxan) promoted B-cell production. The key, of course, remains that it appears to be a promising platelet-elevating agent. The race is on be-tween IL-6 and IL-11; it seems that IL-3 is no longer a strong candidate for the magic platelet agent.—P.J. Quesenberry, M.D.

References

1. Paul SR, et al: *Blood* 77:1723, 1991.
2. Paul SR, et al: *Proc Natl Acad Sci USA* 87:7512, 1990.
3. Delwiche F, et al: *J Clin Invest* 76:137, 1985.
4. Billips LG, et al: *Blood* 75:611, 1990.
5. Yin T, et al: *J Exp Med* 175:211, 1992.
6. Musashi M, et al: *Proc Natl Acad Sci USA* 88:765, 1991.
7. Bruno E, et al: *Exp Hematol* 19:378, 1991.
8. Kawashima I, et al: *FEBS Lett* 2:199, 1991.
9. Goldman S, et al: *Blood* 78:132a, 1991.

Recombinant Interleukin-12 Suppresses the Synthesis of Immuno-globulin E by Interleukin-4 Stimulated Human Lymphocytes

Kiniwa M, Gately M, Gubler U, Chizzonite R, Fargeas C, Delespesse G (Univ of Montreal; Hoffmann La Roche Inc, Nutley, NJ)
J Clin Invest 90:262–266, 1992   2-23

Background.—Synthesis of IgE depends on the balance beween the production of IL-4 and interferon-gamma (IFN-γ) at sites of T- and B-cell interaction. Interleukin-12, is a cytokine that, like IFN-γ and IFN-α, may have a role in protective immunity against infectious agents includ-ing viruses. Interleukin-12 previously was known as natural killer cell stimulatory factor or cytotoxic lymphocyte maturation factor.

Objective.—Whether IL-12 is involved in the selection of immuno-globulin isotypes was examined by determining its effects on the T-cell–dependent synthesis of IgE by IL-4–stimulated peripheral blood mononuclear cells.

Results.—Picomolar amounts of recombinant IL-12 markedly inhib-ited the synthesis of IgE by IL-4–stimulated mononuclear cells. Suppres-sion was observed at both the protein and messengerRNA levels and was isotype specific. Neutralizing monoclonal antibody against IL-12 abol-ished its suppressive effect on IgE synthesis.

Conclusion.—The mechanism by which IL-12 inhibits IgE synthesis in the absence of IFN-γ production remains uncertain, but the present findings suggest that, like interferons, IL-12 may help regulate immuno-globulin isotype selection.

▶ The list of interleukins keeps growing. Recently, IL-13 has been described, and, as noted previously, information on IL-12 is accruing. Interleukin-12 is known as a natural killer cell stimulatory factor or cytoxic lymphocyte matu-ration factor. This article shows that IL-12 inhibits IgE synthesis by IL-4–stimulated monocytes and further suggests the action is not via stimulation of IFN-γ. Interleukin-12, in synergy with IL-2, increases generation of cytoxic T-cells and of lymphokine-activated killer cells (1), increases cytoxic activity of natural killer cells (2), promotes proliferation of activated T-cells and natu-ral killer cells (3), and induces IFN-γ production by resting or activated natural killer cells and T-cells. The action of IL-12 in suppressing IgE synthesis seems to be an indirect one.—P.J. Quesenberry, M.D.

References

1. Gubler U, et al: *Proc Natl Acad Sci USA* 88:4143–4146, 1991.
2. Kobayashi M, et al: *J Exp Med* 170:827–845, 1998.
3. Gately MK, et al: *J Immunol* 147:874–882, 1991.

Cytokine RANTES Released by Thrombin-Stimulated Platelets Is a Potent Attractant for Human Eosinophils
Kameyoshi Y, Dörschner A, Mallet AI, Christophers E, Schröder J-M (Univ of Kiel, Germany; Beiersdorf AG, Hamburg, Germany; St Thomas' Hosp, Lon-don)
J Exp Med 176:587–592, 1992   2–24

Introduction.—Inflammatory disorders are characterized by the immi-gration of different leukocytic subtypes. The stimulation of human plate-lets by thrombin promotes the release of preformed proteinaceous eo-sinophil (Eo)-chemotactic activity. Two Eo-chemotactic polypeptides (EoCPs) were purified chromatographically and exhibited molecular masses close to 8 kD. Amino acid sequencing showed sequences for both polypeptides identical to that of RANTES, a cytokine belonging to the IL-8 family of leukocyte attractants. Whether the the IL-8 family of low-molecular-mass (6–10 kD) cytokines contains Eo-selective attrac-tants was investigated.

Results.—Both the natural forms of RANTES, EoCP-1 and EoCP-2, exhibited strong Eo-chemotactic activity with optimal migration occur-ring at concentrations close to 10 nM. No significant migration was seen with human neutrophils. Chemotactic activity of RANTES for human Eos was affirmed using recombinant material.

Conclusion.—These findings, along with evidence for RANTES gene expression in activated T lymphocytes, suggest that RANTES may have a role in such settings as allergen-induced skin reactions, which are characterized by memory T-cell infiltration and accumulation of Eos, in persons who are atopic or who have asthma.

▶ The cytokine RANTES, which is a member of the IL-8 family of leukocyte attractants, can now be added to the eosinophil-selective attractants IL-5, GM-CSF, and lymphocyte chemotactic factor (1, 2). Interleukin-8 is a polypeptide mediator and a member of a superfamily of structurally related low-molecular-weight cytokines, including melanoma growth stimulatory activity and neutrophil-activating protein 2, both chemotactic for neutrophils and partly for lymphocytes, but not for monocytes or eosinophils. Other members of the subfamily include a monocyte chemotactic protein and monocyte chemotactic inactivating factor chemotactic for monocytes but not for neutrophils. Macrophage inflammatory protein- 1α and -1β, chemotactic for T-lymphocyte subsets, are also members of this family. The present data suggested that RANTES may be one of several cytokines released by T lymphocytes in the setting of response to various allergens.—P.J. Quesenberry, M.D.

References

1. Wang JM, et al: *Eur J Immunol* 19:701, 1989.
2. Rand TH, et al: *J Exp Med* 173:1521, 1991.

Suppressive Effect of Granulocyte-Macrophage Colony-Stimulating Factor on the Generation of Natural Killer Cells In Vitro

Taguchi K, Shibuya A, Inazawa Y, Abe T (Univ of Tsukuba, Ibaraki, Japan)
Blood 79:3227–3232, 1992   2–25

Introduction.—Reductions in both natural killer (NK) cells and their marrow progenitors are described in patients with aplastic anemia and myelodysplastic syndrome who received recombinant human (rh) GM-CSF. Natural killer cells may be cultured from human bone marrow cells in recombinant human IL-2–containing medium after depletion of nylon wool-adherent cells, mature T cells, and NK cells.

Objective.—This culture system was used to determine whether rhGM-CSF suppresses the generation of NK cells in vitro and to clarify the mechanisms underlying this suppressive effect. Marrow and peripheral blood cells were obtained from healthy subjects.

Results.—Exposure to rhGM-CSF significantly suppressed the generation of CD56+cells and NK activity in a dose-dependent manner. The generation of large granular lymphocytes also was suppressed but was unaffected by rhG-CSF. Neither cytokine altered the CD56+count in peripheral blood.

Conclusion.—Treatment with rhGM-CSF might suppress the generation of NK cells in patients who are granulocytopenic.

▶ We continue to expand our knowledge about the potent cytokines, G-CSF and GM-CSF, that currently are being given to many patients with neoplastic diseases (in many cases, I am afraid, inappropriately). Here GM-CSF inhibits NK cell production, whereas G-CSF has no effect. This is important, basic information on the use of these growth factors in a number of settings, especially marrow transplantation. This article also highlights the ignorance with which most practitioners are now proceeding to use these potent biologicals. Many use G-CSF and GM-CSF virtually indistinguishably, disregarding the dramatic differences in toxicity profiles and biological activites. This article suggested that GM-CSF may be of interest in modulating NK cell activity, especially when this activity may result in adverse clinical consequences. This effect will have to be particularly attended to by individuals conducting autologus and allogeneic marrow transplant studies. It seems to have become almost automatic that one of the cytokines, either G-CSF or GM-SCF, gets included in a new transplant protocol. This is quite appropriate if the aim is to study the action and clinical efficacy of the cytokines, but it is not appropriate with regard to the question of patient benefit, because as yet, there have been no data indicating a survival advantage for patients in the transplant setting given these cytokines.—P.J. Quesenberry, M.D.

The Sweet Syndrome During Therapy With Granulocyte Colony-Stimulating Factor

Park JW, Mehrotra B, Barnett BO, Baron AD, Venook AP (Univ of California, San Francisco)
Ann Intern Med 116:996–998, 1992   2–26

Introduction.—The G-CSF, an important new adjunct to cancer chemotherapy, lessens the degree and duration of neutropenia. Although G-CSF therapy is usually well tolerated, the Sweet syndrome (acute febrile neutrophilic dermatosis) developed in 1 patient who was receiving chemotherapy and G-CSF.

Case Report.—Woman, 41, had acute fever and skin rash while receiving chemotherapy and G-CSF for breast cancer. She had started neoadjuvant combination chemotherapy after diagnosis, 2 months previously because of the size of her tumor. The G-CSF therapy (300 μg daily by subcutaneous injection) was initiated before the third cycle of chemotherapy. The patient's symptoms appeared 2 days after discontinuing G-CSF (5 doses had been given). She was hospitalized with a temperature of 38.8°C and erythematous nodules on her extremities. A skin punch biopsy specimen yielded findings consistent with the Sweet syndrome. Corticosteroid treatment was not given because it was believed that the woman's symptoms would resolve in the absence of further G-CSF therapy. The lesions did begin to resolve within several days, and full healing without scarring occurred after the hospital discharge.

Conclusion.—Approximately 20% of cases of the Sweet syndrome are associated with a malignant disease. Patients most often affected have hematologic malignancies, particularly acute myelogenous leukemia. To the authors' knowledge, only 4 cases have been reported in patients with breast cancer. Therapy with G-CSF has been associated with the exacerbation of pre-existing skin disorders. The development of the Sweet syndrome in this patient suggests that G-CSF can also induce an inflammatory process de novo.

Cutaneous Reactions to Granulocyte-Monocyte Colony-Stimulating Factor
Mehregan DR, Fransway AF, Edmonson JH, Leiferman KM (Mayo Clinic and Mayo Found, Rochester, Minn)
Arch Dermatol 128:1055–1059, 1992   2–27

Introduction.—The GM-CSF is a hematopoietic growth factor acting on neutrophils, monocytes, and eosinophils. Reported side effects from intravenous GM-CSF have included fever, bone and muscle pain, thrombophlebitis, headache, dyspnea, and serosal infusions. Cutaneous reactions have been rare.

Series.—Cutaneous reactions developed in 26 of 57 patients given GM-CSF subcutaneously as part of a therapeutic protocol for advanced malignant disease. Ovarian adenocarcinoma was the most common diagnosis.

Clinical Aspects.—Fourteen patients had localized urticarial or angioedematous reactions causing itching or pain. Twenty-one patients had generalized cutaneous reactions during treatment with GM-CSF. None gave a history of dermatologic disease. Most of the patients responded to a smaller dose of GM-CSF or topical treatment. Other side effects included fever, myalgia, bone pain, and nausea. Leukocytosis was a consistent finding, and most patients with generalized reactions had peripheral eosinophilia.

Histology.—Four biopsies from patients with generalized erythrodermic reactions demonstrated perivascular and periadnexal lymphocytic inflammation involving the dermis. Eosinophilia was evident in the same distribution in 2 instances. The major basic protein was present extracellularly in specimens from patients with eosinophilia.

Conclusion.—Cutaneous reactions are common with subcutaneous administration of GM-CSF. Eosinophils, which may release toxic products when activated, may have a role in the cutaneous reactions associated with GM-CSF administration.

▶ These 2 selections (Abstracts 2–26 and 2–27) are grouped as examples of dermatologic reactions to the cytokines, G-CSF and MG-CSF. The association of the Sweet syndrome with G-CSF therapy has raised some controversy, but the former article (Abstract 2–26), along with a number of unpublished anecdotal reports, suggests that this is a real association and complication of G-CSF therapy. This article also raises interesting questions about the possible role of G-CSF in the etiology or progression of leukemias associated with the Sweet syndrome. Ongoing studies determining G-CSF serum levels, messenger RNA expression, and leukemic cytokine responsiveness should help to clarify this important issue.

Abstract 2–27 categorizes the cutaneous reactions to GM-CSF. A relatively extraordinary 26 of 57 patients given GM-CSF subcutaneously had cutaneous reactions. Twenty-one had generalized reactions, and 18 of these 21 had peripheral blood eosinophilia. In previous reports, the cutaneous reactions have been relatively rare, although perhaps ignored given the wide variety of other toxic manifestation of GM-CSF. Some of these skin reactions were rather severe and, at times, long lasting. The authors speculate that eosinophil activation and extracellular deposition of eosinophilic major basic protein may be related to the skin reactions. They note that a similar setting exists with chronic urticaria, solar urticaria, pressure urticaria, Well's syndrome, and episodic angioedema with eosinophilia (1, 2). This association remains speculative.—P.J. Quesenberry, M.D.

References

1. Gleich GJ, et al: N Engl J Med 310:1621–1626, 1984.
2. Leiferman KM: J Am Acad Dermatol 24:1101–1112, 1991.

Increased Serum Levels of Granulocyte Colony-Stimulating Factor After Autologous Bone Marrow or Blood Stem Cell Transplantation
Haas R, Gericke G, Witt B, Cayeux S, Hunstein W (Univ of Heidelberg, Germany)
Exp Hematol 21:109–113, 1993   2–28

Introduction.—The G-CSF is a glycoprotein that promotes the production and activation of neutrophilic granulocytes. The G-CSF has been shown to synergize with IL-3 to recruit quiescent hematopoietic stem cells into active cell cycle.

Method.—The biological role of G-CSF for hematologic reconstitution after autologous bone marrow or stem cell transplantation was evaluated in 48 patients with hematologic malignacies, most often acute myeloid leukemia or malignant lymphoma. Forty patients received autologous marrow and 8 received stem cells.

Observations.—The serum levels of G-CSF increased during marrow aplasia, with peak levels present a median of 5 days after transplantation. Leukocytes and neutrophils recovered faster in patients given autologous blood stem cells than in recipients of marrow transplant. A reverse rank correlation of .76 was noted between serum levels of G-CSF and WBC counts. Febrile patients had much higher levels of G-CSF than others. Patients with fungal septicemia had the highest levels.

Conclusion.—These findings support a central role for G-CSF as a circulating hematopoietin after myeloablation and autologous marrow or stem cell transplantation. Endogenous production of G-CSF increases during times of high demand, such as when fever or infection develops. This may reflect the actions of tumor necrosis factor-α and IL-1 as inflammatory mediators.

▶ This is a nice demonstration of serum G-CSF elevations during the periods of marrow aplasia in patients with marrow transplant. We have seen similar data in our transplant unit. In this setting, IL-6 correlates very closely with G-CSF levels.—P.J. Quesenberry, M.D.

Stem Cell Factor Induction of In Vitro Murine Hematopoietic Colony Formation by "Subliminal" Cytokine Combinations: The Role of "Anchor Factors"

Lowry PA, Deacon D, Whitefield P, McGrath HE, Quesenberry PJ (Univ of Virginia, Charlottesville)
Blood 80:663–669, 1992
2–29

Objective.—Optimal proliferation of early hematopoietic progenitor cells requires high levels of multiple hematopoietic growth factors, raising questions about their role in normal hematopoietic maintenance. Whether using a combination of cytokines to stimulate progenitors allows individual factors to have effects at more physiologically relevant concentrations was evaluated.

Methods.—Combinations of murine hematopoietic growth factors were evaluated through their ability to stimulate both total colonies and high proliferative potential colony-forming cells (HPP-CFCs), an early murine progenitor, in double-layer agar cultures.

Results.—Various combinations of CSF-1, G-CSF, GM-CSF, IL-1, and IL-3 exhibited little or no clonogenic activity when used in low concentration. Plateau levels of stem cell factor (SCF) alone were also ineffective, but when it was combined with the other factors, it produced substantial growth of total colonies and HPP-CFCs. Delayed addition studies indicated that this may reflect the sequential activity of SCF and the other factors.

Conclusion.—In high local concentration on stromal cell surfaces, SCF may "anchor" the response of hematopoietic stem cells to various cytokines in physiologic concentration. Stresses such as infection, inflammation, and cell loss might lead to increased cell production by modulating concentrations of circulating factors, which, in turn, could selectively stimulate clones in selected anchor-factor niches. Alternately, high levels of circulating growth factors might "override" the usual process and induce all early progenitors along a common differentiative pathway.

▶ This contribution, from our own laboratory, indicates that certain cytokines, in this case most prominently Steel factor, can "anchor a synergy," i.e., if present at optimal concentrations, multiple other factors may be able to produce a maximal synergistic stimulation of primitive progenitors (HPP-CFCs) at low or subliminal concentrations. There appears to be a hierarchy to this effect with IL-1α showing some anchoring, GM-CSF and IL-3 less, and G-CSF and CSF-1 essentially none. This type of anchoring may occur in a temporal sequence with Steel factor acting on the earliest progenitor, possibly as a survival factor, and others acting in a temporal sequence (to be defined). Steel may also act as a physical anchor, the membrane form actually binding primitive stem cells to the stromal cell surface. Thus, low-dose interactions, temporal sequence, and physical presentation are probably all key features in the regulation of stem cell proliferation and differentiation. We are just at the beginning of a learning curve in this area of synergistic stem cell stimulation.—P.J. Quesenberry, M.D.

Hepatocyte Growth Factor Is a Synergistic Factor for the Growth of Hematopoietic Progenitor Cells

Kmiecik TE, Keller JR, Rosen E, Vande Woude GF (Natl Cancer Inst, Frederick, Md; Yale Univ, New Haven, Conn)
Blood 80:2454–2457, 1992   2–30

Background.—Hepatocyte growth factor (HGF) is derived from fibroblasts, and it is a critical motigen for generation of liver tissue. In addition to acting on hepatocytes, HGF promotes the growth of melanocytes, epithelial cells, and endothelial cells. The factor exhibits considerable homology with plasminogen. The HGF is a ligand for the c-*met* proto-oncogene, one of the receptor class of tyrosine kinases. Although c-*met* messenger RNA (mRNA) is mainly expressed in epithelial cells, it also has been found in several murine hematopoietic progenitor cell lines.

Objective.—The expression of *met* in myeloid progenitor cell lines prompted a study of whether unfractionated, progenitor-enriched murine marrow cell populations express *met* mRNA and protein.

Findings.—Murine bone marrow cells expressed both *met* mRNA and protein. The HGF acted in synergy with IL-3 and GM-CSF to stimulate the formation of colonies of hematopoietic progenitor cells. Colony formation was enhanced by as much as 60%. The colonies contained macrophages and granulocytes in proportions similar to those obtained using IL-3 or GM-CSF alone.

Interpretation.—There may be a feedback mechanism by which the HGF produced by differentiated myeloid cells stimulates the production of monocytes and macrophages from marrow progenitor cells. It also is possible that HGF modulates the interaction of bone marrow progenitor and stromal cells with the extracellular matrix.

▶ This article outlines another potential stromal-based cytokine system. The HGF or scatter factor is the ligand for the c-*met* proto-oncogene, a protein expressed on murine bone marrow cells. The HGF is expressed on murine stromal cells and appears to represent a membrane-bound form that may be modulated by proteases, i.e., plasmin exposure. Now a number of defined cytokines have membrane forms expressed on stromal cells, including fibroblast growth factor, IL-1, Steel factor, and, most recently, HGF. An intriguing possibility is that protease modulation/activation may be a critical form of regulation in this system. This possibility is highlighted by the observations of Wilson and colleagues that there are relatively high concentrations of plasminogen activator inhibitor in stroma. One can envision a nice system in which the evolution of plasmin activates or exposes different membrame-based cytokines and in which the degree of this is then limited by the plasminogen activator inhibitor. This could be a means for both stimulating and geographically restricting hematopoiesis.—P.J. Quesenberry, M.D.

Granulocyte-Macrophage Colony-Stimulating Factor, Interleukin-3, and Steel Factor Induce Rapid Tyrosine Phosphorylation of p42 and p44 MAP Kinase

Okuda K, Sanghera JS, Pelech SL, Kanakura Y, Hallek M, Griffin JD, Druker BJ (Dana-Farber Cancer Inst, Boston; Harvard Med School, Boston; Univ of British Columbia, Vancouver, Canada)
Blood 79:2880–2887, 1992
2–31

Introduction.—Hematopoietic cell proliferation is known to be induced by GM-CSF, IL 3, and Steel factor (SF) via binding to specific, high-affinity cell-surface receptors. Each of these factors independently can support proliferation of the human MO7 cell line and induce a rapid increase in protein-tyrosyl phosphorylation. The proteins phosphorylated on tyrosine by GM-CSF and IL-3 are similar or identical in MO7 cells. Many proteins phosphorylated on tyrosine after SF are different, but 2 proteins—p42 and p44—are prominently phosphorylated in response to all 3 factors. The p42 and p44 proteins are identified in this report.

Findings.—Tyrosyl phosphorylation of both p42 and p44 was transient in MO7 cells and temperature dependent, unlike many proteins that are tyrosyl phosphorylated in response to GM-CSF, IL-3, and SF. Using monospecific antisera to mitogen-activated protein (MAP) kinase, the p42 protein was identified as p42 MAP kinase (p42^{mapk}) and the p44 protein as a p42^{mapk}-related protein. Assayed in vitro with a myelin basic protein substrate, GM-CSF, IL-3, and SF all induced MAP kinase activity. Even in nonproliferative cells that respond to GM-CSF, this factor induced tyrosyl phosphorylation of both p42 and p44. After GM-CSF stimulation, p42 and p44 were among the most prominently tyrosyl phosphorylated proteins.

Conclusion.—This study identifies p42^mapk and p44 as important transducing molecules in myeloid cells. These kinases probably take part in a sequential "kinase cascade" that links growth factor receptors to mitogenesis and other cellular responses. Comprehension of the signaling pathways of GM-CSF, IL-3, and SF will depend on identification of kinases that phosphorylate MAP kinase and further identification of its substrates.

▶ This solid contribution indicates that p42 and p44 MAP kinase probably represent a connection in the signaling pathway for GM-CSF, IL-3, and Steel factor. However, we are still left with a very large informational void on how cytokines transmit messages to the DNA level. There is now evidence not only for MAP kinase but for MAP-kinase-kinase and MAP-kinase-kinase-kinase. Given the developing complexity of the cytokine reactor system and signaling pathways (7–9 isozymes of protein-kinase C now are known), not to mention the probability (certainty) that many new second messenger pathways may be described, a lot of fun lies ahead. How about conceptualizing 1,000 different second messenger pathways? This article represents a step in the unraveling process.—P.J. Quesenberry, M.D.

Genes, Oncogenes, and Transcription Factors

Bone and Haematopoietic Defects in Mice Lacking c-*fos*

Wang Z-Q, Ovitt C, Grigoriadis AE, Möhle-Steinlein U, Rüther U, Wagner EF (Research Inst of Molecular Pathology, Vienna; EMBL, Heidelberg, Germany)
Nature 360:741–745, 1992   2–32

Background.—The proto-oncogene c-*fos* is the cellular homologue of v-*fos*, originally isolated from murine osteosarcoma. Expression of c-*fos* is observed in murine bones, germ cells, hematopoietic cells, and the CNS. It may contribute to signal transduction as well as cellular proliferation and differentiation. The functions of c-*fos* in vivo were examined by using gene targeting in embryonic murine stem cells to generate animals lacking the gene as well as heterozygotes.

Observations.—Heterozygous *fos* +/− mice appeared normal, but females had an altered transmission frequency. The homozygous *fos* −/ −animals exhibited retarded growth and osteopetrosis developed with deficient bone remodeling. Tooth eruption also was affected, as was hematopoiesis. The frequency of thymic CD3+ cells bearing CD4+ or CD8+ was much increased, and there was a significant reduction of splenic B (B220+) cells. The growth plates of homozygotes had a much reduced zone of proliferating chondrocytes and a very irregular proliferating zone.

Conclusion.—The *fos* gene appears to have a specific function in the development of bone, cartilage, and hematopoietic cells. Mice mutant for c-*fos* should prove useful in studying AP-1–mediated signal transduction as well as skeletogenesis and hematopoiesis.

▶ The *fos*-deficient mice showed impressive abnormalities of bone remodeling, extramedullary hematopoiesis in the spleen, and decreased B220⁺ B cells. *Fos* is a major component of the AP-1 transcription factor complex, which includes members of the Jun family. These results concur with previously reported studies by the same group indicating that overexpression of C-*fos* in transgenic and chimeric mice affected bone, cartilage, and hematopoietic cell development. Osteopetrosis in general appears to be caused by failure of osteoclast resorption, and resorptive abnormalities have been demonstrated in several osteopetrotic mutants and in mice lacking c-src (1–4). —P.J. Quesenberry, M.D.

References

1. Revell PA: *Pathology of Bone.* Berlin, Springer, 1986.
2. Green MC, in Lyon AG, Searle AG (eds): *Genetic Variants and Strains of the Laboratory Mouse,* ed 2. Oxford, Oxford University Press, 1989.
3. Marks SC Jr, et al: *Am J Anat* 186:325–334, 1989.
4. Soriano P, et al: *Cell* 64: 693–702, 1991.

Abnormal Expression of Wild Type p53 Protein in Normal Cells of a Cancer Family Patient

Barnes DM, Hanby AM, Gillett CE, Mohammed S, Hodgson S, Bobrow LG, Leigh IM, Purkis T, MacGeoch C, Spurr NK, Bartek J, Vojtesek B, Picksley SM, Lane DP (Guy's Hosp, London; Royal London Hosp; Inst of Haematology and Blood Transfusion, Prague, Czech Republic; et al)
Lancet 340:259–263, 1992   2–33

Introduction.—Mutations in the p53 gene are a common finding in cancer in humans. Although the p53 protein is not readily detected immunochemically in normal tissues, large amounts accumulate in cells of many tumors and may be demonstrated by simple immunochemical staining.

An Unusual Finding.—A mother and daughter, both of whom had a history of breast cancer, exhibited strong immunohistochemical staining for p53 in their normal epithelial and mesenchymal cells. An infiltrating grade III ductal carcinoma in the daughter's lactating breast contained stained tumor cells and many stromal fibroblasts and endothelial cells. Some ducts in normal breast tissue stained positively. Staining for the p53 protein also was observed in an abdominal wall leiomyosarcoma that developed later, in an in situ ductal carcinoma, and in a benign skin lesion developing in the mother. The mother's breast cancer also stained positively. Extensive studies failed to demonstrate a mutation.

Interpretation.—This family appears to have a new syndrome of inherited cancer susceptibility distinct from the germline mutations found in some Li-Fraumeni families. The syndrome seemingly affects p53 tumor-suppressor function through some indirect mechanism that stablizes normal p53. A mutation of p53 is not necessary for a high level of expression of its protein.

▶ This interesting contribution suggests that a possible new cancer syndrome exists. The authors noted that the mutations in p53 are the most common specific genetic change in human cancer and propose that this family is separate from the Li-Fraumeni families because large quantities of the p53 protein were found in normal epithelial and mesenchymal cells as opposed to the detection of mutations in the coding region of p53 as seen with the Li-Fraumeni syndrome. There is current interest in p53 as potential gene therapy to reverse the progression of various tumors including T-lymphoblastic leukemia. This is, of course, based on the extensive data indicating that loss of function at p53 may relate to the development of tumors or, in many cases, to the evolution of a more aggressive form of a specific tumor. Clearly, there is a great deal more to be learned about the actual role of p53 in neoplastic cell development, and this particular entity with overexpression of normal p53 highlights the challenge for investigators.—P.J. Quesenberry, M.D.

Cloning and Antisense Oligodeoxynucleotide Inhibition of a Human Homolog of *cdc2* Required in Hematopoiesis
Lapidot-Lifson Y, Patinkin D, Prody CA, Ehrlich G, Seidman S, Ben-Aziz R, Benseler F, Eckstein F, Zakut H, Soreq H (Hebrew Univ of Jerusalem; Max Planck Institute fur Experimentelle Medizin, Gottingen, Germany; Tel Aviv Univ, Israel)
Proc Natl Acad Sci U S A 89:579–583, 1992   2–34

Background.—The mechanisms that commit pluripotent marrow stem cells to differentiated lineages remain unknown, but there is evidence that cholinergic signaling is involved. Cell division control (CDC) genes have been implicated in marrow cell proliferation and differentiation.

Objective and Methods.—This study cloned a complementary DNA coding for cholinesterase-related cell division controller (CHED), a human homolog of the *Schizosaccharomyces pombe* cell division cycle 2 (cdc2)–like kinases that are universal controllers of the mitotic cell cycle. The complementary DNA reverse-transcribed from cellular messenger RNA was analyzed by RNA blot hybridization and direct PCR amplification.

Findings.—Multiple tissues, including bone marrow, showed evidence of CHED messenger RNA. The CHED protein included consensus adenosine triphosphate binding and phosphorylation regions typical of kinases, and had as much as 42% identically aligned amino acid residues with other cdc2-related kinases. An antisense oligodeoxynucleotide intended to interrupt the expression of CHED significantly reduced its ratio to actin messenger RNAs and also selectively inhibited megakaryocyte development in murine marrow culture. Other hematopoietic pathways were unaffected.

Conclusion.—These findings affirm a relationship between cholinergic signaling and CDC in hematopoiesis. The relationship may be based on characteristic CDC proteins acting in a cell lineage–specific manner.

▶ Both yeast and *Drosophila* genetics continue to inform us about the mechanisms of growth control in mammalian cells. The mammalian *Drosophila* homeobox gene equivalence, *Hox,* appears to represent transcriptional factors that determine different myeloid differentiation pathways, whereas the cdc2-like kinases described in yeast have been found, not surprisingly, to mediate cytokine (CSF-1)-induced cell cycle progression. This fascinating report ties cholinesterase and cholinergic signaling to hematopoietic cell proliferation and differentiation. The authors point out that cholinergic signaling in hematopoiesis has been inferred from observations that cholinesterase genes amplify in leukemia (1) and that antisense oligodeoxynucleotides complementary to butyrylcholinesterase in RNA block megakaryocyte maturation (2). In addition, acetylcholine stimulates inositol phospholipid hydrolysis in "cholinoceptive" cells (3, 4), inducing phosphorylation of cdc2 kinases and increasing cell proliferation (5–7). The data presented here looked convincing for inhibition of megakaryocyte maturation by antisense to butyrylcholinesterase, although the data indicating megakaryocyte inhibition by antisense to CHED could be questioned because a decrease in the percentage of megakaryocytes was seen concomitantly with an increase in the total number of cells, i.e., no true decrease in total megakaryocyte production. The concept is still fascinating, and the connection between cholinesterase, cdc2, and hematopoietic regulations seems real.—P.J. Quesenberry, M.D.

References

1. Lipidot-Lifson Y, et al: *Proc Natl Acad Sci USA* 86:4715–4719, 1989.
2. Patinkin D, et al: *Mol Cell Biol* 10:6046–6050, 1990.
3. Balduini W, et al: *J Pharmacol Exp Ther* 241: 421–427, 1987.
4. Pearce B, et al: *J Neurochem* 45:15341–1540, 1985.
5. Rozengurt E: *Science* 234:161–166, 1986.
6. Berridge MJ: *Annu Rev Biochem* 56:159–193, 1987.
7. Nishizuka Y: *Nature* 334:661–665, 1988.

Helix-Loop-Helix Transcription Factors E12 and E47 Are Not Essential for Skeletal or Cardiac Myogenesis, Erythropoiesis, Chondrogenesis, or Neurogenesis

Zhuang Y, Kim CG, Bartelmez S, Cheng P, Groudine M, Weintraub H (Fred

Hutchinson Cancer Research Ctr, Seattle; Howard Hughes Med Inst, Seattle)
Proc Natl Acad Sci USA 89:12132–12136, 1992   2–35

Background.—The E2A gene encodes 2 non-tissue-specific helix-loop-helix (HLH) transcription factors, E12 and E47, which appear to participate in regulating differentiation in many tissue types including muscle, blood, and nerve. They achieve this through direct heterodimer interactions with tissue-specific HLH proteins.

Objective.—The functions of E12 and E47 during cell differentiation were studied by mutating both copies of E2A in murine embryonic stem cells and examining the effects of the mutations on differentiation in vitro.

Results.—The embryonic stem cells lacking functional E12 and E47 were capable of differentiating into skeletal muscle, cardiac muscle, erythrocytes, neurons, and cartilage to the same degree as wild-type cells.

Conclusion.—The HLH transcription factors E12 and E47 are not required for the terminal differentiation and various tissues. It remains possible, however, that they have a role in the more subtle in vivo regulation of muscle tissue, cartilage, red cells, and neurons.

▶ Embryonic stem cell knockout experiments have been carried out to assess the function of a number of genes. This "negative" article is representative of a number of studies in which the knockout of genes coding for various proteins thought to have growth control roles has little effect on the final phenotype of an adult mouse. The *MyoD* and *src* knockouts are particularly impressive examples of this lack of dramatic effect. Some suggest that this indicates a great deal of redundancy amongst different genes, with 1 gene product being able to compensate for the absence of another. Perhaps a more likely scenario is that all of these knockouts have significant effects that may not have come within the preview of the investigator's bias. In general, "mother nature does not fool around." I think that we will simply have to work harder to find the true tale of many of these gene products.—P.J. Quesenberry, M.D.

Stochastic Rearrangement of Immunoglobulin Variable-Region Genes in Chicken B-Cell Development

Benatar T, Tkalec L, Ratcliffe MJH (McGill Univ, Montreal)
Proc Natl Acad Sci USA 89:7615–7619, 1992   2–36

Background.—The molecular mechanism underlying the rearrangement of immunoglobulin genes is highly conserved between mammalian and avian species, but, in the latter, an equivalent of the mammalian pre-B cell has not been definitively demonstrated. Such a cell would have undergone immunoglobulin heavy-chain gene rearrangement and would express μ heavy chains in the absence of immunoglobulin light-chain rearrangement. It is not clear whether an orderly progression of gene rearrangement events leads to functional immunoglobulin expression in avian species.

Objective.—The sequence of immunoglobulin gene rearrangement was studied by transforming day-12 chick embryo bursal cells with the retrovirus reticuloendotheliosis virus strain T chick syncytial virus. More than 100 clones were analyzed by the Southern blot and PCR techniques.

Findings.—A majority of the clones studied contained only germline immunoglobulin sequences. Several clones contained complete heavy- and light-chain rearrangements, whereas 13 contained only heavy-chain rearrangements analogous to mammalian B-cell development. Five clones contained rearranged light-chain genes without evidence of complete heavy-chain rearrangement.

Conclusion.—These observations suggest that a stochastic—rather than programmed—sequence of immunoglobin gene rearrangements takes place during the development of avian B cells.

▶ This interesting study shows that light-chain gene rearrangements can occur without heavy-chain gene rearrangements in chicken B-cell development. The authors claim that this can happen but do not establish a stochastic as opposed to a programmed sequential mechanism for immunoglobin gene rearrangements in chickens.—P.J. Quesenberry, M.D.

Mutations in the DNA Ligase I Gene of an Individual With Immunodeficiencies and Cellular Hypersensitivity to DNA-Damaging Agents
Barnes DE, Tomkinson AE, Lehmann AR, Webster ADB, Lindahl T (Clare Hall Labs, South Mimms, England; Univ of Sussex, Brighton, England; Northwick Park Hosp, Harrow, England)
Cell 69:495–503, 1992   2–37

Objective.—The DNA ligase I gene encodes the major DNA ligase in proliferating mammalian cells. Mutations in the structural gene encoding DNA ligase I were sought by analyzing the coding sequence in a human fibroblast strain, 46BR, and Bloom syndrome cell lines. The 46Br cells exhibit a decreased rate of joining of Okazaki fragments during DNA replication. In Bloom syndrome, cells accumulate mainly large replication intermediates of about 20 kb in vivo.

Findings.—Two missense mutations were detected in different alleles of the DNA ligase I gene in 46BR cells from a patient who had symptoms of immunodeficiency as well as retarded growth and solar sensitivity. The genetic defects correlated with an impaired ability of DNA ligase I to form a labeled enzyme-adenylate intermediate.

Conclusion.—Human DNA ligase I is needed to joint Okazaki fragments during lagging-strand DNA synthesis and to complete DNA excision repair.

▶ A number of diseases are characterized by abnormal sensitivity of cells to various cytotoxic agents. Bloom syndrome cells are hypersensitive to several DNA-damaging agents, including mitomycin-C (1, 2) and a number of alkylating agents (3, 4). Ataxia telangiectasia cells are sensitive to ionizing radiation, whereas Fanconi's anemia cells are sensitive to DNA cross-linking agents. These syndromes are associated with both immunodeficiency and increased risk of cancer. The case report here of a possible immunodeficiency associated with DNA ligase I gene mutation has many similarities to Bloom syndrome. The authors argued that it is different because of the much lower spontaneous sister chromatid exchange rates in these cells compared with the typical cells from Bloom disease. The authors further speculated that the immunodeficiencies could be caused by defective DNA ligation during immunoglobulin gene and T-cell receptor gene recombination. As the authors noted, the key experiments will test whether the mutant phenotype of the 46BR cells is corrected with normal human DNA ligase I.—P.J. Quesenberry, M.D.

References

1. Ishizaki K, et al: *Mutat Res* 80:213–219, 1981.
2. Hook GJ, et al: *Mutat Res* 131:223–230, 1984.
3. Krepinsky AB, et al: *Hum Genet* 50:151–156, 1979.
4. Kurihara T, et al: *Mutat Res* 184:147–151, 1987.

Granulocytes and Monocytes

Brief Report: Recurrent Severe Infections Caused by a Novel Leukocyte Adhesion Deficiency

Etzioni A, Frydman M, Pollack S, Avidor I, Phillips ML, Paulson JC, Gershoni-Baruch R (Technion-Israel Inst of Technology, Haifa; Univ of Tel Aviv, Israel; Cytel Corp, San Diego, Calif)
N Engl J Med 327:1789–1792, 1992   2–38

Background.—Congenitally defective adhesion molecules (LFA-1, Mac-1) can lead to a marked deficiency of leukocyte adhesion. The neutrophils are defective in both adhesion and motility, making those patients affected vulnerable to recurrent severe infections.

A New Form.—Two unrelated children were seen with identical anomalies and a defect in the leukocyte adhesion molecule caused by the absence of the Sialyl-Lewis X ligand of E-selectin. This disorder is termed leukocyte adhesion deficiency type 2, as distinct from the previously described (type 1) defect.

Clinical Features.—The boys, aged 3 and 5 years, each came from consanguineous parents. Both were severely mentally retarded and short and had a distinctive facies and the Bombay (hh) blood phenotype. Both have had recurrent bacterial infections, chiefly pneumonia; otitis media; periodontitis; and localized cellulitis without pus formation. Leukocyte counts were as high as 150,000/mm³; there were recurrent infections; and neutrophil motility was markedly defective.

Leukocyte Function.—Phagocyte function was normal, but neutrophil motility was only 10% of normal. Neutrophil levels of CD18 antigen were normal. Sialyl-Lewis X was not expressed on the surface of neutrophils from either patient. Patient neutrophils failed to adhere to E-selectin expressed on activated endothelial cells after activation with IL-1β.

Discussion.—This form of leukocyte adhesion deficiency probably is inherited as an autosomal recessive trait. A number of fucosylated carbohydrates are deficient in these patients. The basic defect in leukocyte adhesion deficiency type 2 probably represents a general defect in fucose metabolism.

▶ The leukocyte adhesion deficiency syndrome has been described in more than 50 patients (1, 2). This disorder is characterized by delayed separation of umbilical cord, impaired formation of pus, severe recurrent bacterial infections, high leukocyte counts, and abnormalities in granulocyte adherence–dependent function. These appear to be caused by the absence or decreased expression of the common beta-subunit (CD18) of the integrin receptor molecules LFA-1 and Mac-1. These members of the integrin family bind to the glycoprotein intracellular adhesion molecule-1 on endothelial cells. This interaction is important for firm adhesion to the blood vessel wall and extravasation into surrounding tissues. This article outlines a similar syndrome but with a different underlying mechanism. The authors have termed this leukocyte adhesion deficiency type 2 to distinguish it from the previously described leukocyte adhesion deficiency. The defect here in leukocyte adhesion molecules appears to be caused by the absence of the Sialyl-Lewis X ligand of E-selectin. The rolling of neutrophils on the blood vessel wall precedent to adhesion and extravasation is mediated by members of the selectin family, including E-selectin and P-selectin, which are expressed in the surface of activated endothelial cells, and L-selectin, which is constitutively expressed on neutrophils (3, 4).—P.J. Quesenberry, M.D.

References

1. Anderson DC, et al: *Annu Rev Med* 38:175–194, 1987.
2. Anderson DC, et al: Leukocyte adhesion deficiency and other disorders of leukocyte motility, in Scriver CR, et al (eds): *The Metabolic Basis of Inherited Disease,* ed 6. New York, McGraw-Hill, 1989, pp 2751–2777.
3. Paulson JC: Selectin/carbohydrate-mediated adhesion of leukocytes, in Harlan JM, Liu DY (eds): *Adhesion: Its Role in Inflammatory Disease.* New York, W.H. Freeman, 1992, pp 19–42.
4. Springer TA, et al: *Nature* 349:196–197, 1991.

Differential Effects of Granulocyte- and Granulocyte-Macrophage Colony-Stimulating Factors (G- and GM-CSF) on Neutrophil Adhesion In Vitro and In Vivo

Yong KL, Linch DC (Univ College and Middlesex School of Medicine, London)

Eur J Haematol 49:251–259, 1992   2–39

Introduction.—The GM-CSF stimulates the proliferation and differentiation of erythroid, megakaryocytic, monocyte, eosinophil, and neutrophil precursors. The G-CSF is a more lineage-specific growth factor acting mainly on neutrophil precursors. The effects of G-CSF and GM-CSF on the expression of adhesion receptors on the phagocyte surface as well as on neutrophil-endothelial interactions were compared.

Methods.—The factors were administered to patients with Hodgkin's disease or non-Hodgkin's lymphoma who were having myeloablative chemotherapy, with or without autologous marrow transplantation. Pulmonary leukostasis was examined, and in vitro studies were done to estimate the adherence of neutrophils to cultured human endothelial cells.

Results.—In vitro studies showed that GM-CSF and G-CSF both upregulated neutrophil CD11b (a $\beta 2$ integrin mediating phagocyte adhesion) by more than 200%. The GM-CSF was more effective in downregulating neturophil leukocyte adhesion molecule-1. In vivo, both factors upregulated neutrophil CD11b but did not alter surface levels of leukocyte adhesion molecule-1 on circulating cells. Only GM-CSF increased neutrophil adhesion to cultured endothelial cells in vitro. Patients had transient leukopenia after factor administration, with peripheral cell counts recovering much more rapidly after G-CSF than when GM-CSF was given.

Conclusion.—Both G-CSF and GM-CSF alter the expression of adhesion receptors on the phagocyte surfce. The G-CSF is a less potent proadhesive agonist for neutrophils than GM-CSF is.

▶ This intriguing article suggests that GM-CSF may be a more potent agent than G-CSF in causing stickiness of neutrophils to endothelial cells. The temptation is too great not to suggest that this might be involved in the differential toxicity of GM-CSF vs. G-CSF. Certainly one can envision that the adherence of activated neutrophils to endothelial cells could set the stage for a capillary leak–like syndrome or local inflammatory reactions. The picture is probably much more complicated.

One additional note, the authors' comments notwithstanding, neither of these factors is truly lineage specific. The G-CSF has a predominant effect on neutrophil lineages, but it has multiple effects, especially in synergy with other factors, on lymphocyte and megakaryocyte lineages and early stem cells (a noninclusive list).—P.J. Quesenberry, M.D.

Interactions of Granulocyte-Macrophage Colony-Stimulating Factor (CSF), Granulocyte CSF, and Tumor Necrosis Factor α in the Priming of the Neutrophil Respiratory Burst

Khwaja A, Carver JE, Linch DC (Univ College and Middlesex School of Medicine, London)
Blood 79:745–753, 1992   2–40

Objective. —Much interest has been shown recently in the clinical use of CSFs to increase the numbers of neutrophils and to enhance their functional activity. Neutrophil response to agonist-induced activation of the respiratory burst is augmented by exposure to a range of cytokines. The effect of systemic GM-CSF administration on the neutrophil respiratory burst was examined. In vivo, cells exposed to this factor still respond appropriately to priming with tumor necrosis factor (TNF)-α.

Methods and Results. —A whole blood flow cytometric assay designed to minimize artefactual activation was used to examine the effects of several cytokines on the priming of N-formyl-methionyl-leucyl-phenylalanine (FMLP) and complement C5a-stimulated neutrophil hydrogen dioxide production. Although both GM-CSF and TNF-α primed the FMLP-stimulated burst in vivo to a similar degree (558% and 581% of the response seen with FMLP alone, respectively), the kinetics were distinctly different—half-maximal response at 20 and 7 minutes. Only a modest priming of 202% was achieved with G-CSF alone; however, combinations of G-CSF, TNF-α, and GM-CSF were highly synergistic, recruiting neutrophils unresponsive to priming by single agents. There was no sigificant difference in priming with GM-CSF and G-CSF compared with GM-CSF alone, and similar results were noted using C5a as the respiratory burst stimulus. In patients receiving GM-CSF infusion, there was significant priming of the FMLP-stimulated respiratory bust—332% of preinfusion response to FMLP. A 152% level of priming was noted in patients receiving G-CSF, but this did not reach statistical significance. The in vivo response to GM-CSF infusion was 48% less than that predicted by the in vitro response, and addition of further GM-CSF ex vivo did not correct the response. Still, these neutrophils responded appropriately to ex vivo priming with TNF-α, doubling their hydrogen dioxide production.

Conclusion. —Cytokines may have synergistic effects on the priming of the neutrophil respiratory burst in whole blood, recruiting previously unresponsive neutrophils and increasing the activity of those cells that do respond. The neutrophil-priming activity of G-CSF in whole blood is modest, but it has a synergistic effect with TNF-α. Neutrophils appear to respond to lower TNF-α concentrations in the presence of systemic GM-CSF.

▶ This article is important, if just to emphasize the complexity of the action of cytokines on neutrophil function. The relatively modest effects of G-CSF compared with GM-CSF may "partly" explain the lack of local tissue reactions with G-CSF compared with GM-CSF, but the observations of synergistic interactions indicate a potential for major in vivo effects that may not have been assessed in the in vitro setting.—P.J. Quesenberry, M.D.

Expansion of a Unique Subpopulation of Cytotoxic T Cells That Express a CαVδ1 T-Cell Receptor Gene in a Patient With Severe Persistent Neutropenia

Bank I, Book M, Cohen L, Kneller A, Rosental E, Pras M, Bassat IB, Ben-Nun A (Tel Aviv Univ, Israel; Weizmann Inst of Science, Rehovot, Israel)
Blood 80:3157–3163, 1992   2–41

Background.—Chronic or relapsing neutropenia may be accompanied by the abnormal expansion of T-cell subsets in the peripheral blood, most often CD8+ T cells. Such expanded T-lymphocyte populations may have a role in suppressing granulopoiesis. Specific oligonucleotides in the PCR were used to amplify complementary DNAs specific for different families of T-cell receptor (TCR) genes in a patient with chronic severe neutropenia.

Case Report.—Man, 55, who had a pustular skin eruption followed by sore throat and signs of subacute thyroiditis. Later candidiasis developed, as well as a skin infection and lymphangitis, and neutropenia was discovered. Marrow biopsy showed few granulocyte precursers and maturation arrest of the granulocyte lineage, as well as a sparse lymphocytic infiltrate in the marrow.

Observations.—Persistent expansion of CD3+CD8+ T lymphocytes was noted, along with a diminished repertoire of TCR Vα and Vβ genes in peripheral blood mononuclear cell preparations. A majority of T lymphocytes expressed an unique TCR structure. From 40% to 60% of T cells stained with anti-Vδ1 monoclonal antibody. The PCR studies showed the Vδ1 gene segment to be rearranged to Cα, rather than to Cδ genes. The expanded CαVδ1+ cells expressed CD8 and were cytotoxic. The CαVδ1 receptor exhibited a functional role in cytotoxicity.

Conclusion.—This first description of expanded cytotoxic CD8+ lymphocytes expressing a functional "hybrid" gene in vivo suggests a pathogenetic role for such cells in some cases of idiopathic neutropenia.

▶ Diagnosis of chronic neutropenia remains a frustrating exercise. This article suggests that the formation of a "hybrid" CαVδ 1 gene may characterize a CD8+ population of T lymphocytes that induces neutropenia presumably through a direct attack on marrow precursors. A number of neutropenic cases have been associated with proliferations of natural killer–like CD3− CD8+ or CD3+ CD8+ T lymphocytes (1–5). Clonal expansion of CD3+ and CD8+ cells expressing αβ-TCR has also been documented (5, 6). In addition, several reports have implicated Vδ1 and πδ T cells as possible suppressors of hematopoietic precursors (7, 8). The major message here is that the work-up of neutropenia is not obviously linked to drug exposure or other disease, and it should include a detailed analysis for typing and clonality of T-cell populations. On second thought, considering that we still do not understand the basic mechanisms underlying most neutropenias, they should probably be included in all neutropenic evaluations.—P.J. Quesenberry, M.D.

References

1. Grillot-Courvalin C, et al: *Blood* 70:1204, 1987.
2. Newland AC, et al: *Br J Haematol* 58:433, 1884.
3. Loughran TP, et al: *Medicine* 66:397, 1987.
4. Chan WC, et al: *Blood* 68:1142, 1987.
5. Pelicci PG, et al: *Blood* 70:1500, 1987.
6. Loughran TP, et al: *Blood* 71:822, 1988.
7. Mami Chouaib R, et al: *J Exp Med* 172:1071, 1990.
8. Hara T, et al: *Blood* 75:941, 1990.

Reactive Hemophagocytic Syndrome—A Clinicopathologic Study of 40 Patients in an Oriental Population
Wong K-F, Chan JKC (Queen Elizabeth Hosp, Kowloon, Hong Kong)
Am J Med 93:177–180, 1992   2–42

Introduction.—The reactive hemophagocytic syndrome (RHS) is characterized by the systemic proliferation of benign hemophagocytic histiocytes, fever, cytopenia, liver dysfunction, and often, coagulopathy. Most reported series are from Western populations. This series included 40 Oriental patients with RHS, 24 males and 16 females with a mean age of 46.5 years.

Clinical Features.—Fever was present in all patients; often a swinging pattern was evident. About one third of patients had an enlarged liver and/or spleen, and 10 had lymphadenopathy. Blood cell counts often fell precipitously. Liver function was abnormal in more than two thirds and one third had coagulation anbormalities. Eleven had evidence of disseminated intravascular coagulation. Eight patients had previous immune suppression. A wide range of associated disease was noted. A malignant lymphoma in 10 of 16 patients was initially manifested as RHS. Infections were documented in 13 patients.

Hematologic Findings.—Cytopenia involved 2 or 3 cell lines. Red cells usually were normochromic and normocytic; reticulocytes were uniformly low. Megakaryocytes were increased in the bone marrow, and normoblastic erythropoiesis was noted, as was active granulopoiesis. Histiocytes ranged from 2% to 15% of nucleated marrow cells, many of which phagocytized red cells, leukocytes, platelets, and erythroblasts.

Outcome.—Most patients required red cell transfusion support, and one third required platelets. Eighteen died of complications fo RHS, such as bleeding and liver failure, of underlying diseases, or of both.

Only 1 of 11 patients with disseminated intravascular coagulation survived. The cell counts recovered within 1–2 weeks in patients surviving an acute episode of RHS.

Discussion.—RHS is as prevalent in Hong Kong as in Western populations. Once it is diagnosed, infection and malignant lymphoma should be sought.

▶ The RHS is one of those disorders that seems to fluctuate in incidence, at least on a routine hematologic counsulting service, depending on whether someone has come across a recent review article or a very dramatic case report on this entity. A fairly large number of diagnostic cells ensues and then taper off with time. However, it clearly is a real finding, and this article indicates that RHS is also present in Hong Kong with a particular association with lymphoma and infection.—P.J. Quesenberry, M.D.

Decay-Accelerating Factor Functions as a Signal Transducing Molecule for Human Monocytes

Shibuya K, Abe T, Fujita T (Univ of Tsukuba, Japan; Fukushima Medical College, Japan)
J Immunol 149:1758–1762, 1992   2–43

Introduction.—The decay-accelerating factor (DAF) is a regulatory protein that prevents damage to host cells by autologous complement activation. Using 1C6 and 5B2 monoclonal antibodies prepared in a laboratory, whether human monocytes are activated via DAF molecules was investigated. The signal transducing pathways used by DAF were also determined. Earlier, 1C6 had completely blocked DAF function, and 5B2 partially blocked it.

Methods.—Monocytes were cultured with 1C6 and 5B2. The glucose content in the supernatant was measured at intervals, and then a calculation of the precentage of glucose consumption was made. Next, monocytes were incubated with increasing amount of 1C6, and glucose consumption was measured after 48 hours.

Results.—In moncytes incubated with 1C6 alone, glucose was consumed in significant amounts. The glucose consumption depended on a 1C6 concentration below 10 μg/mL and reached a plateau of more than 10 μg/mL. The enhanced phagocytosis of latex beads indicated that monocytes had been activated, but the production of monokines, tumor necrosis factor-α, IL-1α, and IL-1β was not enhanced. The F(ab^1)$_2$ fragment of 1C6 activated monocytes, but 5B2 and the Fab fragment of 1C6 did not. In monocytes treated with phosphatidylinositol-specific phospholipase C, the increased glucose consumption and enhanced phagocytic activity by 1C6 was reduced by about 50%. The 1C6 also stimulated the generation of inositol triphosphate.

Conclusion.—The stimulation of DAF on monocytes by anti-DAF monoclonal antibody 1C6 activated the monocytes and resulted in increased glucose consumption and enhanced phagocytosis. The 1C6 had no effect on the secretion of tumor necrosis factor-α, IL-1α, or IL-1β. The signal transmitted via the DAF molecule is capable of stimulating monocytes.

▶ The DAF[3] protein blocks complement action and protects host cells (1–3). It is a glycosylphosphatidylinositol-linked protein (4) that controls classic and alternative C3 convertases by dissociating enzymatically active C2a and Bb from the binding sites (5). In addition, it is a membrane component of erythrocytes (1) neutrophils, lymphocytes, monocytes, platelets, and endothelial cells (6). Recent studies suggest that some glycosylphosphatidylinositol-linked proteins such as Thy-1 or CD59 may participate in signaling events in T cells (7–9). This study indicates that DAF serves as a signaling function in human monocytes and broadens its role in host defense.—P.J. Quesenberry, M.D.

References

1. Nicholson-Weller A, et al: *J Immunol* 129:184, 1982.
2. Pangburn MK, et al: *J Exp Med* 157:1971, 1983.
3. Medof ME, et al: *J Exp Med* 160:1558, 1984.
4. Davitz A, et al: *J Exp Med* 163:1150, 1986.
5. Fujita T, et al: *J Exp Med* 166:1221, 1987.
6. Asch AS, et al: *J Exp Med* 163:221, 1986.
7. MacDonald HR, et al: *Eur J Immunol* 15:495, 1985.
8. Kroczak RA, et al: *J Immunol* 136:4379, 1986.
9. Korty PE, et al: *J Immunol* 146:4092, 1991.

HIV

Role of Human Immunodeficiency Virus Replication in Defective In Vitro Growth of Hematopoietic Progenitors

Louache F, Henri A, Bettaieb A, Oksenhendler E, Raguin G, Tulliez M, Vainchenker W (Hôpital Henri Mondor, Créteil, France; Hôpital Saint Louis, Paris; Hôpital Claude Bernard, Paris; et al)
Blood 80:2991–2999, 1992   2–44

Background.—Patients infected by HIV exhibit a range of hematologic abnormalities including cytopenias affecting a single or several hematopoietic lineages. In most cases, cytopenia is associated with marrow morphologic abnormality and defective growth of progenitor cells. Some maturing marrow cells may express HIV transcripts. Progenitor cell growth was examined in 27 patients with HIV, all of whom exhibited cytopenias.

Findings.—All patients had markedly reduced colony formation by erythroid, granulomacrophagic, and megakaryocytic marrow progenitors. Study of individual colonies by the PCR technique failed to demonstrate HIV-1 DNA. Adding antisense oligonucleotides directed against HIV gene sequences significantly increased colony formation, but no HIV-1–infected colonies were detected after this treatment. Antisense oligomers did not alter the plating efficiency of hematopoietic progenitors derived from CD34+ cells.

Interpretation.—These findings suggest that deficient growth of hematopoietic progenitor cells in the setting of HIV infection is partly related to viral replication outside the progenitor compartment. The altered regulation of hematopoiesis may contribute to the cytopenias associated with HIV infection.

▶ This contribution supports much of the conclusion found in Abstract 2–45, i.e., that progenitor stem cells are not infected with HIV-1, but that some accessory cell population in which HIV replication can occur probably influences colony growth and results in depression of both colony growth and the abnormalities of hematopoiesis.—P.J. Quesenberry, M.D.

Impaired In Vitro Growth of Purified (CD34+) Hematopoietic Progenitors in Human Immunodeficiency Virus-1 Seropositive Thrombocytopenic Individuals

Zauli G, Re MC, Davis B, Sen L, Visani G, Gugliotta L, Furlini G, La Placa M (Univ of Bologna, Italy; Med Research Inst, San Francisco)
Blood 70:2680–2687, 1992   2–45

Objective.—Thrombocytopenia may develop early in the course of HIV-1 infection as the sole hematologic abnormality. The mechanism involved is unknown. Evidence of impaired in vitro growth in samples of enriched hematopoietic stem/progenitor cells was sought from 15 thrombocytopenic individuals who were HIV-1–seropositive. Samples also were taken from 5 nonthrombocytopenic individuals who were HIV-positive, 12 seronegative patients with immune thrombocytopenia purpura, and 15 normal subjects.

Methods.—The CD34+ cells were examined for release of gag p24 antigen in liquid culture and for the presence of HIV-1 proviral DNA to discern a direct interaction between HIV-1 and the hematopoietic stem/progenitor cell compartment. Levels of HIV-1 gag p24 were estimated in bone marrow plasma to see whether the in vitro growth of CD34+ cells correlates with evidence of active viral replication in vivo.

Findings.—Only CD34+ cells from thrombocytopenic seropositive patients exhibited an impaired ability to produce megakaryocyte colonies. Cell numbers declined in liquid culture containing human IL-3. In addition, erythroid and granulocyte/macrophage progenitors declined as did megakaryocyte precursors. No productive infection of CD34+ cells by HIV-1 was observed, and HIV-1 DNA usually was absent from these cells. Reduced numbers of CD34+ cells in culture, however, were associated with the presence of HIV-1 p24 antigen in bone marrow plasma.

Conclusion.—Increased viral replication in the bone marrow may contribute to HIV-associated thrombocytopenia.

▶ The mechanisms underlying hematopoietic suppression patients with AIDS remain elusive. Initial reports indicated that CD34+ progenitors might be directly infected with HIV, but the weight of more recent evidence suggests that this is not the case (1, 2). In general, using very sensitive PCR techniques and evaluation of either CD34+ cells or hematopoietic colonies from patients with HIV investigators have failed to show evidence of HIV DNA. Patients with HIV-associated thrombocytopenia showed no evidence of infection of CD34+ cells, but there were deficiencies of hematopoietic progenitors most pronounced in the megakaryocyte lineage. Zucker-Franklin et al. (3, 4) have found evidence of HIV infection of megakaryocytes, whereas the presence of antiplatelet antibodies in 10 of 15 of these patients with HIV and thrombocytopenia, consistent with other reports (5–10), indicates that the "pure thrombocytopenia" in AIDS is probably multifactorial. As the disease progresses and multiple hematopoietic defects become apparent, infection and drug toxicity also contribute to the cytopenias.

One caveat to all of these studies is that you cannot detect something that is not present, so that if HIV causes lytic destruction of a class of CD34+ progenitors, which could, in this particular study, be accentuated by the overnight incubation, there may be a deficiency of progenitor stem cells without detectable HIV DNA.—P.J. Quesenberry, M.D.

References

1. Von Laer D, et al: *Blood* 76:1281, 1990.
2. Davis BF, et al: *J Virol* 65:1985, 1991.
3. Zucker-Franklin D, et al: *Proc Natl Acad Sci USA* 86:5595, 1989.
4. Zucker-Franklin D, et al: *Blood* 75:1920, 1990.
5. Morris L, et al: *Ann Intern Med* 96:714, 1986.
6. Stricker RB, et al: *N Engl J Med* 313:1375, 1985.
7. Abrams DI, et al: *Ann Intern Med* 104:47, 1986.
8. Murphy MF, et al: *Br J Haematol* 66:337, 1987.
9. Karpatkin S: *Semin Hematol* 25:219, 1988.
10. Ratner L: *Am J Med* 86:194, 1989.

Specific Inhibition of Human Immunodeficiency Virus Type 1 Replication by Antisense Oligonucleotides: An In Vitro Model for Treatment
Lisziewicz J, Sun D, Klotman M, Agrawal S, Zamecnik P, Gallo R (Natl Cancer Inst, Bethesda, Md; Worcester Found for Experimental Biology, Shrewsbury, Mass)
Proc Natl Acad Sci USA 89:11209–11213, 1992   2–46

Introduction.—One approach to antiviral chemotherapy is to use antisense oligonucleotides to inhibit specifically the expression of HIV-1 or other viruses.

Methods.—A culture system simulating in vivo HIV-1 infection was developed to assess antisense oligonucleotide use over the long term. Five oligonucleotide phosphorothioates complementary to different regions of HIV-1 RNA were used to block viral replication in a sequence-specific manner at a concentration of 1 αM.

Observations.—The different oligonucleotides had varying degrees of antiviral activity. Mismatched or random phosphorothioates delayed HIV-1 replication but did not totally inhibit it. After inhibition by a splice-acceptor site antisense oligodeoxynucleotide, breakthrough occurred after 25 days, suggesting that an "escape mutant" had developed. This was not seen when the oligodeoxynucleotides were complementary to the primary-sequence regions of the rev-responsive element and *rev-1* genes. Escape mutants also were prevented by administering multiple antisense oligonucleotides once each.

Conclusion.—Specifically targeted antisense oligonucleotide phosphorothioates may represent an effective means of lowering the viral burden in HIV-1 infection. It may help to target different sequences, either in combination or by sequential administration of differently targeted oligomers.

▶ Antisense approaches to inhibit expression of various messenger RNA species have generated a great deal of information and attempts are now ongoing to apply this in the clinic. Gerwirtz and colleagues (1) have used differential sensitivity of leukemic and normal marrow cells to c-myb to "clean" marrow in vitro, and this article outlines approaches that use antisense to critical HIV proteins to inhibit viral production. These techniques are clearly feasible and may be limited primarily by the ability to deliver antisense to the appropriate target cells in vivo.—P.J. Quesenberry, M.D.

Reference

1. Gerwirtz AM, et al: *Science* 242:1303, 1988.

Human T-Cell Leukemia Virus Type I Infection of Monocytes and Microglial Cells in Primary Human Cultures
Hoffman PM, Dhib-Jalbut S, Mikovits JA, Robbins DS, Wolf AL, Bergey GK, Lohrey NC, Weislow OS, Ruscetti FW (Retrovirus Research Ctr, Baltimore, Md; Univ of Maryland, Baltimore; Natl Cancer Inst, Frederick, Md)
Proc Natl Acad Sci USA 89:11784–11788, 1992   2-47

Background.—Both HTLV-I and HIV can cause CNS pathology, but the pathogenesis of HTLV-I–associated myelopathy tropical spastic paraparesis (HAM/TSP) remains uncertain. Lymphocytes T and B may be naturally infected by HTLV-I, and mononuclear cells are found close to lesions of reactive gliosis in HTLV-I and HIV infections. There is evidence that HIV-infected monocytes release neurotoxins.

Objective.—To determine whether HTLV-I is able to infect cells isolated from primary cultures of human brain tissue, a method of cell-free infection by HTLV-I was used. Brain tissue was taken from patients having partial temporal lobe resection because of intractable epilepsy.

Findings.—It proved possible to infect the human monocyte cell line THP-1 as well as peripheral blood monocytes and isolated microglial cells. Astrocytes and oligodendroglial cells from the adult human brain were not infected by HTLV-I. Infected microglial cells secreted increased amounts of IL-6, but the release of IL-1 by monocytes and microglial cells was not stimulated. Infection of both microglial cells and monocytes by HTLV-I enhanced the production of tumor necrosis factor-α, and this effect was magnified by small amounts of lipopolysaccharide.

Conclusion.—Microglial cells and monocytes infected by HTLV-I may have a role in the pathogenesis of HAM/TSP. Brain macrophages may be involved either directly by infection with HTLV-I or indirectly through activation secondary to HTLV-I binding or the release of soluble tax protein.

▶ These are potentially important observations related to therapeutic strategies for both HTLV-I and HIV. If the neurologic syndromes are caused predominantly by monocyte infection, and if there is continuous turnover of infected CNS monocytes, then various transplant-gene therapy approaches could prove effective. These remain, of course, big "ifs," but this study suggests that monocyte infection may play a critical role in the development of neurologic disease in HTLV-I– and HIV-infected individuals.—P.J. Quesenberry, M.D.

Effects of Cytokines From Activated Immune Cells on Vascular Cell Growth and HIV-1 Gene Expression: Implications for AIDS-Kaposi's Sarcoma Pathogenesis

Barillari G, Buonaguro L, Fiorelli V, Hoffman J, Michaels F, Gallo RC, Ensoli B (Natl Cancer Inst, Bethesda, Md; Biotech Research Labs, Inc, Gaithersburg, Md)
J Immunol 149:3727–3734, 1992   2–48

Background.—Among persons infected with HIV-1, Kaposi's sarcoma (KS) is especially likely to develop in homosexual and bisexual men. Homosexuals frequently are infected with multiple organisms or are vulnerable to other antigenic stiumuli. Kaposi's sarcoma may be evident before there are signs of immune deficiency, suggesting that products of activated immune cells may influence the development of AIDS and KS.

Objective.—Cytokines able to influence events contributing to the pathogenesis of AIDS and KS were sought in conditioned media from activated immune cells. Conditional media were prepared from mitogen-activated or HTLV-II–infected T cells. The AIDS-KS cells, smooth muscle, or endothelial cells were studied. In addition, COS-1 cells were transfected with HIV-1 constructs.

Findings.—Conditioned media from both activated and dysregulated T cells contained various cytokines that promote the growth of KS cells and induced normal vascular cells to resemble KS cells in their "spindle" cell morphology. The latter cells also were responsive to the mitogenic influence of extracellular HIV-1 Tat protein. The same conditioned media promoted HIV-1 gene expression, interrupted HIV-1 latency, and promoted the production of Tat protein. The cytokine effects were enhanced by picomolar concentrations of extracellular Tat protein.

Conclusion.—Cytokines produced by activated immune cells may contribute to the development of KS in the presence of HIV-1 infection. The HIV-1 infection may itself activate the expression of some cytokines that normally are produced after immune stimulation. These findings may help explain the high frequency of AIDS and KS in homosexual and bisexual men, and possibly the few cases of relatively unaggressive KS described in HIV-1–negative homosexual men.

▶ This contribution suggests that KS seen in AIDS may be related to the production of various cytokines, possibly interacting with small concentrations of extracellular HIV Tat protein. Thus, the etiology of KS in patients with HIV infection may relate more to an immune dysregulation with associated cytokine production as opposed to immune deficiency. This is further suggested by observations in other forms of KS, the classic Mediterranean (1) and the endemic African (2), in which there does not appear to be significant immune deficiencies. As the authors point out, a number of infectious pathogens, including cytomegalovirus, human papilloma virus, and amoeba (3–5), have been implicated in the development of KS in both bisexual and homosexual men, and this relationship could possibly be caused by these pathogens. This article suggests that efforts to potentially block various cytokines might be indicated in the treatment of KS.—P.J. Quesenberry, M.D.

References

1. Schwartz RA, et al: *J Surg Oncol* 34:243, 1987.
2. Kestens L, et al: *Int J Cancer* 36:49, 1985.
3. Giraldo G, et al: *Int J Cancer* 26:23, 1980.
4. Huang YQ, et al: *Lancet* 339:515, 1992.
5. Abrams DI: *J Acquir Immune Defic Syndr* 3:44, 1990.

Unexplained Opportunistic Infections and CD4+ T-Lymphocytopenia Without HIV Infection: An Investigation of Cases in the United States

Smith DK, Neal JJ, Holmberg SD, and The Centers for Disease Control Idiopathic CD4+ T-Lymphocytopenia Task Force (Natl Ctr for Infectious Diseases, Atlanta, Ga)
N Engl J Med 328:373–379, 1993   2–49

Introduction.—Severe opportunistic infection and CD4+ T-lymphocytopenia in the absence of HIV infection have recently been found. Out of 230,000 patients, the Centers for Disease Control and Prevention AIDS Reporting System yielded 47 patients with idiopathic CD4+ T-lymphocytopenia, defined as fewer than 300 CD4+ cells/mm³ or a CD4+ count less than 20% of the total T cells on 2 occasions. Thirty-one of those patients and 23 contacts were evaluated.

Findings.—There was no particular age distribution. A majority of patients reported no risk factors for HIV infection. Hemophilia was the most common risk factor. Forty percent of patients had AIDS-defining illnesses. A variety of opportunistic infections were seen. Counts of CD4+ cells ranged from 0 to 37% of total T cells. Most immunoglobulin values were within normal ranges. All contacts were clinically well and HIV-seronegative and had normal counts of Cd4+ T-lymphocytes.

Conclusion.—Idiopathic CD4+ T-lymphocytopenia is a rare disorder not associated with an identified transmissible agent. Low CD4+ cell counts may sometimes reflect a transient response to infection or other disorders, or may even be a normal finding in an asymptomatic person.

▶ This article could be reassuring. Apparently there are cases of CD4+ T-lymphocytopenia that are associated with a risk of infection but are not caused by HIV infection. The assumption that this relatively rare condition is caused by many diseases is probably right, but the dismissal of a possible new infectious disease may be less firmly based. Unfortunately, the official governmental bodies addressing AIDS issues have a rather dismal track record of rushing to inappropriate reassurance. I would not be surprised if a new infectious agent is behind some of these cases.—P.J. Quesenberry, M.D.

The Gelantinous Bone Marrow (Serous Atrophy) in Patients With Acquired Immunodeficiency Syndrome

Mehta K, Gascon P, Robboy S (Univ of Medicine and Dentistry of New Jersey, Newark; Monmouth Med Ctr, Long Branch, NJ; Duke Univ, Durham, NC)
Arch Pathol Lab Med 116:504–508, 1992   2–50

Background.—Gelatinous transformation of the bone marrow consists of the extracellular deposition of gelatinous material in addition to marrow hypoplasia and fat atrophy. The condition, also known as serous atrophy, has been described in patients with AIDS.

Methods.—Seventy-five consecutive marrow biopsies from patients with AIDS were evaluated in a 2-year period. Gelatinous transformation was observed in 22 of the specimens (29%).

Clinical Aspects.—The patients with serous atrophy of the marrow had a mean age of 33 years. A large majority were black men, reflecting the study population and AIDS risk factors. The presenting symptoms were typical of AIDS. Nearly all the patients had at least 1 demonstrable opportunistic infection, with *Candida* and *Pneumocystis carinii* infections being most prevalent.

Blood and Marrow Findings.—All patients were anemic when admitted. One fourth of the group were pancytopenic. Marrow aspirates typically contained gelatinous pink material mixed with few marrow elements. About one third of cases exhibited marked serous atrophy. High magnification revealed the gelatinous material to have a granular and fibrillary composition. Hyaluronic acid and sulfated glycosaminoglycan were identified. Nearby hematopoietic elements were hypoplastic, and focally atypical megakaryoctyes were seen.

Discussion.—A damaged hematopoietic inductive microenvironment in patients with AIDS may lead to failed hematopoiesis and, consequently, to peripheral hematologic abnormalities. Such damage is at least 1 potential cause of anemia in AIDS.

▶ We occasionally encounter gelatinous bone marrow or serous atrophy on the hematology consult service. They have been associated with conditions in which there was chronic wasting or starvation and with malignant disease. This article attempts to implicate glycosaminoglycans with the AIDS-related type of gelatinous marrow. The point is made that in studies of patients with serous atrophy but without AIDS, the gelatinous material appeared to be composed of nonsulfated glycosaminoglycans, i.e., hyaluronic acid, whereas in the AIDS variety, sulfated glycosaminoglycans seem to predominate. The discussions on selective inhibition of erythropoiesis with support of granulopoiesis were not convincing, but the incidence of this phenomenon in these patients is quite striking.—P.J. Quesenberry, M.D.

3 Platelets and Coagulation Factors

Introduction

During the past year, there continued to be a plethora of literature concerned with the problems of bleeding, particularly in the areas of congenital factor deficiency, platelet activation, and thrombus formation. The most significant advances in the area of congenital factor deficiency states have been the availability of factor concentrates, such as recombinant-produced factor VIII, of greater purity and safety. These products, to a considerable extent, have reduced thrombus formation and the serious problem of transmissible diseases. Although the frequency of these conditions is perhaps less than ever before, it has not approached the ideal zero. The frequency of antibodies, induced and directed against factor VIII by the recombinant preparations, has been between 20% to 30% in recipients of these products. We must not completely ignore that these recombinant-produced products are expressed by a variety of different cells in tissue culture and that viral contamination is a possibility, although hopefully never a reality. In the past, 1-deamino-8-D-arginine vasopressin (DDAVP) was reported to be helpful in hemorrhage associated with trauma, surgical intervention, and uremia-azotemia, but it has been reexamined by several investigators and found to be of no benefit when compared with placebo. Furthermore, DDAVP has been associated with hypoatremia and seizures.

A considerable number of publications about antiplatelet agents were seen this year. The efficacy of these agents in the prevention or retardation of thrombus formation remains questionable, but many of these agents continue to be used universally. Undesirable side effects of these agents are being appreciated. One particular agent, 5-[(2-chlorophenyl)-methyl]-4,5,6,7-tetrahydrothieno-[3,2-c] pyridine hydrochloride (ticlopidine hydrochloride) is repeatedly associated with the diagnosis of the thrombotic thrombocytopenic purpura–hemolytic uremic syndrome (TTP-HUS).

Accumulating evidence suggests that the time-honored linear series of the conversion of inactive to active coagulation proteins, the "coagulation cascade," is a limited and inadequate model of the complexity involved in the coagulation process. At present, the initiating step is the exposure of tissue factor (III) on an activated cell from an intra- or extravascular source initiating the binding of VIIa from circulating plasma.

Depending on the degree or amount of activation of the VIIa-III activation complex, the reaction may be stopped by AT-III or protein C/S, or it may continue forward and catalyze the formation of additional factor VIIa, Xa, IXa, and so forth. The quantity of forward reaction depends on the degree of expressed tissue factor and the availability of the surface area of activated membrane. This strategy provides a more realistic understanding of in vivo thrombus formation. Some recent investigation has elucidated that the vascular endothelium synthesizes a number of "thromboprotectine" factors, including prostacyclin, nitric oxide, thrombomodulin, glycosaminoglycans, tissue plasminogen activator, and a variety of ectoenzymes (e.g., adenosine diphosphatase, adenosine triphosphatase, angiotensin-converting enzyme). Thus, when endothelium is damaged, such as in TTP-HUS, the endothelial antithrombotic effect is lost and thrombus formation ensues. Mechanisms controlling the formation and expression of these inhibitors await identification but will be of crucial importance.

Several trials of different low-molecular-weight heparin (LMWH) preparations have been completed. One preparation has been approved by the Food and Drug Administration in the United States. According to some experts, the use of these agents will completely revolutionize the treatment of venous thrombosis. All that will be required are the diagnosis and then subcutaneous LMWH once every 24 hours—no blood specimens for monitoring, hospitalization, or physician care. A nurse or paramedic can periodically visit to relate to the physician that all symptoms and signs have cleared so that he or she can give the order to cease treatment. Time will tell if such an idealistic world can become reality.

William R. Bell, M.D.

Platelet Physiology

Molecular Basis for Glanzmann's Thrombasthenia (GT) in a Compound Heterozygote With Glycoprotein IIb Gene: A Proposal for the Classification of GT Based on the Biosynthetic Pathway of Glycoprotein IIb-IIIa Complex

Kato A, Yamamoto K, Miyazaki S, Jung SM, Moroi M, Aoki N (Tokyo Med and Dental Univ, Japan; Saga Med School, Japan; Kurume Univ, Fukuoka, Japan)

Blood 79:3212–3218, 1992   3–1

Introduction.—Glycoprotein (GP) IIb-IIIa is a heterodimer complex belonging to the family of integrin receptors that contributes to cell-cell and cell-matrix adhesion. On platelet activation, it is able to bind various ligands (e.g., fibrinogen, collagen, and vWF), thereby fulfilling a primary role in thrombus formation at sites of vascular injury. Hereditary defects of this receptor lead to the bleeding disorder Glanzmann's thrombasthenia (GT).

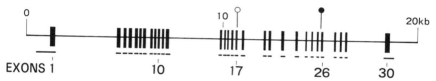

Fig 3–1.—Sequence analysis of the PCR-amplified genomic DNA fragments of the patient's GPIIb gene. *Solid rectangles* represent exons. *Broken lines* (**below**) indicate the nucleotide regions amplified by PCR and sequenced. The positions of 2-point mutations (*open and filled circles*) in the patient's GPIIb gene are indicated. (Courtesy of Kato A, Yamamoto K, Miyazaki S, et al: *Blood* 79:3212–3218, 1992.)

Case Study.—Boy, 8, with a variant of GT had platelets lacking normal GPIIb but containing a trace amount of an abnormal GPIIb. The defective molecule resembles a previously described GPIIb that had a single polypeptide chain lacking the cleavage site needed for proteolytic processing of precursor GPIIb to the mature form. Sequence analysis of PCR-amplified genomic DNA fragments of the patient's GPIIb gene revealed 2-point mutations (Fig 3–1). The defective GPIIb molecule was expressed at about 6% of the control level.

Conclusion.—The defective GPIIb may be rapidly degraded by the endoplasmic reticulum because it is unable to form a stable heterodimer complex, consequent to its misfolded structure. Glycoprotein IIIa may be secondarily reduced because much of it cannot be complex and therefore is vulnerable to proteolysis. The bleeding tendency in GT appears to depend largely on the amount of "functional" GPIIb-IIIa complex on the platelet surface.

▶ The authors have provided solid evidence that identifies the abnormality in GT. It is clearly shown, at least in this 1 patient, that the GPIIb is abnormal in content and results in degradation of the GPIIIa molecule, rendering the GPIIb-IIIa complex nonfunctional in patients with this disease process.—W.R. Bell, M.D.

Role of Fibrinogen α and γ Chain Sites in Platelet Aggregation

Farrell DH, Thiagarajan P, Chung DW, Davie EW (Univ of Washington, Seattle)
Proc Natl Acad Sci USA 89:10729–10732, 1992   3–2

Introduction.—Platelet aggregation is mediated by fibrinogen in interaction with the platelet glycoprotein IIb-IIIa. These interactions are inhibited by peptides containing the amino acid sequence RGD derived from the alpha-chain and the HHLGGAKQAGDV sequence derived from the carboxyl terminus of the gamma-chain of fibrinogen. The importance of these sequences in intact fibrinogen was investigated.

Methods and Results.—The BHK cells were transfected with recombinant human fibrinogen (rFbg), mutant rFbgs with an RGD→ RGE substitution at either position alpha-97 or alpha-574, and an rFbg gamma'-

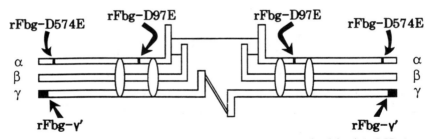

Fig 3–2.—Location of the mutations of Fbg. The RGE mutations in the alpha-chain RGD sites at positions 95–97 and 572–574 are indicated by rFbg-D97E and rFbg-D574E, respectively. The replacement of the gamma-chain with the gamma′ variant chain is indicated by rFbg-gamma′. (Courtesy of Farrell DH, Thiagarajan P, Chung DW, et al: *Proc Natl Acad Sci USA* 89:10729–10732, 1992.)

containing varient with a carboxyl-terminal interruption in the HHLGGAKQAGDV sequence. Site-specific fibrinogen mutants were expressed with mutations in the putative binding domains for the platelet receptor GPIIb-IIIa (Fig 3–2). Reduced polyacrylamide gel electro-

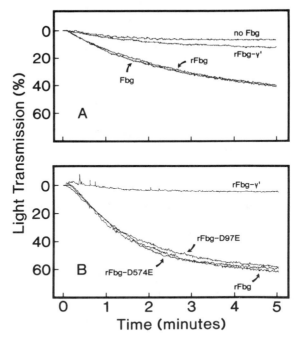

Fig 3–3.—Platelet aggregation. Platelets were incubated at 37°C with the indicated types of Fbg while stirring at 1,000 rpm in a 4-channel aggregometer. Aggregation was induced by adding adenosine diphosphate at 10 μM to the reaction mixture, and the extent of aggregation was measured at the increase in light transmission through the cuvette. **A,** no Fbg, plasma Fbg, rFbg, and rFbg-gamma′. **B,** rFbg, rFbg-D97E, rFbg-D574E, and rFbg-gamma′. (Courtesy of Farrell DH, Thiagarajan P, Chung DW, et al: *Proc Natl Acad Sci USA* 89:10729–10732, 1992.)

phoresis showed that the purified rFbgs had the proper complement of alpha-, beta-, and gamma-chains. Platelet aggregation was much less effectively mediated by rFbg-gamma' than by either rFbg or plasma fibrinogen (Fig 3–3).

Conclusion.—The carboxyl-terminal region of the gamma-chain of fibrinogen appears to be vital to optimal platelet aggregation. In contrast, the alpha-chain RGD sequences are neither essential nor adequate for platelet aggregation. The RGD peptides in intact fibrinogen may simply block gamma-chain binding, which would explain their inhibition of platelet aggregation.

▶ This very thorough and complete study clearly establishes that the carboxyl-terminal region of the gamma-chain of fibrinogen is essential for optimal platelet aggregation. Also, it is clear that RGD peptide sequences are neither necessary nor sufficient to support platelet aggregation. This is critically important information, because many investigators and manufacturers of antiaggregating agents are making antibodies and agents that inhibit RGD sequences. This, of course, will not be of therapeutic benefit because the major site of binding is not associated with RGD peptide, but is found in the carboxyl-terminal region of the gamma-chain.—W.R. Bell, M.D.

The Residues AGDV of Recombinant γ Chains of Human Fibrinogen Must Be Carboxy-Terminal to Support Human Platelet Aggregation
Hettasch JM, Bolyard MG, Lord ST (Univ of North Carolina, Chapel Hill; Southern Illinois Univ, Edwardsville)
Thromb Haemost 68:701–706, 1992   3–3

Background.—The carboxy-terminal of the gamma-chain of fibrinogen has a sequence that interacts with glycoprotein (GP) IIb/IIIa to support platelet aggregation. A normal variant of fibrinogen (γ'), in which the 4 carboxy-terminal amino acids are replaced by 20 amino acids, reportedly binds less effectively to platelets.

Objective.—Site-directed mutagenesis was used to determine the exact differences in amino acid sequences of γ and γ' that might explain the difference in the ability to support platelet aggregation.

Methods.—The gamma-chain complementary DNA in a bacterial plasmid expression vector was modified by oligonucleotide-directed mutagenesis to produce recombinant gamma-chains having different amino acid sequences in the carboxy terminus. Three novel gamma-chains and a recombinant γ' variant were produced.

Results.—The recombinant gamma-chain with an unchanged carboxy-terminus supported platelet aggregation as well as intact fibrinogen. Neither the recombinant γ' variant nor a variant where the 16-amino acid γ' extension was added to the carboxy terminus supported aggregation nearly as well. A variant lacking the 4 carboxy-terminal amino acids was

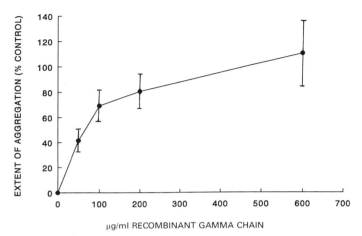

μg/ml RECOMBINANT GAMMA CHAIN

Fig 3–4.—Effect of gamma-chain concentration on adenosine diphosphate–induced platelet aggregation. The aggregation response is expressed as a percentage of the maximal aggregation response obtained with intact fibrinogen (420 μg/ml). The results represent the mean ± SEM for 4 experiments. (Courtesy of Hettasch JM, Bolyard MG, Lord ST: *Thromb Haemost* 68:701–706, 1992.)

incapable of supporting platelet aggregation. The influence of the gamma-chain concentration on adenosine diphosphate–induced platelet aggregation is shown in Figure 3–4.

Conclusion.—The 4 carboxy-terminal residues in the gamma-chain of human fibrinogen are essential for supporting platelet aggregation.

▶ The authors convincingly showed that binding to GPIIb/IIIa is accomplished by a sequence near the carboxy-terminal portion of the gamma-chain of human fibrinogen. They reported that similar sequences in other places in the molecule do not support platelet aggregation and, thus, do not bind to GPIIb/IIIa. Therefore, it would be important for inhibitors to block this attachment, but they must have a property to disturb those residues associated near the carboxy terminus.—W.R. Bell, M.D.

Antiplatelet Agents

Antiplatelet Drugs and Generation of Thrombin in Clotting Blood
Szczeklik A, Krzanowski M, Góra P, Radwan J (Copernicus Academy of Medicine, Krakow, Poland; Jagiellonian Univ, Krakow, Poland)
Blood 80:2006–2011, 1992   3–4

Background.—Platelets provide an initial hemostatic mechanism at sites of vascular injury. Because they also participate in formation of thrombin, it seemed possible that drugs inhibit platelet function might influence the process of thrombin generation.

Study Plan.—The generation of thrombin was examined in vitro and ex vivo before an after oral administration of an antiplatelet drug or a

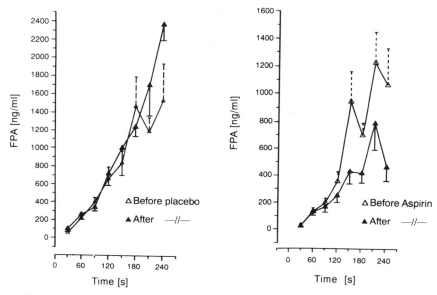

Fig 3–5.—Generation of thrombin ex vivo (*open triangles*) before and (*filled triangles*) 2 hours after ingestion of 500 mg of aspirin (A, *n* = 17) or placebo (R, *n* = 5). Data represent means ± SE of fibrinopeptide A concentrations in blood samples collected within subsequent 30-second periods. (Courtesy of Szczeklik A, Krzanowski M, Góra P, et al: *Blood* 80:2006-2011, 1992.)

lactose placebo. Ticlopidine, aspirin, and indomethacin were used. Fifty-four healthy volunteers, aged 19–63 years, most of them male, participated in the in vitro study, and 58 similar subjects took part in the ex vivo study.

Methods.—The generation of thrombin in recalcified plasma was monitored by assays for fibrinogen clotting time and for amidolytic activity toward a chromogenic substrate. The generation of thrombin ex vivo was estimated by measuring fibrinopeptide A.

Results.—Both in vitro and ex vivo formation of thrombin were significantly impaired 2 hours after the ingestion of 500 mg of aspirin (Fig 3-5), but they were unchanged after ingestion of indomethacin, placebo, or the thromboxane synthase inhibitor OKY-046. Ticlopidine did not alter the generation of thrombin even after administration of 500 mg daily for 5 days.

Conclusion.—Unlike other antiplatelet drugs, aspirin depresses the formation of thrombin in clotting blood. This may reflect the acetylation of prothrombin or macromolecules of platelet membrane, or both. Impairment of the formation of thrombin may help explain the efficacy of aspirin in patients with thrombogenic disorders.

▶ The authors have carefully demonstrated that the ingestion of aspirin reduces the amount of thrombin in clotted blood. For many years it has been known that high doses of aspirin actually inhibit the production of prothrombin by hepatocytes. It is instructive to learn that other antiplatelet agents do not share this property. If aspirin is efficacious in the treatment of in vivo thrombus formation, this pathway may be of critical importance.—W.R. Bell, M.D.

Aspirin Inhibits Platelet Activity But Does Not Attenuate Experimental Atherosclerosis
Sun Y-P, Zhu B-Q, Sievers RE, Isenberg WM, Parmley WW (Univ of California, San Francisco)
Am Heart J 125:79–86, 1993   3–5

Objective.—Because platelet inhibition is helpful in the treatment of atherosclerotic disease, the value of aspirin was examined in lipid-fed rabbits.

Methods.—Rabbits were fed a .3% cholesterol diet that included 3% soybean oil for 12 weeks. Treated animals received aspirin by gavage in a daily dose of 1, 10, 30, or 60 mg/kg for the same period.

Findings.—Aspirin treatment increased the bleeding time from 58 seconds to 75 seconds on average, but only the highest dose significantly inhibited platelet aggregation. When aortic endothelial injury was produced with a balloon catheter, treatment with aspirin in a dose of 40 mg/kg daily did not significantly lessen the amount of surface that exhibited lesions or the thickness of lesions in the aorta and pulmonary artery. Lesions in the aorta correlated with the number of cholesterol-weeks.

Conclusion.—Doses of aspirin that exerted an antiplatelet effect did not significantly lessen atherosclerosis in this study of cholesterol-fed rabbits.

▶ Several times each month, individuals are referred to our group who have been taking aspirin for more than 10 years, yet they arrive at the hospital with totally occluded coronary artery disease. Often we have to see these individuals because they are experiencing hemorrhage secondary to aspirin therapy. It is apparent that the bleeding problem inherent with the administration of aspirin secondary to platelet dysfunction does not prevent the atherogenic process. This article does not suggest that it even retards the atherogenic process. Considerable attention should now be given to these findings.—W.R. Bell, M.D.

Thrombocytopenia

IMMUNE-MEDIATED THROMBOCYTOPENIA

A Multicenter Study of the Treatment of Childhood Chronic Idiopathic Thrombocytopenic Purpura With Anti-D
Andrew M, Blanchette VS, Adams M, Ali K, Barnard D, Chan KW, DeVeber

LB, Esseltine D, Israels S, Korbrinsky N, Luke B, Milner RA, Woloski BMR, Vegh P (McMaster Univ, Hamilton, Ont, Canada; Hosp for Sick Children, Toronto; Janeway Child Health Ctr, St John's, Newfoundland, Canada; et al)
J Pediatr 120:522–527, 1992   3–6

Background.—Chronic idiopathic thrombocytopenic purpura (ITP) in children can be treated effectively with corticosteroids or intravenously administered immunoglobulin, but the former causes side effects and the latter is expensive. There is evidence that intravenously administered anti-D is an effective treatment. Because the most effective dose, duration of response, and side effects in children have not been determined, the responses of children with ITP to escalating doses of intravenous anti-D therapy were evaluated.

Patients and Methods.—This multicenter prospective cohort study involved 25 Rh-positive children, aged 1–18, who had ITP of more than 6 months' duration with a platelet count of $< 50 \times 10^9$ cells/L. Anti-D was administered intravenously on an outpatient basis in escalating doses of 25 μg/kg on day 1, 25 μg/kg on day 2, 35 μg/kg on day 7, 45 μg/kg on day 14, and 55 μg/kg on day 21. Treatment was terminated at this point, or earlier, when the platelet count increased to $> 150 \times 10^9$ cells/L or the hemoglobin level decreased to 100 gm/L. A response was defined as a doubling of the pretreatment platelet count and a level $> 50 \times 10^9$ cells/L.

Results.—The median platelet count at entry was 34×10^9 cells/L. By day 7, 92% of children responded, and 72% of children had platelet counts $> 150 \times 10^9$ cells/L. The response ranged in duration from 1 to 24 weeks, with a median duration of 5 weeks. Side effects included an average decrease in the hemoglobin level of 13.7 g/L, but only in 1 child did hemoglobin levels decrease to < 100 g/L. Second responses occurred in 18 of 21 children after decreases of platelet counts to baseline values. Sixteen children received additional doses during several months with the same success rate.

Conclusion.—Intravenously administered anti-D in a single dose of 50 μg/kg seems to provide a safe, convenient, inexpensive, and effective therapy for childhood chronic ITP. The response lasts several weeks and is repeatable with retreatment.

▶ The frequency of response to this form of therapy with an increase in the platelet count is reasonably impressive. The duration of response is of some concern because it is relatively short in most patients. The mechanism whereby this agent induces a response in the platelet count needs to be identified. Is it simply reticuloendothelial system blockade that prevents altered platelets from being removed from the circulation prematurely? Furthermore, it must be asked whether any other problems can be transmitted with this form of treatment.—W.R. Bell, M.D.

Splenic Radiation for Corticosteroid-Resistant Immune Thrombocytopenia

Calverley DC, Jones GW, Kelton JG (McMaster Univ, Hamilton, Ont, Canada; Hamilton Regional Cancer Ctr, Ont, Canada; Canadian Red Cross Blood Transfusion Service, Hamilton, Ont)

Ann Intern Med 116:977–981, 1992   3–7

Introduction.—Splenectomy often is effective in patients with idiopathic thrombocytopenic purpura (ITP) but can produce serious morbidity, including infection, bleeding, thromboembolism, and pulmonary complications. As an alternative, 11 older patients with ITP and 8 patients with secondary immune thrombocytopenia, who were resistant to steroid therapy but were not good surgical candidates, received a brief course of splenic irradiation.

Treatment.—A dose ranging from 75 to 1,370 centigray was delivered to the spleen during 1–6 weeks. The most frequent regimen was 600 centigray in 6 doses during 3 weeks. Treatment volumes were increased in patients with splenic enlargement.

Results.—Platelet counts rose impressively after splenic irradiation in the patients with ITP (table). No radiation toxicity occurred, even with 2 courses of irradiation, and there were no hyposplenism-related changes in erythrocyte morphology. Only 1 patient with secondary immune thrombocytopenia had a significant—but short-lived—increase in platelets. Toxicity also was lacking in this group.

Conclusion.—Splenic irradiation is a safe treatment that frequently increases the platelet count in older patients with steroid-resistant ITP. Splenectomy may be done later if indicated.

Mean Platelet Count Before and After Splenic Radiation in
Patients With Idiopathic Thrombocytopenic Purpura

Response Category	Patients	Platelet Count before Radiation Treatment*	Months after Completion of Radiation	
			2	6
	n	$\times 10^{-9}/L$		
Good long term	3	12	153	128
Good	3	20	150	150
Partial	2	20	45	45
No response	3	17	67	73

*Pretreatment platelet count was the average of several determinations recorded before the patient was treated with corticosteroids and before radiation therapy.

(Courtesy of Calverley DC, Jones GW, Kelton JG: Ann Intern Med 116:977–981, 1992.)

▶ The authors reported that in a total of 11 patients with ITP, irradiation of the spleen alone resulted in satisfactory treatment. This treatment has been tried on many occasions, and there are several reports, none of which identify a beneficial effect. The explanation for these different results vs. the older literature is not apparent. Perhaps a greater amount of radiation more selectively focused into the spleen is more effective than what could be achieved by radiation techniques in the past.—W.R. Bell, M.D.

DRUG-INDUCED THROMBOCYTOPENIA

Antenatal Treatment of Alloimmune Thrombocytopenia
Lynch L, Bussel JB, McFarland JG, Chitkara U, Berkowitz RL (Mount Sinai Med Ctr, New York; Cornell Univ Med Ctr—New York Hosp, New York; Blood Ctr of Southeastern Wisconsin, Milwaukee)
Obstet Gynecol 80:67–71, 1992   3–8

Background.—Incompatibility of platelet antigens between the mother and fetus results in neonatal alloimmune thrombocytopenia. The fetus may have severe thrombocytopenia, which leads to intracranial hemorrhage at birth or before. Gamma-globulin was used for in utero treatment of neonatal alloimmune thrombocytopenia to prevent these hemorrhages.

Patients and Methods.—Eighteen mother-fetus pairs were treated during a 5-year period. In each case, the mother had given birth to an infant with neonatal alloimmune thrombocytopenia, and all of the previous siblings had platelet counts less than 40,000/μL during the neonatal period. The treatment with weekly infusions of intravenous gamma-globulin (IVGG) (Table 1) was begun if the fetal blood count decreased to less than 100,000/μL at a dose of 1 g/kg of body weight per week in most cases. Nine patients received supplemental corticosteroids (Table 2). Treatment was continued until birth occurred.

Results.—The median platelet count before treatment was 32,000/μL and at birth was 60,000/μL. An intracranial hemorrhage did not occur in any of the treated infants, compared with 48% of their untreated siblings. Platelet counts of less than 30,000/μL occurred in only 3 of the treated siblings vs. 16 of 20 untreated siblings. There were 2 failures in the IVGG-only group, 1 in a fetus with very severe thrombocytopenia who required platelet transfusion, and the other in an obese woman who received a lower dose of IVGG. There was 1 failure in the IVGG plus steroid group.

Conclusion.—Weekly IVGG therapy before birth in fetuses with alloimmune thrombocytopenia can improve fetal platelet count and prevent intracranial hemorrhage. The mechanism of action is unclear; it may involve IgG crystalline fragment (Fc)-receptor blockade in the fetal reticuloendothelial system in addition to reduced maternal antibody production. A trial is under way to compare IVGG with and without

TABLE 1.—Patients Treated With IVGG Alone

Patient no.	IVGG dose	Platelet count (GA)			Platelet count at birth	Intracranial hemorrhage	Untreated sibling	
		First	Second	Third			Platelet count	Intracranial hemorrhage
1	1 g	32×10^9 (23)			38×10^9	No	30×10^9	Yes
2	1 g	1×10^9 (30)	6×10^9 (36)		39×10^9	No	20×10^9 18×10^9	Yes Yes
3	1 g	150×10^9 (22)	45×10^9 (28)	140×10^9 (34)	215×10^9	No	38×10^9	No
4	1 g	18×10^9 (20)	51×10^9 (25)	50×10^9 (32)	85×10^9	No	15×10^9	Yes (AN)
5	1 g	129×10^9 (22)	28×10^9 (27)	79×10^9 (32)	140×10^9	No	15×10^9	No
6	1 g	65×10^9 (28)	309×10^9 (36)		322×10^9	No	8×10^9	No
7	1 g	32×10^9 (22)			43×10^9	No	9×10^9	Yes (AN)
8	1 g	55×10^9 (36)			57×10^9	No	7×10^9	No
9	0.5 g	12×10^9 (32)			12×10^9	No	25×10^9	Yes (AN)
							Uncertain	Yes (AN)

Abbreviations: GA, weeks of gestational age; AN, antenatal.
(Courtesy of Lynch L, Bussel J, McFarland JG, et al: *Obstet Gynecol* 80:67–71, 1992.)

TABLE 2.—Patients Treated With IVGG and Corticosteroids

Patient no.	Treatment	Platelet count (GA)			Platelet count at birth	Intracranial hemorrhage	Untreated sibling	
		First	Second	Third			Platelet count	Intracranial hemorrhage
10	IVGG (1 g) Dex (5 mg)				30×10^9	No	3×10^9	Yes (AN)
11	IVGG (1 g) Dex (5 mg)	36×10^9 (20)	193×10^9 (25)	108×10^9 (32)	64×10^9	No	30×10^9	No
12	IVGG (1 g) Dex (5 mg)	92×10^9 (31)	237×10^9 (37)		235×10^9	No	10×10^9	No
13	IVGG (1 g) Dex (3 mg)	13×10^9 (27)	26×10^9 (32)		42×10^9	No	11×10^9	No
14	IVGG (1 g) Dex (3 mg)	14×10^9 (22)			50×10^9	No	2×10^9	Yes (AN)
15	IVGG (1 g) Dex (1.5 mg)	159×10^9 (23)	78×10^9 (32)		134×10^9	No	20×10^9	No
16	IVGG (1 g) Dex (1.5 mg)	25×10^9 (22)	43×10^9 (28)		204×10^9	No	18×10^9	No
17	IVGG (1 g) Predn (10 mg)	2×10^9 (28)	10×10^9 (39)		17×10^9	No	40×10^9 14×10^9	No Yes
18	IVGG (1 g) Predn (10 mg)	96×10^9 (27)	92×10^9 (32)		200×10^9	No	5×10^9	No

Abbreviations: GA, weeks of gestational age; AN, antenatal; *Dex,* dexamethasone; *Predn,* prednisone.
(Courtesy of Lynch L, Bussel J, McFarland JG, et al: *Obstet Gynecol* 80:67–71, 1992.)

dexamethasone and should also address the mechanism and the issue of fetal risk.

▶ Infant delivery from a patient who is experiencing idiopathic thrombocytopenic purpura has been a major dilemma during the past several decades. The use of gamma-globulin may be helpful, particularly in making it possible to avoid cesarean section (1).—W.R. Bell, M.D.

Reference

1. Pearlman SA, et al: *Am J Perinatol* 9:448–451, 1992.

Thrombotic Thrombocytopenia Purpura

Calpain Activity in Patients With Thrombotic Thrombocytopenic Purpura Is Associated With Platelet Microparticles

Kelton JG, Warkentin TE, Hayward CPM, Murphy WG, Moore JC (McMaster Univ, Hamilton, Ont, Canada; Canadian Red Cross Blood Transfusion Service, Hamilton, Ont; Univ of Edinburgh, Scotland)
Blood 80:2246–2251, 1992   3–9

Background.—A platelet-aggregating factor has been proposed as a pathogenetic component of thrombotic thrombocytopenic purpura (TTP). Affected patients reportedly have calpain (calcium-dependent protease) activity in their serum. Calpain is an intracellular enzyme normally present in many tissues, including platelets. Its activity is neutralized by several plasma factors including high-molecular-weight kininogen.

Objective.—Calpain was sought in soluble and particulate fractions of TTP plasma. Samples from 10 untreated patients with TTP were used.

Methods.—The presence of calpain was estimated by using a bioassay for enzyme activity and also by immunoblotting with anticalpain monoclonal antibody. Plasma samples were subjected to ultrafiltration and ultracentrifugation to determine whether calpain is associated with microparticles in plasma.

Findings.—Calpain was detected both antigenically and functionally in acute TTP samples of serum and plasma, but not in control specimens. An exception was a patient who had a cardiopulmonary bypass; the patient's sample contained antigenic calpain. Calpain was associated with membrane material in microparticles. It was removed by monoclonal antibodies against platelet membrane glycoproteins, but not by antibody against red cell membrane glycophorin.

Conclusion.—Active calpain is present on platelet microparticles in plasma from patients with TTP. Calpain activity resists inhibition by cysteine protease inhibitors in normal plasma.

▶ This is a very potentially important observation with respect to calpain and its presence in patients with TTP. It must be asked whether this is a primary event associated with this illness or a secondary event that results from cellular damage as platelets interact with damaged and subendothelial surfaces. The sample size of the patients studied needs to be considerably increased to substantiate this observation.—W.R. Bell, M.D.

Coagulation Factors

Hageman Factor and Risk of Myocardial Infarction in Middle-Aged Men

Kelleher CC, Mitropoulos KA, Imeson J, Meade TW, Martin JC, Reeves BEA, Hughes LO (Med College of St Bartholomew's Hosp, London; Northwick Park Hosp, Harrow, England)
Atherosclerosis 97:67–73, 1992

3–10

Background.—Factors that dispose to increased activation of factor VII, and thereby to hypercoagulability, are probably important in the development of coronary heart disease. In addition to its classic activation by the extrinsic pathway, factor VII may be directly activated by factor XIIa. Men with a history of myocardial infarction reportedly have higher levels of XII coagulant activity (Hageman factor) than control subjects.

Subjects.—Plasma factor estimates were made in 51 men, aged 45–69 years, who had had a documented myocardial infarction. Thirty-one others who were seen at a cardiovascular screening clinic served as a control group.

Findings.—The plasma level of fibrinogen and total cholesterol were significantly higher in the infarct group than in control subjects (table). The mean level of factor VIIc tended to be higher in control subjects. Differences in coagulant activities were not statistically significant. A his-

Principal Results (Mean ± SD) in 82 Subjects			
Variable	Cases 51	Controls 31	*P*-value
Factor XIIc (%st)	83 (27)	89 (21)	0.18
Fibrinogen (g/l)	3.00 (0.53)	2.71 (0.43)	0.02 †
Factor VIIc (%st)	107 (27)	114 (37)	0.5
Total cholesterol (mmol/l)	7.0 (1.3)	6.4 (1.3)	0.03 †
Total triglycerides (mmol/l)	2.1 (1.1)	1.9 (1.0)	0.30
Oestradiol (pmol/l) *	141 (63)	122 (37)	0.30
Prolactin (mIU/l) *	124 (113)	96 (60)	0.30

*Comparison is between 44 cases and 28 controls.
†Statistically significant difference between the 2 groups.
(Courtesy of Kelleher CC, Mitropoulos KA, Imeson J, et al: *Atherosclerosis* 97:67–73, 1992.)

tory of infarction did not significantly predict the activation of factor VIIc after overnight incubation of plasma at 4°C. All measures of factor XII concentration correlated positively with factor VIIc after cold activation. In addition, factor XIIa correlated closely with many lipoprotein variables, especially very-low-density lipoprotein cholesterol and triglycerides.

Conclusion.—Increased flux within the contact system could result in increased factor VIIc and thereby contribute to an acute thrombotic event such as myocardial infarction.

▶ The authors point out a potential pathway that may be responsible for thrombus formation in the coronary arteries. These studies support the contention that increased levels of activated factor XII are present and can, in turn, activate factor VII, leading directly to thrombus formation via the extrinsic pathway. The correlation with plasma fibrinogen and cholesterol is instructive. This finding should be examined in much larger populations to substantiate this potential treatable mechanism.—W.R. Bell, M.D.

Factor XII (Hageman) Deficiency in Women With Habitual Abortion: New Subpopulation of Recurrent Aborters?
Braulke I, Hinney B, Pruggmayer M, Köstering H, Melloh P, Günther E (Univ of Göttingen, Germany)
Fertil Steril 59:98–101, 1993   3–11

Background.—Although patients deficient in factor XII do not generally experience increased bleeding, some do have thrombotic complications. Patients with elevated phospholipid antibodies may also experience an excessive thrombophilia. Both of these conditions reportedly increase both vascular and placenta thromboses and, thus, may be associated with recurrent abortions. The relationship between factor XII levels and patients with repeated abortions was investigated.

Patients and Methods.—Forty-three women, 26–35 years old, who had experienced 3 or more abortions were examined. Of these women, 17 had at least 1 pregnancy longer than 28 weeks. Factor XII activity was determined by clotting assay, and circulating levels were measured by rocket immunoelectrophoresis. Levels of antiphospholipid antibodies were calculated by enzyme-linked immunosorbent assay. Eight women were subsequently excluded because of high anticardiolipin antibodies.

Results.—Of the remaining 37 women, 8 were identified with reduced factor XIIc activity. These deficiencies occurred in 4 of 28 women with 3 abortions, and in 4 of 9 women with more than 3 abortions. Six of these patients also had reduced factor XII antigen.

Conclusion.—The occurrence of factor XII defects in this group of recurrent aborters is highly significant. However, further study is needed to demonstrate that factor XII defects can identify a subset of patients with recurrent abortions.

▶ These authors clearly demonstrate evidence that suggests the possibility of recurrent abortion associated with factor XII deficiency. This finding needs confirmation in other thoroughly prospectively conducted studies.—W.R. Bell, M.D.

Hemostatic Abnormalities in Total Artificial Heart Patients as Detected by Specific Blood Markers
Walenga JM, Hoppensteadt D, Fareed J, Pifarré R (Loyola Univ, Maywood, Ill)
Ann Thorac Surg 53:844–850, 1992   3–12

Introduction.—At the Loyola University Medical Center in Maywood, Illinois, the Jarvik 7-70 total artificial heart (TAH) is used in patients with end-stage heart failure who are awaiting a human donor heart. Overall outcome with the TAH has been successful, but hemostatic abnormalities continue to be a problem. The hemostatic system of 13 patients during implantation of the Jarvik 7-70 TAH was retrospectively evaluated.

Patients and Methods.—The patient group had a mean age of 40 years; the range of time with TAH support was 2–35 days. One patient had a failed heart transplant, 1 had giant-cell myocarditis, and 11 had a diagnosis of cardiomyopathy. All received intravenously administered heparin sodium and dipyridamole during TAH support. Blood samples were obtained for measurement of variables specific for coagulation and fibrinolytic, platelet, or endothelial activation.

Results.—Five patients had hemorrhagic complications while on the TAH and required an exploratory operation. When no definite bleeding site was identified, the diagnosis was a generalized coagulation disorder. The remaining 8 patients had no major hemostatic abnormalities. All underwent heart transplantation, and 9 of 13 have survived for more than 1 year. Routine coagulation assays during TAH showed slight abnormalities but no correlation to hemorrhagic or thrombotic events. The activation of the fibrinolytic system was marked in all patients. Decreased fibrinolysis, in addition to a hypercoagulable state and platelet activation, appeared to result from the TAH, and they were associated with thrombosis. The hemostatic activation returned to normal within a day of removal of the TAH.

Conclusion.—In addition to routine coagulation assays, patients with a TAH should be evaluated by more sensitive plasma markers specific for coagulation, fibrinolytic, and platelet activation. The fibrinogen, protein C, thrombin-antithrombin, tissue plasminogen activator, plasminogen activator inhibitor, D-dimer, and thromboxane B_2 assays are especially useful in monitoring these patients for both thrombotic and hemorrhagic complications.

▶ These studies clearly indicate that individuals who are maintained on a TAH require intensive monitoring of the coagulation and fibrinolytic systems. Somewhat disturbing is the observation that these individuals may have a coagulation disorder leading to bleeding as well as a coagulable state that may result in thrombosis. It appears, however, that these states can be defined and appropriately counteracted with proper therapy.—W.R. Bell, M.D.

Desmopressin Has No Beneficial Effect on Excessive Postoperative Bleeding or Blood Product Requirements Associated With Cardiopulmonary Bypass
de Prost D, Barbier-Boehm G, Hazebroucq J, Ibrahim H, Bielsky MC, Hvass U, Lacombe C, Français JL, Desmonts JM (CHU Xavier Bichat, Paris; ETEST, Paris)
Thromb Haemost 68:106–110, 1992   3–13

Background.—Cardiopulmonary bypass during open heart surgery may be associated with excessive perioperative bleeding. Desmopressin acetate, a synthetic vasopressin analogue, has hemostatic properties and has been used to reduce blood product needs in patients who bleed excessively, with mixed results.

Objective and Methods.—A double-blind, placebo-controlled trial of desmopressin was carried out in 92 adult patients with open heart surgery who had significant mediastinal bleeding within 6 hours of surgery as well as a prolonged template bleeding time. Treated patients received .3 μg of desmopressin per kg in physiologic solution during 30 minutes by infusion.

Results.—The degree of bleeding was similar in the treatment and placebo groups before infusion (Table 1). In the first 24 hours after treatment, blood losses did not differ significantly in the 2 groups (Table 2). Blood loss after infusion correlated with the amount of initial loss. More placebo patients required reoperation for bleeding, but the difference

TABLE 1.—Inclusion Criteria

	Desmopressin	Placebo	*p* value
Blood loss (ml h^{-1} m^{-2})	130 ± 54	121 ± 51	0.56
(ml/h)	229 ± 92	217 ± 87	0.50
Bleeding time (min)	18 ± 3	18 ± 3	0.85

(Courtesy of de Prost D, Barbier-Boehm G, Hazebroucq J, et al: *Thromb Haemost* 68:106–110, 1992.)

TABLE 2.—Post-Treatment Bleeding, Reoperation Rates, Blood
Product Use, and Prescription of Hemostatic Drugs in Desmopressin
and Placebo Groups During the First 24 Hours
After Treatment

	Desmopressin ($n = 47$)	Placebo ($n = 45$)	p value
Blood loss	($n = 44$)*)	($n = 37$)*)	
ml/m†	582 ± 410	465 ± 303	0.15
Reoperation for			
hemorrhage	3 (6.4%)	8 (17.8%)	0.12
Localized bleeding	3	7/8	
Hematocrit (%) at 24 h	31 ± 4	31 ± 4	0.80
Blood product utilization (units/patient)			
red cells	3.4 ± 2.6	3.2 ± 2.4	0.71
fresh frozen plasma	1.6 ± 2.1	1.4 ± 1.8	0.66
platelets	2.4 ± 3.4	2.2 ± 3.4	0.74
macromolecules†) (ml/patient)	1,202 ± 697	1,156 ± 858	0.78
Haemostatic drugs			
additional protamine	13 (27.7%)	11 (24.4%)	0.81
aprotinin	5 (10.6%)	6 (13.3%)	0.76

*Blood loss was measured only in patients who were not reoperated on.
†Macromolecules were 4% albumin in saline solution or modified gelatin fluid.
(Courtesy of de Prost D, Barbier-Boehm G, Hazebroucq J, et al: *Thromb Haemost* 68:106–110, 1992.)

was not significant. Bleeding times declined in both groups after infusion, whereas levels of vWF and factor VIII:C increased significantly.

Conclusion.—Desmopressin has no apparent value in patients who bleed overtly immediately after cardiopulmonary bypass.

▶ In a reasonably-sized patient population, the authors have very clearly identified the failure of 1-deamino-8-D-arginine vasopressin (DDAVP) in reducing bleeding and the need for transfusion products after a cardiopulmonary bypass. This is in sharp contrast to previously published reports. Never has there been a physiologic explanation as to why DDAVP should be helpful in this situation. In addition, DDAVP is known to increase von Willebrand's protein concentration in the circulating blood by stimulating its release from endothelial cells. In all patients after cardiopulmonary bypass, the von Willebrand protein concentration is normal or supranormal when the DDAVP is administered. This now makes the von Willebrand protein concentration 3 or 4, instead of 1 or 2, times the normal value. At my institution, we have noted that DDAVP repeatedly fails to improve postcardiopulmonary bypass bleeding. Before this article appeared, we had discontinued using DDAVP in this situation (1–4).—W.R. Bell, M.D.

References

1. Hackmann T, et al: N Engl J Med 321:1437–1443, 1989.
2. Salzman EW, et al: N Engl J Med 314:1402–1406, 1986.
3. Rocha E, et al: Circulation 77:1319–1323, 1988.
4. Czer LSC, et al: J Am Coll Cardiol 9:1139–1147, 1987.

Valproate Therapy Induces von Willebrand Disease Type I
Kreuz W, Linde R, Funk M, Meyer-Schrod R, Föll E, Nowak-Göttl U, Jacobi G, Vigh Z, Scharrer I (Klinikum der Johann Wolfgang Goethe-Universität, Frankfurt am Main, Germany)
Epilepsia 33:178–184, 1992   3–14

Background.—Valproate (VPA), used widely to treat seizure disorders, may produce hematologic reactions including thrombocytopenia, platelet dysfunction, decreased fibrinogen, and hemorrhagic diathesis.

Study Group.—Observations in 83 children given VPA therapy showed that hemorrhage was fairly frequent and sometimes correlated with a reduction in levels of factor VIII/vWF complex. Thirty children, aged 1–18 years, were followed closely during treatment with 20–30 mg of VPA per kg daily. The duration of treatment ranged from 6 months to 14 years.

Observations.—Fibrinogen levels and platelet counts, as well as levels of factor VIII complex, declined during VPA treatment. Most treated children had reductions in vWF and ristocetin-cofactor activity. A diagnosis of von Willebrand's syndrome type I was made in two thirds of patients having VPA treatment. Sixty-three percent of the patients had a history of bleeding. Reduced coagulation factor levels did not correlate with either the dose of VPA or the time of treatment.

Conclusion.—It is important to consider the risk of von Willebrand's disease developing in patients treated with VPA, particularly after trauma or when surgery is contemplated.

▶ For a considerable time, bleeding problems have been a recognized associated, undesirable effect of VAT. Several studies have attributed this to dysfunction of platelets and, in some instances, to thrombocytopenia. The authors of this study really showed progressive reduction in von Willebrand's protein simultaneous with treatment by this agent in a sizable patient population. If a patient requires this type of therapy, it is reasonable to follow the von Willebrand protein levels.—W.R. Bell, M.D.

Effects of Oral and Intramuscular Vitamin K Prophylaxis on Vitamin K₁, PIVKA-II, and Clotting Factors in Breast Fed Infants
Cornelissen EAM, Kollée LAA, De Abreu RA, van Baal JM, Motohara K, Verbruggen B, Monnens LAH (Univ of Nijmegen, The Netherlands; Amakusa-

Sumoto Hosp, Kumamoto, Japan)
Arch Dis Child 67:1250–1254, 1992

3–15

Introduction.—Vitamin K deficiency is implicated in hemorrhagic disease of the newborn, including fatal intracranial bleeding. Vitamin K prophylaxis has been widely recommended to prevent deficiency, but the best way of providing effective prophylaxis remains uncertain.

Objective and Methods.—The efficacy of administering vitamin K orally was compared with that of intramuscular dosing for preventing vitamin K deficiency after the first week of life in breast-fed infants. A total of 331 infants with a gestational age of 37 weeks or more were randomized to receive 1 mg of vitamin K_1 orally or the same dose intramuscularly on the first or second day of life.

Results.—None of the infants had an obvious bleeding diathesis or significantly disordered coagulation parameters. Blood coagulability and factor VII and X activities were comparable in the 2 treatment groups at all times of study (Fig 3–6). Levels of PIVKA-II (inert precursors of prothrombin) also were similar. Plasma levels of vitamin K_1 declined significantly during follow-up in both treatment groups, but they initially were significantly higher in the intramuscularly treated infants.

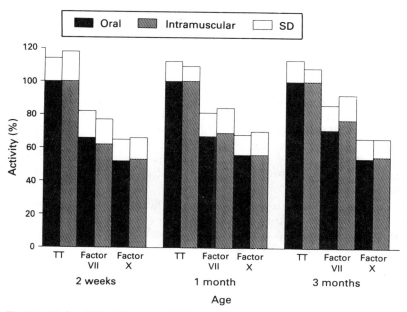

Fig 3–6.—Median (SD) of blood coagulability (thrombotest, TT) values and activities of clotting factors VII and X in breast-fed infants at age 2 weeks, 1 month, and 3 months after either oral or intramuscular vitamin K prophylaxis at birth. Values are expressed as percentage of normal adult pooled plasma. (Courtesy of Cornelissen EAM, Kollée LAA, De Abreu RA, et al: *Arch Dis Child* 67:1250–1254, 1992.)

Conclusion.—Repeated oral administration of vitamin K₁ appears necessary to fully protect breast-fed infants against late hemorrhagic disease of the newborn.

▶ Recently, some studies have suggested that the administration of vitamin K in the newborn is either unhelpful or unnecessary. This rather substantial finding in more than 300 infants clearly supports the contention that supplemental vitamin K administration is necessary in the newborn.—W.R. Bell, M.D.

Congenital Coagulation Factor Deficiency

Incidence of Development of Factor VIII and Factor IX Inhibitors in Haemophiliacs

Ehrenforth S, Kreuz W, Scharrer I, Linde R, Funk M, Güngör T, Krackhardt B, Kornhuber B (Univ Hosp, Frankfurt am Main, Germany)
Lancet 339:594–598, 1992   3–16

Background.—One of the most serious complications of repeated transfusion in patients with hemophilia A is the development of inhibitors to factor VIII:C. The reported frequency of this occurrence has ranged from 3.6% to 25% and may be rising, but these data have been derived mainly retrospectively from all known persons with hemophilia rather than from those truly at risk. The risk and incidence of the development of inhibitor in treated patients with hemophilia were assessed, and whether the type of purified factor VIII product used was related to inhibitor formation was tested.

Patients and Methods.—This prospective study included 46 children born after 1970 with moderate or severe hemophilia A who had received factor VIII concentrates, and 13 children with hemophilia B who had received factor IX concentrates. Children were enrolled from 1976 through 1991, and they received factor concentrates of various purities from various manufacturers. Seventeen children with mild hemophilia A were also studied.

Results.—Inhibitors developed only in children who had received factor VIII products. Factor VIII inhibitors developed in 33% of the patients with hemophilia A who received factor VIII products, including 14 of 27 (52%) patients with severe hemophilia, but only 1 of 19 patients with moderate hemophilia. Inhibitors developed in 24% of all patients with hemophilia A seen, including those with mild hemophilia. The incidence of inhibitor formation was 15 per 383 patient-years of observation or 39.1 per 1,000 patient-years. Twelve of 15 patients with inhibitors had high titers and anamnestic responses after administration of factor VIII, whereas 3 had low titers of inhibitors. Inhibitors were first detected at .08 years of age, and they had developed in 33% of patients by age 1 year, in 73% of patients by the age of 2.6 years, and in all patients by the age of 5.2 years. No individual factor VIII product seemed more likely than another to induce inhibitor formation.

Conclusion.—The risk of acquiring factor VIII inhibitors seems higher than previously reported. This complication occurs mainly in infants and children, and it seems to be about 4 times higher for children younger than age 5 years than for older patients.

▶ The development of an inhibitor in a patient with hemophilia A is a dreaded complication. Although a number of studies have documented the occurrence of inhibitors to be as high as 25% in hemophiliac populations, most hematologists would probably select a figure closer to 10% for the risk of inhibitor development. The recent availability of recombinant factor VIII products has made the issue of inhibitors more prominent, because studies of inhibitor development in patients receiving recombinant therapy suggest a risk as high as 29% (1). If a high rate of inhibitor development can be attributed to the use of recombinant factor VIII, enthusiasm for its use must be tempered, particularly since monoclonal products have no apparent risk of disease transmission. The current study suggests that 33% of patients have inhibitors develop. Two important points deserve emphasis: it is important to distinguish whether inhibitor development is recorded as incidence or prevalence in a population; and concurrent controlled prospective studies are the only valid way to assess this type of risk.—P.M. Ness, M.D.

Reference

1. Schwartz RS, et al: *N Engl J Med* 323:1799–1805, 1990.

Twenty-Five Years' Experience of Prophylactic Treatment in Severe Haemophilia A and B
Nilsson IM, Berntorp E, Löfqvist T, Pettersson H (Malmö Gen Hosp, Sweden; Univ Hosp, Lund, Sweden)
J Intern Med 232:25–32, 1992   3–17

Introduction.—Joint defects caused by frequent bleeding are common in patients with severe hemophilia. In an attempt to convert the disease from a severe to a milder form, thereby preventing the development of chronic arthropathy, Swedish physicians have used factor VIII or IX prophylactically in boys with severe hemophilia. The outcome of 60 patients treated for 2 to 25 years was reported.

Patients and Methods.—The patients ranged in age from 3 to 32 years. Fifty-two patients had severe hemophilia A and 8 patients had severe hemophilia B. Between 1960 and 1975, hemophilia A patients received factor VIII concentrates at a dosage of 10 to 20 units kg^{-1} body weight, usually at intervals of 3 to 5 days. Hemophilia B patients received factor IX concentrates since 1972 at a dosage of 15 to 20 units kg^{-1} body weight at intervals of 5 to 7 days. Starting in 1976, the prophylactic treatment was intensified. Boys entered treatment at the age of 1 to 3 years and continued at least until the age of 20. Patients who received regular treatments were compared with control groups of boys with severe hemophilia who had received only sporadic therapy.

Results.—The 2 youngest groups of patients (ages 3 to 12 years) who started the treatment at 1 to 2 years of age have had virtually no bleedings. All had orthopedic and radiologic joint scores of zero. Older boys (ages 13 to 17 years) who started at lower dosages have experienced some joint bleeding. However, 14 of 20 had orthopedic joint scores of zero, and 11 had radiologic scores of zero. The oldest group (ages 24 to 32 years) received factor VIII at considerably lower doses for 10 years. Some had joint defects at the start of treatment. They have improved over the years, however, in both bleeding incidence and joint scores. Differences in orthopedic scores between treatment and control groups were striking.

Conclusion.—With the present high-dosage regimen, patients have mild to moderate hemophilia and lead normal lives. By preventing the VIII:C or IX:C concentration from decreasing to less than 1% of normal, bleedings and arthropathy are almost entirely eliminated. Side effects have been relatively minor.

▶ This report indicated that continuous prophylaxis from an early age is effective in preventing hemophilic arthropathy. It is instructive to learn that, despite the frequency with which treatment was given in this study, many patients still experienced hemorrhage. However, apparently the volume of hemorrhage was minimal. The frequency of the induction of circulating anticoagulants was slightly less than 10%, which is noteworthy and at the present time appears to be acceptable. This is in contrast to a recent report (1) where the frequency of inhibitors reached a high of 52% in some patient populations.—W.R. Bell, M.D.

Reference

1. Ehrenforth S, et al: *Lancet* 339:594–598, 1992.

Purified Factor IX Using Monoclonal Immunoaffinity Technique: Clinical Trials in Hemophilia B and Comparison to Prothrombin Complex Concentrates
Kim HC, McMillan CW, White GC, Bergman GE, Horton MW, Saidi P (UMDNJ-Robert Wood Johnson Med School, New Brunswick, NJ; Univ of North Carolina at Chapel Hill; Rorer Central Research, Horsham, Pa; et al)
Blood 79:568–575, 1992   3–18

Objective.—Because the use of prothrombin complex concentrate (PCC) may cause thromboembolism or transmit viral infection when used as replacement therapy for hemophilia B (factor IX deficiency), a

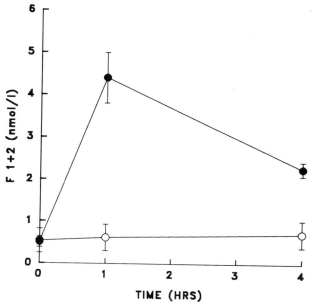

Fig 3–7.—Prothrombin activation fragment F_{1+2} measured preinfusion, and 1 hour and 4 hours postinfusion of Mononine (*open circles*) or PCC (*filled circles*). (Courtesy of Kim HC, McMillan CW, White GC, et al: *Blood* 79:568–575, 1992.)

highly purified monoclonal antibody–purified factor IX (Mononine) was studied as an alternative. Mononine lacks other vitamin K–dependent factors.

Trial.—Ten patients with factor IX deficiency, aged 11–60 years, underwent in vivo recovery studies at entry and 6 months later after receiving about 25 units of Mononine concentrate per kg. Six patients received infusions of PCC at least 2 weeks after the 6-month Mononine infusion.

Results.—The recovery of factor IX was .67 units/dL for each 1 unit of Mononine per kg infused. Its biological half-life was 22.6 hours. Mononine infusion did not alter levels of other vitamin K–dependent factors or prothrombin activation fragment (F_{1+2}), in contrast to PCC infusion (Fig 3-7). Patients using Mononine alone for 1 year exhibited an excellent hemostatic response during bleeding episodes. Antibody against murine IgG or an increase in IX inhibitor did not appear in any patient.

Discussion.—Mononine is less thrombogenic than less purified forms of factor IX concentrate and involves less exposure to allogeneic protein. It is costly, however, and adverse reactions to small amounts of contaminating murine protein are a possibility.

▶ Because of considerable frequency of thrombogenic problems associated with factor IX concentrates (PCC), efforts have been made recently to identify a factor IX concentration preparation that would avoid these very serious and disabling therapeutic complications. This thorough study in a reasonably sized patient population identified a newer isolated factor IX concentrate preparation that can be safely used and that provides equal efficacy with respect to factor IX replacement as former and older preparations did.—W.R. Bell, M.D.

Comparison of Four Virus-Inactivated Plasma Concentrates for Treatment of Severe von Willebrand Disease: A Cross-Over Randomized Trial
Mannucci PM, Tenconi PM, Castaman G, Rodeghiero F (IRCCS Policlinico Hosp, Milan, Italy; Hosp of Vicenza, Italy)
Blood 79:3130–3137, 1992   3–19

Introduction.—The main focus of treatment for von Willebrand's disease (vWD) is to alleviate the plasma factor VIII coagulant (VIII:C) activity deficiency. Until recently, cryoprecipitate has accomplished this goal, but it could still carry and transmit deadly viruses (e.g., HIV). Now, plasma concentrates containing factor VIII:C and vWF undergo antiviral purification methods and have become safer for routine use. Four virus-inactivated concentrates were examined in 10 patients with severe vWD.

Methods.—At the initiation of the study, none of the 10 patients with vWD were bleeding and the patients received no replacement treatment. Each patient randomly received a single infusion of 1 of 4 concentrates, and they crossed over to a single infusion of the remaining 3 treatments after at least 15 days. The 4 concentrates included hemate P, 8Y, very-high-purity vWF, and alpha-VIII, reflecting an intermediate-purity, pasteurized factor VIII-vWF concentrate; an intermediate-purity, dry-heated factor VIII-vWF concentrate; a solvent/detergent–treated vWF concentrate with a low level factor of VIII; and a high-purity solvent/detergent–treated factor VIII-vWF concentrate.

Results.—All 4 concentrates equally produced normal and sustained amounts of factor VIII:C after injection. The vWF concentrate required more time to reach peak levels, however. One hour after the hemate P (pasteurized factor VIII-vWF) infusion, the prolonged bleeding time corrected in 3 of 10 patients, partially corrected in 5, and did not correct in 2 (Fig 3–8), the vWF concentrate did not correct the bleeding time in any patient. The bleeding time outcomes did not correlate with the plasma concentrations of the ristocetin cofactor activity reached after infusion.

Conclusion.—None of the concentrates tested consistently corrected the bleeding time in this group of nonbleeding patients with vWD.

▶ The therapy of patients with vWD usually requires cryoprecipitate because factor VIII concentrates do not contain the larger multimers needed to

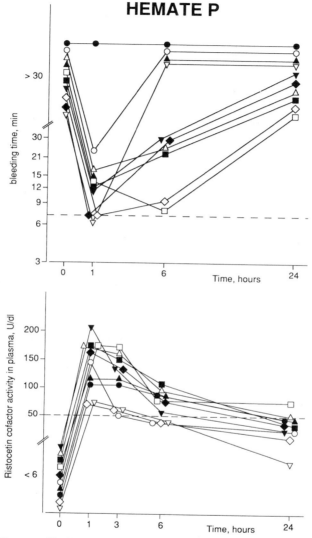

Fig 3–8.—Changes in bleeding time (**upper panel**) and Ricof (**lower panel**) in 10 patients with severe vWD before and after Hemate P. The *horizontal broken lines* indicate the upper limits of normal laboratory ranges. Each patient is identified by a different symbol. The scale of the vertical axis is logarithmic, that of the horizontal axis is arbitrary. (Courtesy of Mannucci PM, Tenconi PM, Castaman G, et al: *Blood* 79:3130–3137, 1992.)

correct the bleeding time as well as the factor VIII coagulant deficiency. A number of anecdotal reports suggest that some of the virus-inactivated concentrates may correct the bleeding time, perhaps because of some unknown manipulation of the coagulant proteins, and thus be of use in patients with vWD. This study compared 4 of the candidate factor VIII concentrates in patients with vWD. Although several concentrates produced transient correction of the bleeding time, none of them consistently corrected the bleeding time to justify their representation as useful therapy for vWD.—P.M. Ness, M.D.

Human Immunodeficiency Virus Infection Due to Clotting Factor Concentrates: Results of the Seroconversion Surveillance Project

Fricke W, Augustyniak L, Lawrence D, Brownstein A, Kramer A, Evatt B (Natl Insts of Allergy and Infectious Disease, Bethesda, Md; Natl Hemophilia Found, New York; Centers for Disease Control, Atlanta, Ga)
Transfusion 32:707–709, 1992   3–20

Background.—Efforts to reduce HIV infection risks include inactivation or elimination of viruses during the fractionation process and donor screening. In vitro studies have not satisfactorily predicted residual risk of infection, which has necessitated the use of surveillance projects in infection identifications. An ongoing surveillance project designed to detect new HIV infection in patients receiving clotting factor concentrates was introduced.

Methods.—A total of 131 hemophilia treatment centers supplied information on 9,496 patients with hemophilia and related disorders. When seroconversions were identified, additional data were collected, including dates and results of all HIV-antibody testing, history of clotting factor and other blood component use, and the presence of other risk factors.

Results.—Of the 9,496 patients, 4,366 (46%) are seropositive, and 37 (.39%) new seroconversions have been identified. Nine (.095%) of these seroconversions met Centers for Disease Control guidelines for seroconversion associated with blood factor products. However, no new HIV infections were found in patients who received only concentrates derived from screened blood pretreated to remove viral particles.

Conclusion.—These results show that the risk of HIV infection from currently treated clotting factor concentrates is extremely low. However, these results should be interpreted cautiously for several reasons: incomplete data gathering, undetected positive seroconversions, testing policy differences among participating agencies, and insufficient study sizes.

▶ This interesting report described an ongoing mechanism whereby clotting factor concentrates are monitored by collaborative efforts of hemophilia treaters and the Food and Drug Administration. These data collectively show that about 50% of patients are now HIV infected but offer some reassurance that newer concentrates used to inactivate viruses such as HIV have not been associated with seroconversions.—P.M. Ness, M.D.

Immune Status of Asymptomatic HIV-Infected Hemophiliacs: Randomized, Prospective, Two-Year Comparison of Treatment With a High-Purity or an Intermediate-Purity Factor VIII Concentrate

Mannucci PM, Gringeri A, de Biasi R, Baudo F, Morfini M, Ciavarella N (IRCCS Maggiore Hosp, Milan, Italy; Pellegrini Hosp, Naples, Italy; Cà Granda Hosp, Milan, Italy; et al)

Thromb Haemost 67:310–313, 1992   3–21

Introduction.—Patients with hemophilia require plasma-derived factor VIII to maintain a normal bleeding time. Recently, it has been suggested that a high-purity factor VIII product may cause less deterioration of the immune system in patients with hemophilia infected with HIV. Patients with hemophilia who received a licensed intermediate-purity factor VIII concentrate and a nonlicensed high-purity product for 2 years were studied.

Patients and Methods.—Thirty-three patients with hemophilia A, HIV seropositive but asymptomatic (Centers for Disease Control stages II–III) and currently receiving intermediate-purity factor VIII concentrate, participated in the study. Patients were first stratified by CD4 cell counts, then 17 continued to receive the intermediate-purity product while 16 began receiving the high-purity concentrate. Follow-up continued for 24 months.

Results.—The yearly concentrate usage was the same for both patient groups during the 2-year follow-up. Five patients withdrew from the trial, 4 from the intermediate-purity group (usually because they began to receive zidovudine therapy). The CD4 cell counts varied but tended to

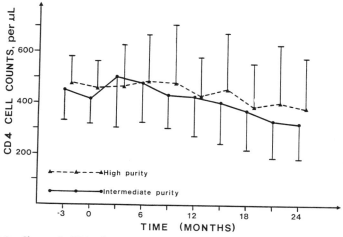

Fig 3–9.—Changes in CD4 cell counts in patients with hemophilia treated with high-purity or intermediate-purity factor VIII concentrates for 24 months. Data are given as means and 1 SD. (Courtesy of Mannucci PM, Gringeri A, de Biasi R, et al: *Thromb Haemost* 67:310–313, 1992.)

decrease from the baseline values at the same rate for both treatments (Fig 3–9). Baseline measurements demonstrated 7 patients with high-purity concentrate and 5 patients with intermediate-purity concentrate anergic to all recall antigens. At 24 months, 8 patients with high-purity concentrate and 6 patients with intermediate-purity concentrate appeared anergic. Four patients had HIV infection symptoms: 3 in the intermediate-purity product group and 1 in the high-purity product group.

Conclusion.—The immune system of patients with asymptomatic HIV-positive hemophilia derives no particular benefit from using a high-purity factor VIII concentrate during a period of 2 years.

▶ Factor VIII preparations of varying purity have been available for many years. Concentrates of higher purity tend to be more expensive for the patient and their yield from plasma is smaller, so the total availability of factor VIII products is reduced by the production of high-purity products from plasma. The advantages of higher purity have been difficult to establish clinically, although the virtues of purity in general are undebatable. It has been suggested that high-purity factor VIII concentrates may be advantageous to the hemophiliac with HIV because the impurities in other concentrates may lead to more rapid immunosuppression and disease progression. This 2-year study failed to show the advantage of higher-purity products, but longer scrutiny may be required to resolve this issue.—P.M. Ness, M.D.

Effect of Age on Human Immunodeficiency Virus Type 1-Induced Changes in Lymphocyte Populations Among Persons With Congenital Clotting Disorders

Fletcher MA, Mosley JW, Hassett J, Gjerset GF, Kaplan J, Parker JW, Donegan E, Lusher JM, Lee H, and The Transfusion Safety Study Group (Univ of Miami, Fla; Univ of Southern California, Los Angeles; Mt Sinai Med Ctr, New York; et al)
Blood 80:831–840, 1992   3–22

Background.—Past the neonatal period, children infected with HIV-1 have low rates of progression to AIDS. The effect of age on HIV-1–induced changes in lymphocyte populations was determined among persons with congenital clotting disorders.

Methods and Results.—Pair-wise comparisons of uninfected and HIV-infected boys and adults with hemophilia were used to determine whether the HIV-1 impact on peripheral blood mononuclear cell subpopulations differed with age. Infected children had smaller decreases in total lymphocytes than did adults. However, children had proportionately lower numbers of CD2+, CD4+, CD2+CD26+, and CD4+CD29+ counts. The CD4+CD45RA+ cell counts were more than two-fold greater in uninfected and infected children than in adults. The CD4+CD45RA+/CD4+ proportion rose by 1.4-fold with infection in adults but remained the same in children. Infected adults had very significant increases in total CD8+ counts. Both children and adults had increased CD8+HLA-DR+ counts. Children with infection had significantly greater total B-cell counts than adults with infection and a disproportionately lower number of resting B cells. In 2 years of follow-up, infected children and adults had lymphocyte changes in the same directions that were proportionately equal.

Conclusion.—Children's lower rate of HIV-1 progression may be partly associated with differences in lymphocyte populations compared with adults. The functional properties of immune cells may be equally or more important.

▶ A number of studies have documented that children infected with HIV tend to progress to symptomatic AIDS more slowly than older patients; cohorts of hemophiliacs and other transfusion recipients who were infected in the early 1980s have been well studied to demonstrate this point. The explanation for these observations is not as clear-cut. This article demonstrates that differences in lymphocyte subpopulations may afford at least a partial answer to this dilemma.—P.M. Ness, M.D.

Hemophilia B Caused by Five Different Nondeletion Mutations in the Protease Domain of Factor IX
Ludwig M, Sabharwal AK, Brackmann HH, Olek K, Smith KJ, Birktoft JJ, Bajaj SP (Inst of Experimental Haematology and Blood Transfusion, Bonn, Germany; St Louis Univ, Mo; Inst of Clinical Chemistry, Bonn, Germany; et al)
Blood 79:1225–1232, 1992   3–23

Background.—Hemophilia B is a X-linked recessive disease characterized by a deficiency in factor IX activity. This factor is a multidomain protein and the proenzyme of a serine protease, factor IXa. The point mutations found in the factor IX gene of 5 patients with hemophilia B were studied.

Materials.—Genomic DNA was isolated from blood leukocytes of 5 patients. The factor IX gene was amplified by PCR and sequenced.

Results.—Two patients had serine-365 point mutations. In 1 patient, the change was to isoleucine. The other patient had a mutation to glycine, and this patient also had antibodies to factor IX during replacement therapy. Another patient had point mutation nearby at Asp364His. The remaining 2 mutations were also grouped close together, occurring at Glu245Val in 1 patient and Arg248Gln in the other (table). Additionally, the Arg248Gln mutant did not react to a normal factor IX antibody, whereas the Glu245Val mutant did.

Conclusion.—The effects of the mutations occurring at positions 364 and 365 are readily explained. The aspartate carboxyl group is thought to form an ion pair with a distant valine, forming the substrate-binding pocket. In this context, the serine residues are important in the charged

Summary of Mutations in the Factor IX Variants Investigated

Patient	Mutant	Nucleotide No.	Nucleotide Change	Amino Acid Change	IX:C	IX:Ag	Inhibitor Bethesda Units
A	IX$_{Schmallenberg}$	31,215	G → T	Ser-365 → Ile	<1	80	Negative
B	IX$_{Varel}$	31,214	A → G	Ser-365 → Gly	<1	86	8.1
		31,213	T → C	Silent			
C	IX$_{Mechtal}$	31,211	G → C	Asp-364 → His	<1	100	Negative
D	IX$_{Dreihacken}$	30,864	G → A	Arg-248 → Gln	~2–3	~4	Negative
E	IX$_{Monschau}$	30,855	A → T	Glu-2 45 → Val	~3–5	40	Negative

(Courtesy of Ludwig M, Sabharwal AK, Brackmann HH, et al: *Blood* 79:1225–1232, 1992.)

relay triad, aspartate-Histidine-serine, common to serine proteases. The lack of these active-site amino acids prevents the formation of the binding pocket. In an interesting aside, the development of antibodies to factor IX by the patient with the Ser365Gly mutation shows that deletion of factor IX is not required for antibody formation. The lowered factor IX activity exhibited by the last 2 mutations may be explained by a reduction in calcium^{2+} affinity. The binding site of the normal factor IX antibody encompasses a high-affinity calcium binding site, putatively located at glucose-248. This mutant is inactive because of deficient calcium binding. The arginine-248 mutant also has reduced activity (40%); however, the major cause for hemophilia in this patient is probably a result of a lack of circulating protein.

▶ The authors of this study have provided a detailed and reasonable explanation for the disease entity of hemophilia B. The causative mutations have been found in the protease domain of the factor IX molecule in each of their patients. These authors have also identified that the domain where the mutations have been identified is, in its normal state, critically important as a calcium-binding ligand (1).—W.R. Bell, M.D.

Reference

1. Bajaj SP, et al: *Proc Natl Acad Sci USA* 89:152–156, 1992.

Human Parvovirus B19 Infection in Hemophiliacs First Infused With Two High-Purity, Virally Attenuated Factor VIII Concentrates

Azzi A, Ciappi S, Zakvrzewska K, Morfini M, Mariani G, Mannucci PM (Univ of Florence, Italy; Univ Hosp of Florence, Italy; Univ of Rome; et al)
Am J Hematol 39:228–230, 1992   3–24

Introduction.—Infection by parvovirus B19 is frequent in childhood; as many as half of adults have anti-B19 antibodies. The virus may be transmitted by coagulation factor concentrates, and it is highly resistant to conventional viricidal measures. Whether removing virus chromatographically during the manufacture of high-purity concentrates lowers the risk of transmitting B19 was determined.

Antibodies to Human Parvovirus B19 in Patients With Hemophilia First Infused With High-Purity, Virally Attenuated Factor VIII Concentrates

Concentrates (virucidal methods)	Anti-B19 status	No. of patients before infusion showing anti-B19 IgG	No. of patients after infusion showing anti-B19	
			IgM	IgG
Beriate P	Positive	6	—	—
(pasteurization)	Negative	13	2	4
	Unknown	9	2	4
Emoclot Octa VI	Positive	2	—	—
(solvent/detergent)	Negative	7	5	5

(Courtesy of Azzi A, Ciappi S, Zakvrzewska K, et al: *Am J Hematol* 39:228–230, 1992.)

Treatment.—Nineteen patients with previously untreated hemophilia were treated exclusively with Beriate P, a pasteurized factor VIII concentrate purified by ion-exchange chromatography. Nine other untreated patients were treated with Emoclot Octa VI, a factor VIII concentrate purified by ion-exchange chromatography and treated with a solvent-detergent mixture (tri-[n-butyl]-phosphate and polysorbate 80).

Results.—Four of 13 anti-B19–negative patients seroconverted after treatment with Beriate P (table). Two patients exhibited both anti-B19 IgM and IgG after 6–8 weeks, indicating acute B19 infection. Five of 7 anti-B19–negative patients given Emoclot Octa VI exhibited IgM and IgG antibodies against B19 8–12 weeks after infusion.

Conclusion.—Even modern factor VIII concentrates may transmit parvovirus B19, indicating that further efforts are needed to develop ways of inactivating this virus.

▶ Despite a steadily increasing number of tests and techniques used to purify and decontaminate procoagulant factors, an ever-increasing list of newer contaminants can be found even in the most crystalline pure preparations. This fact should be borne in mind before one adopts an ad-lib, uncontrolled administration of such concentrates to patients.—W.R. Bell, M.D.

Hemophilia A Due to Mutations That Create New N-Glycosylation Sites

Aly AM, Higuchi M, Kasper CK, Kazazian HH Jr, Antonarakis SE, Hoyer LW (Holland Lab, Rockville, Md; Johns Hopkins Univ, Baltimore, Md; Orthopedic Hosp, Los Angeles)
Proc Natl Acad Sci USA 89:4933–4937, 1992   3–25

Introduction.—Hemophilia A is caused by a deficiency of factor VIII procoagulant activity (VIII:C). Many factor VIII gene mutations have been described, most of them presumably being point mutations. Five percent of hemophilic plasma contain nonfunctional factor VIII-like protein, which is detected by immunoradiometric assay, and are said to be cross-reacting material–positive.

Patients.—Among 24 unrelated patients with cross-reacting material–positive hemophilia A, 2 had abnormal nonfunctional factor VIII–like protein with slow-moving heavy or light chains. Both these patients had less than 1% of normal factor VIII activity but a normal plasma level of factor VIII antigen.

Mutations.—When gel electrophoretic screening of PCR-amplified products of the factor VIII–coding DNA sequence was carried out, 1 patient had a methionine-to-threonine substitution at position 1772 in the factor VIII light chain, creating a potential new N-glycosylation site at asparagine-1770. The other patient had an isoleucine-to-threonine substitution at position 566, creating a potential new N-glycosylation site at

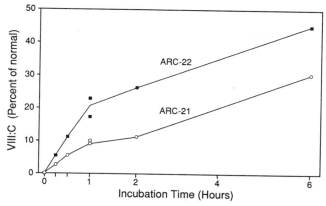

Fig 3–10.—Effect of N-glycanase on factor VIII:C. Aliquots (100 μL) of cross-reacting material-positive plasma were incubated with 1 unit N-glycanase for as long as 6 hours. Factor VIII:C of the sample (determined by a 1-stage clotting assay) was then compared with that of normal pooled plasma that had been incubated with the enzyme for the same period of time. (Courtesy of Aly AM, Higuchi M, Kasper CK, et al: *Proc Natl Acad Sci USA* 89:4933–4937, 1992.)

asparagine-564 in the A2 domain of the factor VIII heavy chain. Incubation of patient plasmas with N-glycanase led to increased procoagulant activity (Fig 3–10), suggesting that post-translational glycosylation led to a loss of factor VIII function.

Conclusion.—Some cases of severe hemophilia A may reflect abnormal N-glycosylation that blocks VIII:C activity.

▶ The authors have presented convincing data that suggest abnormal N-glycosylation is capable of blocking the procoagulant activity of factor VIII:C. This abnormal glycosylation results from a mutation in the factor VIII gene. The most convincing evidence provided is that when the factor VIII molecule was incubated with N-glycanase, there was a progressive increase in the amount of factor VIII activity identified. One must be absolutely certain, however, that the N-glycanase does not in some way unfold, alter, or denature the molecule that results in an apparent in vitro increase in coagulant activity.—W.R. Bell, M.D.

Recovery From Hemophilia B Leyden: An Androgen-Responsive Element in the Factor IX Promoter
Crossley M, Ludwig M, Stowell KM, De Vos P, Olek K, Brownlee GG (Univ of Oxford, England; Univ of Bonn, Germany; Catholic Univ, Leuven, Belgium)
Science 257:377–379, 1992   3–26

Introduction.—Patients with hemophilia B Leyden have severe bleeding as children and have less than 1% of normal plasma factor IX. Symptoms lessen after puberty, when the plasma factor IX increases to 60% of normal. The first patient had a T-to-A mutation at -20 in the factor IX promoter, and other patients have had point mutations at various nucleotides.

A New Case.—A patient who failed to improve after puberty had a G-to-C mutation at -26 in the promoter region. He had less than 1% of normal factor IX clotting activity before puberty but, unlike classic Leyden patients, factor IX clotting remained low and clinical recovery did not ensue. Both the -26 and -20 mutations were shown to markedly impair transcription from the factor IX promoter by disrupting the binding site for the liver-enriched transcription factor LF-A1/HNF4. Only the -26 mutation disrupted an androgen-responsive element that overlapped the LF-A1/HNF4 site.

Conclusion.—The presence of an additional disruption of an androgen-responsive element in the -26 mutation may explain why patients so affected fail to improve clinically after puberty.

▶ These authors have very neatly identified that patients with this particular type of hemophilia B possess within their genetic makeup an androgen-responsive element in the promoter of factor IX production. The information as to how to insert this type of androgen-responsive promoter in other types of hemophilia genes is needed.—W.R. Bell, M.D.

Antenatal Diagnosis of Haemophilia B by Amplification and Electrophoresis of an Exon Fragment With a Short Deletion
Ljung R, Green P, Sjörin E, Giannelli F, Nilsson IM (Malmö Gen Hosp, Sweden; Guy's Hosp, London)
Eur J Haematol 49:215–218, 1992   3–27

Background.—Hemophilia B is a X-linked disease characterized by a factor IX deficiency. The sequencing and characterization of the factor IX gene has provided a powerful tool in prenatal diagnosis and counseling of female carriers. The most common techniques used to determine the existence of a mutated gene are restriction fragment length polymorphism (RFLP) or direct sequencing of the gene. However, not all mutations are detectable by RFLP, and direct sequencing can be difficult. A diagnostic technique based PCR amplification of the mutated region has been used in prenatal screening.

Method.—Two sisters were seen for prenatal diagnosis. Blood samples were taken from both sisters and 2 distant relatives with hemophilia B. Direct genomic sequencing of the affected family members identified an 8-base pair deletion in exon h. Polymerase chain reaction primers were generated, amplifying the mutated region. Chorionic villi sampling was used to obtain fetal blood. Peripheral leukocyte DNA was amplified using the generated PCR primers and separated on a polyacrylamide gel.

Results. —The PCR primers chosen allowed a size-based separation of the normal and deleted fragments on the polyacrylamide gel. Both sisters were determined to be carriers. One fetus, female, was also determined to be a carrier, whereas the other, male, was found to have the mutated gene.

Conclusion. —A simplified, direct gene diagnosis may be beneficial in conditions where RFLP is not informational.

▶ These authors demonstrated the feasibility and usefulness of cytogenetics in identifying carriers in affected individuals with factor IX deficiency. This is an important advance and allows the accurate detection of this condition.—W.R. Bell, M.D.

Circulating Anticoagulants

Lupus Anticoagulant in Systemic Lupus Erythematosus: A Clinical and Renal Pathological Study

Farrugia E, Torres VE, Gastineau D, Michet CJ, Holley KE (Mayo Clinic and Mayo Found, Rochester, Minn)
Am J Kidney Dis 20:463–471, 1992   3–28

Objective. —Circulating lupus anticoagulants (LAs), a group of immunoglobulins that interfere in various phospholipid-dependent coagulation reactions, may be associated with thrombosis in both large and small vessels. Only small numbers of highly selected patients have been used to address this issue.

Patients and Methods. —The association between the presence of LA and thrombosis in the renal microcirculation was evaluated in 33 patients with systemic lupus erythematosus (SLE), renal dysfunction, and documented circulating LA. They accounted for 7% of biopsy-proven

TABLE 1.—Thromboembolic and Bleeding Events

No. of Patients With:	LA	C	*P* Value
Thrombosis	13/33 (39%)*	4/32 (13%)‡	0.014
Bleeding	7/33 (21%)†	6/32 (19%)§	NS

*Includes deep vein thrombosis, lower extremities (9), cerebrovascular accident (3), pulmonary embolus (1), axillary artery occlusion (1), anterior spinal artery thrombosis (1).
†Includes bleeding from ear, nose, and throat (2), gut (1), skin (2), and postrenal biopsy (3).
‡Includes deep vein thrombosis, lower extremities (3), pulmonary embolus (1), cerebrovascular accident (3).
§Includes bleeding from gut (2); uterus (2); ear, nose, and throat (2); and postrenal biopsy (3).
(Courtesy of Farrugia E, Torres VE, Gastineau D, et al: *Am J Kidney Dis* 20:463–471, 1992.)

TABLE 2.—Vascular Lesions by Light Microscopy

Interlobular Arteries

	Intimal Sclerosis		Medial Hypertrophy		Arteriolar Sclerosis	
	LA	C	LA	C	LA	C
Mild	14 (42)*	10 (31)	10 (30)	7 (22)	14 (42)	12 (38)
Moderate	4 (12)	3 (9)	2 (6)	1 (3)	3 (9)	1 (3)
Severe	3 (9)	1 (3)	0	1 (3)	1 (3)	1 (3)
Nil	12 (36)	18 (56)	21 (70)	22 (69)	15 (45)	18 (56)

*Percentage of total in each group (LA = 33, C = 22) is given in parentheses. Glomerular and/or anteriolar thrombi were detected only in patients with LA.
(Courtesy of Farrugia E, Torres VE, Gastineau D, et al: Am J Kidney Dis 20:463–471, 1992.)

lupus nephritis patients identified during 25 years. They were matched for age, sex, and biopsy timing to a control group of 32 patients with SLE and a normal gross coagulation screen.

Findings.—The 2 groups were comparable in their prevalence of serositis, neuropsychiatric illness, leukopenia, thrombocytopenia, hemolysis, anti–double-stranded DNA elevation, and complement reduction. The LA group was more likely to have biological false-positive syphilis serology but less likely to have arthritis. Thrombotic events were present in 39% of the LA group vs. 13% of the control group. Their incidence of bleeding episodes was similar (Table 1). At biopsy, the 2 groups had similar hypertension, serum creatinine, and proteinuria. There were also no significant differences in lesions, as assessed by World Health Organization class, activity, and chronicity indexes or by immunofluorescence and electron microscopy findings (Table 2). Five of the LA group had occlusive glomerular, anteriolar, and arterial fibrin thrombi, as well as varying degrees of renal thrombotic microangiopathy, vs. none of the control group. Shortly after biopsy, 3 of 5 patients had died.

Conclusion.—The renal morphologic findings of most patients with SLE, renal dysfunction, and LA appear to be little different from those without LA. A subset of patients with LA had thrombotic microangiopathy at biopsy; this group had a worse prognosis. Although steroid treatment may lead to the disappearance of LAs, it does not eliminate the thrombotic risk in patients with SLE and LA; low-dose aspirin might benefit these patients.

▶ This thorough, detailed study indicates that in certain individuals with a lupus anticoagulant, definite glomerular lesions that are thrombotic in nature can be identified. These lesions also correlate with a deterioration in renal function. Thus, an individual with this illness who demonstrates the presence of a lupus anticoagulant should be thoroughly anticoagulated so long as the LA is present in the circulation, particularly if renal dysfunction or borderline renal function is present.—W.R. Bell, M.D.

Fibrinolytic Balance and Lupus Anticoagulant in Patients With Repeated Spontaneous Fetal Loss

Ferro D, Violi F, Quintarelli C, Sebastianelli A, D'Amelio R, Zichella L, Balsano F (Univ di Roma)
BMJ 305:504–505, 1992

3–29

Background.—Placental infarction is sometimes associated with recurrent pregnancy losses in women without genetic, anatomical, and endocrine abnormalities. Lupus anticoagulant may be present in such cases. Other risk factors include thrombocythemia and deficient fibrinolytic activity.

Subjects.—Fibrinolytic balance was examined in 38 women with 2 or more first- or second-trimester fetal losses. Eighteen were positive for lupus anticoagulant, and 13 of 18 had systemic lupus erythematosus. Studies were carried out at least 3 months after the last fetal loss. Fourteen healthy women and 15 with systemic lupus but no history of abortion also were evaluated.

Findings.—The levels of tissue plasminogen activator were similar in both groups of recurrent aborters and in the healthy subjects. Significantly increased values of plasminogen activator inhibitor antigen and activity were found in the lupus anticoagulant–positive women. Women with systemic lupus who were negative for lupus anticoagulant had fibrinolytic parameters resembling those of healthy subjects.

Conclusion.—Fibrinolytic imbalance is not characteristic of women with recurrent fetal losses who are negative for lupus anticoagulant. However, in women positive for lupus anticoagulant, repeated abortion may be associated with a high circulating level of plasminogen activator inhibitor.

▶ The studies performed by these authors to identify in vivo activity of the fibrinolytic system are inadequate. The in vitro determinations, even if markedly elevated, do not identify that plasmin, which is the final and absolute end point for the fibrinolytic system, is produced in vivo. These results must be considered with this in mind (1).—W.R. Bell, M.D.

Reference

1. Karp JE, Bell WR: *Am J Physiol* 227:1212–1215, 1974.

Comparison Between a One-Point Dilute Phospholipid APTT and the Dilute Russell Viper Venom Time for Verification of Lupus Anticoagulants

Alving BM, Barr CF, Johansen LE, Tang DB (Walter Reed Army Inst of Research, Washington, DC)
Thromb Haemost 67:672–678, 1992   3–30

Background.—A prolonged activated partial thromboplastin time (APTT) may result from the presence of a lupus anticoagulant, which is an antiphospholipid antibody inhibitory in a phospholipid-dependent coagulation assay. Some patients with such antibodies may be at an increased risk for thrombosis or recurrent abortion. Lupus anticoagulant is confirmed by either neutralizing the anticoagulant effect of the antibody by increasing the level of phospholipid in the assay or enhancing its effect by diluting or removing the phospholipid.

Methods.—Two phospholipid dilution procedures, the dilute phospholipid APTT (PL-APTT) and the dilute Russell viper venom time (RVVT), were modified. The modified assays were compared for detecting antiphospholipid antibodies in plasmas from 49 subjects having normal APTT values, and from 72 patients having prolonged APTTs who did not receive heparin and did not have inhibitors against specific factors. Modifications included a single dilution of either bovine brain thromboplastin (Thrombofax) or liposomes consisting of phosphatidylcholine/phosphatidylserine. In addition, the results were expressed as a ratio of the clotting time of the mixture of patient and normal plasmas to that of normal plasma.

Results.—Correlation between the assay results with liposomes and Thrombofax was .88 in the RVVT and .68 in the PL-APTT (Fig 3–11). A positive result was defined as a ratio of 1.3 or more for the PL-APTT with liposomes, and a ratio of 1.2 or higher for the PL-APTT with Thrombofax and for the RVVT with either material. Apart from the source of phospholipid, the PL-APTT was the most sensitive test for antiphospholipid antibody, whereas the RVVT was more specific.

Conclusion.—Assessment of patients with a history of thrombosis, who may have lupus anticoagulant, should include a dilute phospholipid assay and also an estimate of antiphospholipid antibody in a solid-phase enzyme-linked immunosorbent assay.

▶ With the prevalence of the lupus anticoagulant or lupus-like inhibitor in the patient population at the present time, it is critically important that the most sensitive, reliable, and reproducible technique be identified. Comparative studies, such as performed by the authors, clearly identify that the dilute RVVT is the optimal test for the detection of this antiphospholipid inhibitor. The importance of this inhibitor can only be appreciated when its presence is precisely known (1).—W.R. Bell, M.D.

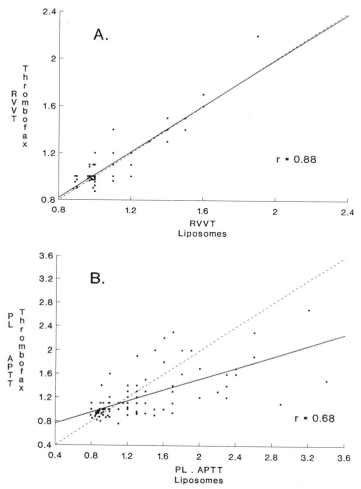

Fig 3–11.—A, correlation between RVVT with Thrombofax and RVVT with PC/PS liposomes. **B,** correlation between 1-point PL-APTT with Thrombofax and with PC/PS liposomes (*n* = 121). The *solid line* is the actual slope defining the relationship between the assays, and the *dashed line* is the expected slope of 1. (Courtesy of Alving BM, Barr CF, Johansen LE, et al: *Thromb Haemost* 67:672–678, 1992.)

Reference

1. Oosting JD, et al: *Thromb Haemost* 67:499–502, 1992.

Relationship of Antiphospholipid Antibodies to Pregnancy Loss in Patients With Systemic Lupus Erythematosus: A Cross-Sectional Study

Ginsberg JS, Brill-Edwards P, Johnston M, Denburg JA, Andrew M, Burrows RF, Bensen W, Cividino A, Long AA (McMaster Univ, Hamilton, Ont, Canada)
Blood 80:975–980, 1992   3–31

Introduction.—The presence of antiphospholipid antibodies has been implicated as an independent risk factor for pregnancy loss, but no such association has been confirmed. Whether antiphospholipid antibodies in women with systemic lupus erythematosus (SLE) are related to spontaneous abortion or stillbirth was investigated.

Methods.—The 42 study participants all had SLE and a history of at least 1 pregnancy. Blood samples were obtained on the patient's initial visit to the rheumatology clinic and at a follow-up visit at least 3 months later. On both occasions, 5 tests of the lupus anticoagulant and an enzyme-linked immunosorbent assay to measure IgG anticardiolipin antibodies were performed.

Results.—The rate of pregnancy loss was high (26.2%) in this patient group. Thirty of the 122 pregnancies had resulted in spontaneous abortion and 2 resulted in stillbirth. One woman had lost 6 of 12 pregnancies. Fifteen women, including all 7 who experienced multiple pregnancy losses, were repeatedly positive for the lupus anticoagulant (Table 1). Transient positivity was less strongly associated with fetal loss (Table 2).

TABLE 1.—Pregnancy Loss and Antiphospholipid
Antibody Results

	No. of Episodes of Pregnancy Loss per Patient		
	>1	1	0
APLA test results			
LA+ ACLA+	4	1	0
LA+ ACLA−	3	2	5
LA− ACLA+	0	0	0
LA− ACLA−	0	8	19
Total	7	11	24

Abbreviations: APLA, antiphospholipid antibody; LA, lupus anticoagulant; ACLA, anticardiolipin antibody; +, repeatedly positive; −, negative or transiently positive.
(Courtesy of Ginsberg JS, Brill-Edwards P, Johnston M, et al: *Blood* 80:975–980, 1992.)

TABLE 2.—Relationship Between Antiphospholipid
Antibodies and Pregnancy Loss

	No. of Episodes of Pregnancy Loss per Patient		
	≥1	0	
LA +	10	5	(OR, 4.8; 95% CI, 1.0-23.6; *P* = .05*)
−	8	19	
ACLA +	5	0	(OR, 20.0; 95% CI, 1.3-97.0; *P* = .01†)
−	13	24	

Abbreviations: OR, odds ratio. For others, see Table 1.
*λ^2 test.
†Fisher exact test.
(Courtesy of Ginsberg JS, Brill-Edwards P, Johnston M, et al: *Blood* 80:975–980, 1992.)

All 5 women who were positive at both blood-sampling periods for anticardiolipin antibodies had 1 or more previous losses.

Conclusion.—Significant associations were noted between repeat lupus anticoagulant and anticardiolipin antibody positivity and previous pregnancy loss in women with SLE. Positivity at repeat testing and on several assays for lupus anticoagulant yields greater sensitivity than a single test or assay. Studies that have not found the associations described here may have relied on the results of a single test.

▶ Although only small numbers of patients were studied, these findings support the suggestion that more than 1 type of antibody is present in patients with the "lupus type" anticoagulant. Clearly, more than simply coagulation studies are needed to identify these various antibodies. No single test is adequate for study. In addition to the type of antibodies that alter the function of coagulation proteins, the presence of an anticardiolipin antibody must be searched for with a different technique.

For additional studies concerning the frequency and clinical course of patients with the lupus-type anticoagulant and/or anticardiolipin antibodies, please see reference 1.—W.R. Bell, M.D.

Reference

1. Rosove MH, Brewer PM: *Ann Intern Med* 117:303–308, 1992.

The Correlation Between Lupus Anticoagulant and Autoantibodies

Gleicher N, Harlow L, El-Roeiy A (Mt Sinai Hosp Med Ctr of Chicago; Rush Medical College, Chicago)
Mt Sinai J Med 59:32–37, 1992   3–32

Background.—A positive lupus anticoagulant (LA) test has been associated with pregnancy wastage, and patients with repeated wastage who were LA-positive have exhibited significant autoantibody abnormalities involving anti-phospholipids. The serologic findings were examined in 326 patients with reproductive failure who had LA studies and also a broad-based autoantibody screen. Lupus anticoagulant was assessed by the tissue thromboplastin inhibition (TTI) test and the activated partial thromboplastin time (APTT).

Findings.—The presence of LA correlated with 12 of 45 autoantibody isotypes investigated, as assessed by TTI, but only 9 of them using the

Autoantibody	Lupus TTI	Anti-coagulant† APTT
Significant Correlation Between LA (By TTI and APTT) and Autoantibodies		
Phospholipids		
IgG anticardiolipin		0.05
IgA anticardiolipin	0.032	
IgG antiphosphatidylserine		0.01
IgG antiphosphatidic acid	0.007	0.034
IgA antiphosphatidic acid	0.006	
IgA antiphosphatidyl-ethanolamine	0.007	0.009
IgG antiphosphatidylglycerol	0.001	
IgA antiphosphatidylinositol	0.042	0.0001
Histones		
IgG anti-H1	0.0001	0.0001
IgA anti-H1	0.0009	
IgA anti-H2A		0.018
IgA anti-H2B	0.017	
IgG anti-H4	0.0001	0.0001
Polynucleotides		
IgA anti-poly I	0.0001	
IgG anti-poly(dt)		
IgM anti-poly(dt)		

Note: Only significant correlations with 6 antiphospholipids, 5 antihistones, and 4 antipolynucleotides are shown.
†Numbers indicate P value.
(Courtesy of Gleicher N, Harlow L, El-Roeiy A: *Mt Sinai J Med* 59:32–37, 1992.)

APTT (table). Five autoantibodies correlated significantly with both the TTI and APTT. With both methods, LA correlated primarily with IgG and IgA autoantibodies. At abnormal levels of LA, correlation was closer with IgM autoantibodies to histones and polynucleotides than with antibodies to phospholipids.

Conclusion.—Correlations between LA and specific autoantibodies are not especially strong. Screening for LA is not an efficient way of detecting abnormal B-cell function in women suspected of having reproductive failure caused by abnormal autoimmunity. Instead, polyclonal B-cell abnormalities should be sought using a broad-based antibody screen.

▶ These findings suggest that antibody produced in the various connective tissue disease states, such as systemic lupus erythematosus, that renders the serologic test for syphilis, venereal disease reference test, and others positive, that prolongs in vitro coagulation tests, that can be identified as an antiphospholipid and/or an anticardiolipin, antibody is not a single molecule. These data support the idea that there is most likely more than 1 autoantibody—probably a family of autoantibodies—present in such individuals that induces positivity in these various serologic tests.

A symposium held in San Francisco in 1991 (1) provides an excellent update on the status of antiphospholipid antibodies, the antiphospholipid syndrome, and other associated antiphospholipid cofactors and thrombotic diseases.—W.R. Bell, M.D.

Reference

1. Kittner SJ, Goelich PB: The antiphospholipid antibodies in stroke (APASS Symposium). *Stroke* 23:119–22, 1992.

Hypercoagulable States and Intravascular Coagulation

Niacin-Induced Clotting Factor Synthesis Deficiency With Coagulopathy

Dearing BD, Lavie CJ, Lohmann TP, Genton E (Ochsner Med Institutions, New Orleans, La)
Arch Intern Med 152:861–863, 1992   3–33

Background.—Niacin is a water-soluble B vitamin that may be an ideal lipid-lowering agent. Short-term adverse effects are troublesome but usually do not threaten life, and niacin has proved safe for long-term use. Hepatotoxicity has occurred, but no changes in clotting factor synthesis or coagulopathy have been noted without significant hepatotoxic effects.

Patients and Findings.—Three patients with coronary artery disease were using sustained-release niacin, 1,000 mg, 2 or 3 times daily, when they were found to have coagulopathy, with a prothrombin time of more than 1.5 times control, and significant deficiency in clotting factor synthesis. Factor assays in 1 case showed a marked reduction in factor VII and a borderline decrease in factor II but normal levels of factors IX and X. Increases in levels of aminotransferase were mild and did not exceed twice the normal value. All abnormalities resolved promptly when niacin was discontinued. In 1 patient, the syndrome recurred on rechallenge with sustained-release niacin, but in another patient the coagulopathy did not recur.

Discussion.—Reduced factor synthesis rather than hepatocellular injury may be responsible for this niacin-induced coagulopathy. Prothrombin time should be measured if even a mild rise in the level of aminotransferase occurs during treatment with sustained-release niacin.

▶ The use of nicotinic acid as a lipid-lowering agent is greater than ever before. This observation strongly supports the statement that any patient receiving nicotinic acid, or any compound that contains this agent, should have their prothrombin time monitored at some reasonable degree of frequency. Hopefully, major and fatal disasters can be avoided. For additional information in this area, please see reference 1.—W.R. Bell, M.D.

Reference

1.   Bussey HI, et al: *Arch Intern Med* 152:278–282, 1992.

Low Accuracy of Color Doppler Ultrasound in the Detection of Proximal Leg Vein Thrombosis in Asymptomatic High-Risk Patients
Davidson BL, for the RD Heparin Arthroplasty Group (Wyeth-Ayerst Research, Philadelphia; Univ of Pennsylvania, Philadelphia; Univ of Utah, Salt Lake City; et al)
Ann Intern Med 117:735–738, 1992   3–34

Background.—Because venous thromboembolism adds substantial morbidity for patients hospitalized for other reasons, it is important to detect proximal deep venous thrombosis (DVT) in patients at risk who are asymptomatic. The advantages claimed for color Doppler ultrasonography prompted a study of its accuracy in detecting proximal DVT in adults having hip and knee replacement surgery.

Study Design.—Seven medical centers that participated in a trial of low-molecular-weight heparin for the prevention of DVT were compared. Contrast venography served as the comparison examination. The subjects were 385 consecutive patients having elective unilateral hip or knee replacement surgery. The results of color Doppler ultrasound studies were interpreted in a blind manner before contrast venography.

Results.—Deep venous thrombosis was detected by contrast venography in 80 of 319 evaluable patients (25%). The proximal veins were in-

Accuracy of Color Doppler Ultrasound for Diagnosis of
Proximal DVT

		Venography	
		Proximal DVT	No Proximal DVT
Color Doppler Ultrasound *	Abnormal	8	23
	Normal	13	275

*Sensitivity, 38%; specificity, 92%; positive predictive value, 26%; negative predictive value, 95%.
(Courtesy of Davidson BL, for the RD Heparin Arthroplasty Group: *Ann Intern Med* 117:735–738, 1992.)

volved in 21 patients, and the color Doppler study detected proximal DVT in 38% of these patients (table). The study was 92% specific and had a positive predictive value of 26% for proximal DVT. Deep venous thrombosis was diagnosed by ultrasonography in 3 of 4 patients with occlusive thrombi. The sensitivity of the Doppler study was 20% for detecting DVT at any site.

Conclusion.—Color Doppler ultrasonography is not sensitive enough to reliably detect DVT in asymptomatic, high-risk patients.

▶ The results of this study are somewhat astonishing when compared with several other reports that have appeared in the past 2–3 years concerning the accuracy of color Doppler ultrasound in the detection of proximal DVT. Although one may use the excuse that this is in asymptomatic individuals, if the thrombus is present as demonstrated by angiography and is not detected in this setting, then clearly the accuracy of this technique is not as good as currently considered by many students of noninvasive thrombosis detection techniques.—W.R. Bell, M.D.

Limitations of Impedance Plethysmography in the Diagnosis of Clinically Suspected Deep-Vein Thrombosis
Anderson DR, Lensing AWA, Wells PS, Levine MN, Weitz JI, Hirsh J (Hamilton Civic Hosps, Ont, Canada; McMaster Univ, Hamilton, Ont, Canada)
Ann Intern Med 118:25–30, 1993   3–35

Introduction.—As many as one fourth of symptomatic patients with proximal venous thrombosis have normal impedance plethysmography (IPG) findings; it is not necessarily safe to withhold anticoagulant therapy from patients whose IPG studies are negative. The accuracy of IPG

	Proximal DVT Present	Proximal DVT Absent	
IPG Abnormal	37*	20**	57
IPG Normal	19***	****	327
	56	****	384

Fig 3–12.—Impedance plethysmographic results in analyzed patients confirmed to have proximal vein thrombosis. Sensitivity, 37/56 (66%) (95% confidence interval, 52% to 78%); positive predictive value, 37/57 (65%). *Seven patients had a diagnosis with proximal vein thrombosis by compression ultrasound. **Two patients had proximal deep vein thrombosis excluded with compression ultrasound. ***Two patients had proximal vein thrombosis diagnosed by compression ultrasound. ****Two hundred forty-two patients did not undergo venography (or compression ultrasound). Thus, a true figure for the total number of patients in whom proximal vein thrombosis was absent cannot be determined. (Courtesy of Anderson DR, Lensing AWA, Wells PS, et al: *Ann Intern Med* 118:25–30, 1993.)

for detecting proximal vein thrombosis in symptomatic outpatients was reexamined.

Study Plan.—Adequate IPG tests were carried out in 386 of 390 patients (mean age, 60.7 years) evaluated for suspected symptomatic deep venous thrombosis. Two different IPG instruments were used. All patients with abnormal IPG findings underwent venography or compression ultrasonography.

Results.—Initial IPG findings were abnormal in 13.7% of those examined. Five patients had an abnormal IPG on serial testing. Proximal venous thrombosis was confirmed in 37 of 58 patients with abnormal IPG findings. Of 73 patients with normal IPG tests but clinical features highly suggestive of deep venous thrombosis, 12 were found to have proximal vein thrombosis. An abnormal IPG had a positive predictive value of 65% for proximal vein thrombosis (Fig 3–12). Nonocclusive thrombosis was more frequent in patients with normal IPG findings.

Conclusion.—It no longer seems wise to rely on a normal IPG result in symptomatic patients. Compression ultrasonography is a better initial test for deep venous thrombosis. If IPG is used, some patients with normal findings should undergo venography to check the sensitivity of the equipment.

▶ This is a very instructive article. Particularly of concern is that the same authors from the same group of investigators have published several previous reports stating the absolute accuracy of impedance plethysmography. They have repeatedly pointed out that this avoids the need for doing invasive venography. The results of this present article are much more in keeping with what has been observed by many workers in this field during the past decade. It is important to recognize that there is now reasonably uniform agreement that IPG is not a substitute for venography in making the diagnosis of deep venous thrombosis.—W.R. Bell, M.D.

Increased Risk of Venous Thrombosis in Carriers of Hereditary Protein C Deficiency Defect

Allaart CF, Poort SR, Rosendaal FR, Reitsma PH, Bertina RM, Briët E (Univ Hosp Leiden, The Netherlands)

Lancet 341:134–138, 1993

3–36

Introduction.—There is debate about hereditary protein C deficiency as a risk factor for venous thrombosis because symptom-free heterozygotes have been identified among blood donors and relatives of homozygotes. Thus, clinicians cannot know whether patients with protein C deficiency and their families need prophylactic measures.

Patients and Methods.—Thrombosis-free survival was compared in 24 families with at least 1 heterozygous patient with known venous thrombosis and protein C deficiency. A total of 161 heterozygous and normal family members was studied for the influence of heterozygosity and other putative risk factors on the incidence of thrombotic events. Each subject underwent measurement of protein C activities; however, the diagnosis of heterozygosity was based on the presence of the specific mutation in 1 of the protein C genes in the proband.

Results.—Seventy-seven family members were heterozygous, and 84 were normal. Thrombosis-free survival curves showed that 50% of heterozygotes would have venous thrombosis by the age of 45, compared with only 10% of the normal subjects. The presence of the mutation and an increased risk of thrombosis were clearly associated. When a patient had been immobile for more than 1 week or had undergone surgery, thrombosis was more likely in that year. The other risk factors investigated demonstrated no significant influence. No predisposing factor was noted for about 50% of first episodes of thrombosis and 65% of recurrent episodes among the heterozygous subjects. They were at no increased risk of arterial occlusion.

Conclusion.—Heterozygous family members of a symptomatic patient with hereditary protein C deficiency appear to be at increased risk of venous thrombotic events compared with their normal family members. Therefore, the heterozygous family members should be considered for prophylaxis, regardless of whether they are symptomatic. This decision should be made on an individual basis, considering the risks and benefits of anticoagulant therapy.

▶ The authors provided substantial evidence that carriers of protein C deficiency are at risk for venous thrombosis. This information should signal physicians to study all known family members for patients with this defect.—W.R. Bell, M.D.

Treatment of Venous Thromboembolism in Patients With Congenital Deficiency of Antithrombin III
Schulman S, Tengborn L (Karolinska Hosp, Stockholm; Sahlgren's Hosp, Gothenburg, Sweden)
Thromb Haemost 68:634–636, 1992   3–37

Background.—Heparin therapy has not always proved effective in patients with hereditary deficiency of antithrombin (AT III). In some patients, heparin lowers circulating levels of AT III to the degree that it cannot function as an efficient cofactor. Treatment with AT III concentrate is very expensive and would require testing for AT III in all patients admitted with thrombosis. The efficacy of treatment was reviewed in 57 patients with congenital AT III deficiency who had a total of 111 thromboembolic events from 1940 to 1989. Deep venous thrombosis was the most common event. Information on treatment was available in 70 instances.

Findings.—The median peak dose of heparin was 39,500 IU, and the median peak activated partial thromboplastin time (APTT) was 100 seconds. The maximum dose did not correlate significantly with the longest APTT. A peak APTT of 50 seconds or longer (about 1.5 times the upper normal limit) was achieved in 30 of 33 cases. Thrombosis progressed during treatment in 5 patients, and 3 others had pulmonary embolism develop while being treated for deep venous thrombosis.

Conclusion.—Heparin therapy is adequate in a large majority of patients with congenital AT III deficiency who have acute venous thromboembolism develop. The use of AT III concentrate probably is warranted only for special reasons, such as mesenteric vein thrombosis and resistance to heparin.

▶ The authors have very thoughtfully evaluated patients with congenital AT III deficiency and have found, as has been the experience of many specialists who treat venous and arterial thrombosis, that AT III is not commonly associated with heparin resistance or heparin failure. The authors astutely noted that the use of AT III concentrates for the treatment of this illness is not only unnecessary but is an obvious misuse of medical funds.—W.R. Bell, M.D.

Fibrinogen and Viscosity as Risk Factors for Subsequent Cardiovascular Events in Stroke Survivors
Resch KL, Ernst E, Matrai A, Paulsen HF (Univ of Vienna; Buchberg-Klinik, Bad Tölz, Germany)
Ann Intern Med 117:371–375, 1992   3–38

Background.—The rheologic properties of blood among stroke patients in both the acute and rehabilitation phases are abnormal. Furthermore, hypoperfusion could occur in stroke survivors, which may predis-

Odds Ratios of Risk Factors for Further Cardiovascular Events

Parameter (dimension)	Predefined Values for Dichotomization	Number of Matched Pairs	Unadjusted Odds Ratio	95% CI
Native blood viscosity				
at shear rate 0.7 s^{-1}	32.5 mPa · s	58	2.00	0.79 to 5.31
Plasma viscosity	1.31 mPa · s	58	2.86	1.06 to 8.43
Fibrinogen	3.5 g/L	53	3.67	1.31 to 11.69
Total cholesterol	6.2 mmol/L	58	1.25	0.51 to 3.08
Triglycerides	4.4 mmol/L	58	0.86	0.34 to 2.12
Leukocytes	8 × 10^9/L	58	1.44	0.53 to 4.07
Red cell aggregation	10 mPa · s	53	1.44	0.53 to 4.07
Hematocrit	0.47	58	1.58	0.69 to 3.74
Body mass index	26 kg/cm^2	58	0.43	0.13 to 1.31
Systolic blood pressure	160 mm Hg	59	0.78	0.34 to 1.74
Diastolic blood pressure	90 mm Hg	59	0.92	0.34 to 2.42
Blood glucose	8.9 mmol/L	55	1.10	0.40 to 3.09

(Courtesy of Resch KL, Ernst E, Matrai A, et al: *Ann Intern Med* 117:371–375, 1992.)

pose them to further strokes. Stroke survivors were studied to determine whether blood viscosity variables measured during the rehabilitation phase can predict subsequent cardiovascular events.

Patients and Methods.—A total of 625 patients from a stroke rehabilitation unit was followed for an average of 2 years. Blood samples were taken the day after each patient was admitted. The types of blood tests performed were native and hematocrit-standardized blood viscosity at 3 shear rates, hematocrit, plasma viscosity, fibrinogen, erythrocyte sedimentation rate, total leukocyte count, and the matching variables. A 2-year follow-up was planned. Any patient who experienced a re-event was paired with a patient from the study group who had not had one.

Results.—Eighty-five patients experienced a subsequent cardiovascular event. Of these, 53 had a second stroke, 13 had a myocardial infarction, 1 had both a second stroke and a myocardial infarction, and 18 experienced other circulatory events. Matching was possible in 60 cases. Blood viscosity measurements showed that both plasma viscosity (odds ratio 2.86) and fibrinogen (odds ratio 3.67) were statistically significant risk factors for re-events. In addition, native blood viscosity (odds ratio 2) showed a trend toward higher risks. All other measured blood variables were not associated with increased future cardiovascular event risks (table).

Conclusion.—When comparisons were made of the matched-pair stroke survivors, plasma viscosity and fibrinogen were risk factors for a second cardiovascular event. Drugs taken by the stroke survivors did not appear to be implicated in second cardiovascular events or in raising blood viscosity or fibrinogen levels. Future studies might confirm a definite link of plasma viscosity and/or blood fibrinogen with second cardiovascular events after an initial stroke.

▶ This article is one of the growing number of publications that cite fibrinogen as a risk factor for thrombotic events. In this study, hyperfibrinogenemia is clearly an independent risk factor for cardiovascular events after stroke. For additional information on this topic, please see references 1–3.—W.R. Bell, M.D.

References

1. Yarnell JW, et al: *Circulation* 83:836–844, 1991.
2. Di Minno G, Mancini M: *Arteriosclerosis* 10:1–7, 1990.
3. Ernst E: *BMJ* 303:596–597, 1991.

Incidence of Thrombotic Complications in Adult Patients With Acute Lymphoblastic Leukaemia Receiving L-asparaginase During Induction Therapy: A Retrospective Study

Gugliotta L, Mazzucconi MG, Leone G, Mattioli-Belmonte M, Defazio D, Annino L, Tura S, Mandelli F, and The GIMEMA Group (Istituto di Ematologia, Bologna, Italy)
Eur J Haematol 49:63–66, 1992   3–39

Introduction.—L-asparaginase (L-ase) has an established therapeutic effect in acute lymphoblastic leukemia (ALL), but it has toxic effects on the liver, pancreas, kidneys, and CNS. L-asparaginase also has been implicated in a hemostatic defect that sometimes is associated with thrombotic events.

Patients and Methods.—Coagulation was investigated in 238 adult patients with ALL who received *Escherichia coli*–derived L-ase during induction treatment. A dose of 6000 U/m² was given daily, subcutaneously or intramuscularly, for 1 week.

Findings.—Treatment with L-ase was withdrawn in 4 patients because of cerebral thrombosis, epistaxis related to severe hypofibrinogenemia, liver failure, and fatal cerebral toxicity, respectively. Ten patients had thrombotic complications during or shortly after treatment with L-ase. The dural sinus was involved in 5 cases. Thrombosis led to 5 deaths. The only risk factor for thrombosis was oral contraceptive use by 1 patient. Six patients had a platelet count more than 100×10^9/L at the time of thrombosis. Four patients had plasma fibrinogen levels greater than 400 mg/dL, and 3 had levels less than 70 mg/dL.

Conclusion.—Treatment with L-ase, even in relatively low dosages, is associated with a significant risk of thrombotic complications that may be fatal. The high expectation of ALL remitting makes this risk difficult to accept.

▶ Even though L-ase reduces the plasma fibrinogen concentration, this does not protect the patient from the complications of thrombosis. The problem appears to be directly associated with the administration of this agent or with one of its metabolites. Somewhat disturbing is the high frequency of thrombotic events within the CNS as well as within the hepatic veins of the liver. Such a complication must be recognized by those administering this compound.—W.R. Bell, M.D.

Evidence That Postoperative Fibrinolytic Shutdown Is Mediated by Plasma Factors That Stimulate Endothelial Cell Type I Plasminogen Activator Inhibitor Biosynthesis
Kassis J, Hirsh J, Podor TJ (McMaster Univ, Hamilton, Ont, Canada; Hamilton Civic Hosps Research Ctr, Ont, Canada)
Blood 80:1758–1764, 1992

3–40

Introduction.—Impaired fibrinolytic activity may have a role in the increased risk of thromboembolism in patients who have major surgery. Plasma levels of type 1 plasminogen activator inhibitor (PAI-1) are elevated after surgery and possibly contribute importantly to fibrinolytic shutdown.

Methods.—Cultured human umbilical vein endothelial cells (HUVECs) were used to determine whether a plasma mediator that stimulates PAI-1 synthesis and secretion by vascular endothelium contributes to the postoperative increase in PAI-1. Plasma was collected from 11 patients before and after total hip replacement surgery. The samples were

PAI-1 Antigen and Activity Levels in Patient Plasma and in
Plasma-Treated HUVEC Conditioned Medium

Sample	PAI-1 Assay	[PAI-1] (ng/mL) Pre-op	Post-op	Mean % Increment	P Value
Plasma	PAI-1 Ag	37 ± 6	103 ± 25	225 ± 44	$P = .003$
	PAI-1 Act	23 ± 4	57 ± 8	190 ± 67	$P = .04$
HUVEC CM	PAI-1 Ag	1,270 ± 259	2,169 ± 404	99 ± 19	$P = .001$
	PAI-1 Act	337 ± 66	548 ± 103	66 ± 24	$P = .002$

Note: HUVECs were incubated overnight (16 hours) with 5% preoperative or postoperative (18 hours) patient plasma ($n = 11$), and PAI-1 antigen and activity in the conditioned media were analyzed.
(Courtesy of Kassis J, Hirsh J, Podor TJ: *Blood* 80:1758–1764, 1992.)

assayed for endogenous plasma PAI-1 antigen and activity. They also were incubated with HUVECs, and PAI-1 antigen and activity were estimated in the conditioned medium using an immunoradiometric assay.

Results.—Endogenous plasma levels of PAI-1 antigen were increased by 225% at 18 hours after surgery, and PAI-1 activity was increased 190%. Plasma taken after surgery increased the HUVEC secretion of PAI-1 antigen by 99% and PAI-1 activity by 66% (table). Both the expression of PAI-1 messenger RNA and protein synthesis were increased. The plasma factor that stimulated PAI-1 biosynthesis had a molecular weight of approximately 30–100 Kd and was heat labile.

Conclusion.—After major surgery, the plasma contains a factor (or factors) that may stimulate synthesis of PAI-1 by endothelial cells in vivo, thereby mediating fibrinolytic shutdown. The endothelial changes may be a major reason for the increased risk of venous thrombosis noted in the postoperative state.

▶ These authors have provided a sufficient explanation for the increased frequency of postoperative thrombosis. In addition to the problems of immobility and reduction in blood flow, there is an apparent increase in PAI-1 activity. This increased activity results in a decrease in the capacity of the plasminogen/plasmin proteolytic enzyme system to bring about resolution of thrombi and emboli. The sample size of this study needs to be expanded, and these findings should be confirmed by a larger group.—W.R. Bell, M.D.

Role of Endothelin in Disseminated Intravascular Coagulation
Asakura H, Jokaji H, Saito M, Uotani C, Kumabashiri I, Morishita E, Yamazaki M, Matsuda T (Kanazawa Univ, Japan)
Am J Hematol 41:71–75, 1992   3–41

Introduction.—Endothelin (ET)-1 is a potent vasoconstrictor peptide that may have an important role in such states as acute myocardial infarction, hypertension, chronic renal failure, and intrauterine growth retardation. An attempt was made to follow changes in plasma ET-1 in disseminated intravascular coagulation (DIC) secondary to various underlying disorders.

Patients.—The 47 patients with DIC included 13 with acute promyelocytic leukemia, 14 with other forms of acute leukemia, and 6 with chronic myelogenous leukemia in blastic crisis. In addition, 5 patients with non-Hodgkin's lymphoma, 5 with solid cancers, and 4 with sepsis were studied.

Methods.—Plasma levels of soluble thermodulin, which reflects the degree of endothelial damage, were measured by an enzyme-linked immunosorbent assay. Plasma ET-1 was estimated by radioimmunoassay.

Findings.—Plasma ET levels were significantly increased in patients with DIC secondary to myelogenous leukemia in blastic crisis, cancer,

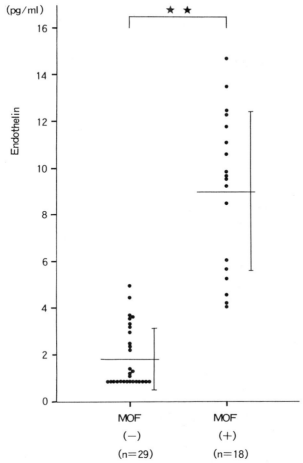

Fig 3–13.—Plasma levels of ET-1 in cases of DIC with (+) or without (−) multiple organ failure (MOF). *Horizontal lines* indicate the mean ± SD values for each group. XX, *P* < .01 significance of difference. (Courtesy of Asakura H, Jokaji H, Saito M, et al: *Am J Hematol* 41:71-75, 1992.)

and sepsis. Patients in all diagnostic groups who had multiple organ failure were at increased risk of having an elevated plasma ET-1 level (Fig 3–13). In most instances, the ET-1 level declined as patients improved clinically but continued to increase in those who died. Levels of ET-1 were directly proportional to both thermodulin and plasminogen activator inhibitor-1.

Conclusion.—These findings support an important role for ET-1 in the multiple organ failure associated with vasoconstrictive and microcirculatory disorders.

▶ The authors identified the presence of yet another transmembrane endothelial cell protein, designated endothelin. That this protein is elevated in the blood should not be unexpected because endothelial cells are known to be altered in the process of DIC. This report clearly indicates that endothelin may be very important with respect to its vasoconstricting properties and may be a major influence on organ failure.—W.R. Bell, M.D.

Comparison of the Effects of Bezafibrate and Acipimox on the Lipid Pattern and Plasma Fibrinogen in Hyperlipidaemic Type 2 (Non-Insulin-Dependent) Diabetic Patients
Niort G, Cassader M, Gambino R, Pagano G (Univ of Torino, Italy)
Diabete Metab 18:221–228, 1992   3–42

Introduction.—The reduction of lipids is an acknowledged means of preventing cardiovascular disease. Patients with diabetes are at particular risk for vascular problems and may require medical control of hyperlipidemia. The effects of 2 widely used drugs on the lipid profile and plasma fibrinogen of non-insulin–dependent (NID) diabetics were compared.

Methods.—The 16 patients who entered the study had good metabolic control of their disease. Hyperlipidemia was resistant to diet in the group. Patients were randomized to a single dose of 400 mg/day of Bezafibrate (BZF) for 1 month, followed by a 2-month wash-out and a 1-month administration of 500 mg/day of Acipimox (APX), or vice versa. Current diabetic treatment, diet, and level of physical activity were continued during the trial.

Results.—Both treatments brought about a nonsignificant improvement in metabolic control; body weight remained stable. Both BZF and APX produced a 14% decrease in total cholesterol, (CHOL), but BZF was more effective in reducing triglycerides (Tg) (-37% vs. -15%). Apolipoprotein B decreased proportionately with BZF and apolipoprotein AI increased significantly; total high-density lipoprotein (HDL), HDL2, and HDL3-CHOL also increased. The treatment with APX increased only HDL2-CHOL. Both drugs reduced very-low-density lipoprotein (VLDL)-CHOL and VLDL-Tg, but the reductions were greater with BZF.

Conclusion.—Both treatments produce favorable changes in NID diabetics with hyperlipidemia. The mechanism of action of BZF is more extensive, acting on plasma fibrinogen and its correlated hemorrheologic parameters, circulating lipids, and HDL-CHOL.

▶ Several recent reports have identified the value of lipid-lowering agents in the treatment of hypertension. This article noted that these agents reduce plasma fibrinogen concentration. Many other reports have also found a lower plasma fibrinogen concentration when these agents are used. Thus, the preventive mechanism may not be necessarily related to lipid lowering but may be caused by a reduction in plasma fibrinogen. For additional findings by other investigators, please see reference 1.—W.R. Bell, M.D.

Reference

1. Pazzucconi F, et al: *Eur J Clin Pharmacol* 43:219–223, 1992.

Update on Fibrinogen as a Cardiovascular Risk Factor
Kannel WB, D'Agostino RB, Belanger AJ (Framingham Heart Study, Mass; Boston Univ)
Ann Epidemiol 2:457–466, 1992   3–43

Background.—There appears to be some causal relationship between high-normal levels of fibrinogen and the occurrence of atherosclerotic cardiovascular disease (CVD). Atherosclerosis and the onset of clinical manifestations have an obvious thrombogenic component. The importance of fibrinogen measurement as a risk factor for CVD was determined.

Methods.—Satisfactory fibrinogen measurements were obtained for 1,247 participants in the Framingham Study who had had no cardiovascular event or cancer. During 18 years of follow-up, 455 of these had some clinical manifestation of atherosclerotic CVD, including 270 coronary events. The association of the fibrinogen level with the development of peripheral arterial disease and cardiac failure was examined.

Findings.—A significant age-associated relationship was noted between the fibrinogen level, coronary heart disease, and CVD in both men and women. There was also a significant relationship to cardiac failure and peripheral arterial disease, but not to stroke, in women. In both sexes, the fibrinogen level was related to age-adjusted cardiovascular, all-cause, and coronary heart disease mortality. The greatest effect of this relationship was in stroke for men and coronary heart disease in women; for both, the absolute risk for an elevated fibrinogen level was greatest for coronary heart diseases. Women and subjects with other risk factors—hypertension, cigarette smoking, diabetes, obesity, and elevated hematocrit—had higher average fibrinogen levels. On adjustment for concomitant risk factors, however, fibrinogen independently contributed to CVD in general and coronary disease in particular. The risk of CVD was increased by fibrinogen in patients with hypertension and diabetes and in cigarette smokers. Higher fibrinogen levels appear to account for about half the cardiovascular risk of cigarette smoking. Excess CVD has been documented in subjects with high-normal fibrinogen levels, with each 1-SD increase bringing increments of coronary heart disease of 30% in men and 40% in women.

Conclusion.—Fibrinogen is an important risk factor for CVD, rivaling that of the other, well-accepted risk factors. Research into fibrinogen-lowering treatment for high-risk coronary candidates is needed.

▶ This review strongly supports a suggestion that attention should be given to the circulating level of plasma fibrinogen in patients who are at risk for CVD. Hypertension, diabetes mellitus, and tobacco use are risk factors. Somewhat instructive is the increased frequency of predictability of this risk factor in females, as opposed to males.—W.R. Bell, M.D.

Fibrinogen Genotype and Risk of Peripheral Atherosclerosis
Fowkes FGR, Connor JM, Smith FB, Wood J, Donnan PT, Lowe GDO (Univ of Edinburgh, Scotland; Western Infirmary, Glasgow, Scotland; Univ of Glasgow, Scotland)
Lancet 339:693–696, 1992   3–44

Introduction.—Variation at the β-fibrinogen locus in relation to the concentration of fibrinogen has been reported in some populations, but the influence of the fibrinogen genotype on plasma concentrations of fibrinogen and on atherosclerotic disease remains uncertain. Whether certain fibrinogen genotypes correlate with an increased risk of peripheral atherosclerotic disease was investigated.

Patients.—A total of 121 patients with peripheral arterial disease and 126 healthy control subjects was matched for age and gender from a population sample in the Edinburgh Artery Study. The men and women were aged 55–74 years.

TABLE 1.—Plasma Fibrinogen and Cigarette Smoking

	Cases (n=121)	Controls (n=126)	p
Mean fibrinogen concentration (g/l)*			
Clotting method	3·12 (2·99–3·26)	2·75 (2·64–2·85)	<0·001
Nephelometric method	4·48 (4·31–4·65)	3·91 (3·74–4·06)	<0·001
Cigarette smoking			
% current smokers	44	20	⎫
% ex-smokers	42	30	⎬ <0·001
% non-smokers	14	50	⎭
Mean √pack years (SE)	4·82 (0·22)	2·04 (0·20)	<0·001

* 95% confidence interval in parentheses.
(Courtesy of Fowkes FGR, Connor JM, Smith FB, et al: *Lancet* 339:693–696, 1992.)

TABLE 2.—Fibrinogen Genotype and Haplotypes

—	Cases (n = 115)	Controls (n = 120)	p*	p†
Genotype α				
2·4/2·4	56	59		
2·4/1·6	41	32	} 0·11	..
1·6/1·6	4	9		
Genotype β				
5·3/5·3	65	82		
5·3/4·2	31	18	} 0·01	..
4·2/4·2	4	1		
Genotype γ				
11/11	60	59		
14/11	37	33	} 0·37	..
14/14	4	8		
Haplotype				
1:α2·4/2·4; β5·3/5·3; γ11/11	42	58		0·18
2:α2·4/1·6; β5·3/5·3; γ14/11	29	36		0·56
3:α2·4/2·4; β5·3/4·2; γ11/11	24	19		0·30
4:α2·4/1·6; β5·3/5·3; γ11/11	7	5	} 0·14	0·47
5:α2·4/1·6; β5·3/4·2; γ14/11	14	5		0·03
6:α1·6/1·6; β5·3/5·3; γ14/14	5	10		0·27
Others	10	10		0·73

* Significance of overall association between genotype-haplotype and peripheral arterial disease.
† Significance of difference between each haplotype and every other haplotype.
(Courtesy of Fowkes FGR, Connor JM, Smith FB, et al: *Lancet* 339:693–696, 1992.)

Findings.—The mean concentration of fibrinogen was significantly higher in the group with arterial disease (Table 1). More patients than controls had ever smoked, but alcohol consumption was lower in patients than in controls. A significant excess of the β-genotype was found in patients (Table 2). The frequency of an allele at the β-locus was .197 in cases and .097 in controls. The haplotype had no marked effect on the association of the plasma level of fibrinogen with disease. Cigarette smoking was a more prominent factor than haplotype.

Conclusion.—Variation at the β-fibrinogen locus appears to be correlated with an increased risk of peripheral atherosclerotic disease, but not simply through an increased level of fibrinogen. A structurally variant fibrinogen or linkage disequilibrium with a nearby gene may be responsible.

▶ The plasma fibrinogen concentration continues to be frequently evaluated as a major risk factor for atherosclerosis, peripheral vascular disease, coronary artery disease, and vascular occlusive diseases of all types. Many publications suggest that above-normal levels of plasma fibrinogen highly correlate with increased peripheral vascular diseases of all types. The authors pointed out that there may be a particular abnormality in the fibrinogen molecule, namely, a particular locus in the beta-chain. A reasonable-size cohort of patients was examined. Further attention must be given to this finding.—W.R. Bell, M.D.

Anticoagulation Therapy

Antithrombotic Properties of Dermatan Sulphate (MF 701) in Haemodialysis for Chronic Renal Failure

Ryan KE, Lane DA, Flynn A, Ireland H, Boisclair M, Shepperd J, Curtis JR (Charing Cross and Westminster Hosp and Med School, London)
Thromb Haemost 68:563–569, 1992   3–45

Background.—Dermatan sulfate (DS) is a glycosaminoglycan seen in connective tissues that accelerates the inhibition of thrombin by heparin cofactor II. Dermatan sulfate inhibits thrombus formation in animals, but its therapeutic potential as an antithrombotic agent in humans remains to be demonstrated.

Objective and Methods.—Dose-ranging studies were performed in groups of 6–8 patients on hemodialysis for chronic renal failure. Two types of dialyzer membrane were used. Plasma levels of fibrinopeptide A (FPA) and thrombin-antithrombin served as markers of fibrin formation and thrombin generation. Bolus doses of 2–6 mg of DS per kg were administered to patients on dialysis with polyacrylonitrile hollow fiber membranes or cuprophane hollow fiber membranes. In some studies, a bolus dose of DS was followed by an infusion of .6 or 1 mg/kg/hr.

Findings.—When dialysis used polyacrylonitrile membranes, additional unfractionated heparin usually was necessary to complete a normal 6-hour session. Dermatan sulfate failed to prevent thrombin and fibrin formation. When cuprophane membranes were used, increasing doses of DS permitted longer sessions of dialysis. Levels of FPA increased compared with the unfractionated heparin regimen, but levels of thrombin-antithrombin did not. When DS levels were maintained at 72–83 $\mu g/mL$ by infusing DS at a rate of 1 mg/kg/hr, dialysis was consistently effective and FPA was suppressed to nearly the normal range.

Conclusion.—Dermatan sulfate can be an effective anticoagulant/antithrombotic agent in patients undergoing hemodialysis for renal failure.

▶ Recently, a sizable number of reports investigated substitutes for heparin in the performance of extracorporeal hemodialysis. This thorough article clearly indicates the potential efficacy of DS (MF701), which appears to exert its inhibitory effect by the inhibition of thrombin, which results in decreased fibrin formation. For additional reports on other agents that can be used instead of heparin for hemodialysis, please see references 1–3.—W.R. Bell, M.D.

References

1. *ASAIO Trans* 38:560M–563M, 1992.

2. Filimberti E, et al: *Int J Artif Organs* 15:590–594, 1992.
3. Kinugasa E, et al: *Int J Artif Organs* 15:595–600, 1992.

Highly Variable Anticoagulant Response After Subcutaneous Administration of High-Dose (12,500 IU) Heparin in Patients With Myocardial Infarction and Healthy Volunteers

Kroon C, ten Hove WR, de Boer A, Kroon JM, van der Pol JMJ, Harthoorn-Lasthuizen EJ, Schoemaker HC, van der Meer FJM, Cohen AF (Univ Hosp, Leiden, The Netherlands; Groot Ziekengasthuis, Den Bosch, The Netherlands)
Circulation 86:1370–1375, 1992   3–46

Introduction.—The use of fixed subcutaneous doses of heparin is convenient, but doubt has been raised about how consistently heparin given in this way is absorbed. The anticoagulant response to a 12,500-IU subcutaneous dose of heparin was examined in 8 patients with suspected or definite acute myocardial infarction. In addition, 10 healthy men received injections of calcium heparin in the lateral abdominal wall by using either a 23-g (.6 × 25 mm) or a 25-g (.5 × 16 mm) needle.

Results.—The individual area under the curve values of plasma anti-Xa activity, anti-IIa activity, activated partial thromboplastin time (APTT), anti-Xa$_{max}$, and APTT$_{max}$ is shown in the table. There was virtually no increase in the APTT after heparin injection in the infarction group. Only 1 patient had a maximum APTT 1.5-fold higher than that of control values at any time. Increases in anti-Xa activity and anti-IIa activity were small. The length of the injecting needle did not influence the anticoagulant effects of heparin.

Area Under APTT, Anti-IIa, and Anti-Xa Curves and APTT$_{max}$ of 8 Patients After Subcutaneous Administration of 12,500 IU of Heparin

Patient	AUC APTT (sec · min/10²)	AUC anti-IIa (min · IU/ml)	AUC anti-Xa (min · IU/ml)	APTT$_{max}$ (seconds)	Anti-Xa$_{max}$ (IU/ml)
1	8.8	43.6	46.7	32.7	0.16
2	38.4	64.8	75.2	44.9	0.35
3	50.5	27.3	28.2	70.7	0.24
4	0	2.7	2.4	30.4	0.05
5	24.6	34.5	29.7	39.4	0.16
6	5.7	2.1	1	42.4	0.02
7	49.6	49.8	26.8	42.4	0.10
8	31.0	22.6	16.7	37.7	0.09
Mean	26.1	30.9	28.3	42.6	0.15
SD	19.7	22.0	24.2	12.4	0.11

Abbreviation: AUC, area under curve.
(Courtesy of Kroon C, ten Hove WR, de Boer A, et al: *Circulation* 86:1370–1375, 1992.)

Conclusion.—Subcutaneous injection of a fixed dose of heparin, even a high dose, may not produce therapeutic or prophylactic levels of anticoagulation. Heparin should be administered in adjusted doses based on body weight and its anticoagulant effect in a given patient.

▶ As was demonstrated a number of years ago, low-dose heparin given for the prophylaxis of venous thrombosis can result in excessive anticoagulation. Such degrees of systemic anticoagulation may be sufficient to actually induce hemorrhage. The response to heparin is thus highly variable from patient to patient. Therefore, when high-dose heparin is given subcutaneously, it is important to periodically evaluate the degree of anticoagulation achieved with the APTT or whole-blood clotting time. Some patients (on a fixed-dose regimen) may become excessively anticoagulated whereas others may not have achieved the therapeutic range.—W.R. Bell, M.D.

Optimum Duration of Anticoagulation for Deep-Vein Thrombosis and Pulmonary Embolism

(Research Committee of the British Thoracic Society; Sully Hosp, Cardiff, Wales)
Lancet 340:873–876, 1992   3–47

Objective.—The optimal duration of anticoagulation therapy for deep venous thrombosis (DVT) and pulmonary embolism (PE) remains uncertain. The effect of anticoagulation treatment for 4 weeks or 3 months was compared in patients who had acute DVT or PE, or both.

Patients and Methods.—A total of 358 patients was assigned to anticoagulant therapy for 4 weeks, and 354 others were to be treated for 3 months. The diagnosis was objectively confirmed in 71% of cases. Standard treatment was used when possible. Heparin was given for 5 to 7 days and warfarin therapy started on day 3.

Results.—Pulmonary embolism caused 7 deaths and contributed to 4 others, with no significant difference between the 2 treatment groups. Persistence of symptoms and signs and nonfatal recurrences were more prevalent in the 4-week group. Failure to resolve was infrequent among patients in whom DVT or PE developed after surgery. In neither treatment group were failures and recurrences more frequent among patients with poorer anticoagulant control. Adverse effects were rare; 1 patient died of bleeding when anticoagulation was out of control.

Conclusion.—Anticoagulation for 4 weeks should suffice if venous thromboembolism develops after surgery. Patients who have a new DVT or PE, or both, with no apparent underlying cause or risk factor should be anticoagulated for 3 months.

▶ Although this study was certainly thoughtfully performed in considerable detail by a large number of investigators, the results have been placed into 2 very broad categories with the final recommendation stating that if the patient had a surgical procedure and experienced DVT or PE, 4 weeks of anticoagulation were sufficient. It is important to point out that the authors actually stated that it is likely to be sufficient, and if the patient did not have a surgical procedure or had DVT or PE from any other cause, 3 months of anticoagulation were required. Such broad categorization and the use of phrases such as "likely to be adequate," are unscientific and actually not helpful for the individual patient. Another serious problem with this study is that the diagnosis in many of the patients was rendered without substantiation by venography. Several patients had a diagnosis based on Doppler or radiolabeled fibrinogen scanning and lung ventilation/perfusion scanning. The nonvenographic techniques are well known to have a very high error rate. Thus, the results and recommendation of this study have to be considered with the knowledge of how the diagnosis was made in the patients.—W.R. Bell, M.D.

Subcutaneous Low Molecular Weight Heparin Versus Subcutaneous Unfractionated Heparin in the Treatment of Deep Vein Thrombosis: A Polish Multicenter Trial

Lopaciuk S, Meissner AJ, Filipecki S, Zawilska K, Sowier J, Ciesielski L, Bielawiec M, Glowinski S, Czestochowska E, et al (Inst of Hematology, Warsaw; Inst of Tuberculosis and Lung Diseases, Warsaw; Med School, Poznan, Poland; et al)
Thromb Haemost 68:14–18, 1992

                                                                    3–48

Introduction.—Subcutaneous unfractionated heparin (UFH) is a safe, effective, and easily administered alternative to continuous intravenous UFH in the treatment of deep vein thrombosis (DVT). Low-molecular-weight (LMW) heparins have recently been found suitable for subcutaneous use, offering a longer half-life and increased bioavailability compared with UFH. The LMW heparin CY 216 (Fraxiparine) was compared with UFH, both administered subcutaneously, as initial treatment for DVT of the lower limbs.

Methods.—The prospective trial enrolled 149 consecutive patients from 6 centers. Once the diagnosis was confirmed by phlebography, patients were stratified according to whether they had a proximal or calf DVT and then randomly allocated to Fraxiparine or UFH. Pre- and post-treatment phlebograms were assessed blindly by a panel of 3 experts.

Results.—Twelve patients were excluded from efficacy analysis for various reasons. After 10 days of treatment, the mean phlebographic score was significantly decreased in both groups. Improvement was noted in 45 of 68 patients (66%) in the Fraxiparine group and in 32 of 66 patients (48%) in the UFH group. The thrombus size increased at similar rates in the 2 groups (15% and 18%, respectively). There was 1 major bleeding episode and 1 symptomatic nonfatal pulmonary embolism in the UFH group. Three months of follow-up found 2 cases of rethrombosis in the UFH group and none in the Fraxiparine group.

Conclusion.—There was no significant difference in efficacy between the 2 heparins. Fraxiparine, however, has some practical advantages in the initial treatment of DVT. The LMW heparin offers equal therapeutic benefits and can be administered without laboratory monitoring.

▶ This article represents another study using a LMW heparin preparation. It is instructive to note that the authors conclude, as do most others, that it is as effective as the standard UFH. The plea is made that the lower-molecular-weight material can be given only once a day and, therefore, is optimal for outpatient therapy, thus avoiding the need for hospitalization for the treatment of venous thrombosis. It will be instructive to learn whether this low-molecular-weight preparation eliminates the need for hospitalization in patients with venous thrombosis. For additional work in this area, please see references 1 and 2.—W.R. Bell, M.D.

References

1. Turpie AG, et al: *Ann Intern Med* 117:353–357, 1992.
2. Drakos PE, et al: *Cancer* 70:1895–1898, 1992.

Low-Molecular-Weight Heparin Versus Standard Heparin in General and Orthopaedic Surgery: A Meta-Analysis
Nurmohamed MT, Rosendaal FR, Büller HR, Dekker E, Hommes DW, Vandenbroucke JP, Briët E (Academic Med Ctr, Amsterdam; Univ Hosp Leiden, The Netherlands)
Lancet 340:152–156, 1992   3–49

Introduction.—Prophylaxis is strongly recommended for patients having major orthopedic or general surgery because of the high risk of venous thrombosis. Low-molecular-weight heparins (LMWHs) have several theoretical advantages over standard heparin in this setting, and numerous trials of LMWHs have been carried out in surgical patients since 1984.

Analysis.—A meta-analysis was done of studies reported in 1984–1991 in which LMWHs were compared with standard heparin in the prevention of venous thrombosis in surgical patients. General surgery trials where fibrinogen leg scanning was done expectantly were included, along with orthopedic surgery trials where venography was done routinely to establish the presence or absence of deep venous thrombosis (DVT).

Findings.—The relative risk of DVT with LMWH administration, compared with standard heparin, was .74. The risk of pulmonary embolism was .43, and that of major bleeding was .98. Similar relative risk values were obtained in the general surgery and orthopedic surgery studies. Less favorable results were obtained when only general surgery studies with strong methodology were examined; the relative risk of DVT was .91.

Conclusion.—The value of LMWH compared with standard heparin is not yet totally clear. Some clinicians may believe that an overall reduction in risk of DVT makes LMWH preferable, despite the lack of a strong effect on bleeding frequency. Others may believe that LMWH has little added prophylactic effect and that the risk of bleeding may be higher in general surgery patients.

▶ Thoughtful analysis of an appreciable number of studies examining a very large patient population size clearly shows that for prophylaxis in the general surgical patient, no convincing evidence presently exists that this type of heparin has a better improvement in the benefit-risk ratio than standard unfractionated heparin does. This finding for the prophylactic use of LMWH is different from the recently reported studies indicating that LMWH fractions may actually be better than standard unfractionated heparin for the treatment of venous thrombosis. It is very difficult to understand why LMWH fractions are better for treatment but are no better for prophylaxis than standard unfractionated heparin. Additional information is needed to resolve this dilemma.—W.R. Bell, M.D.

Subcutaneous Low-Molecular-Weight Heparin Compared With Continuous Intravenous Heparin in the Treatment of Proximal-Vein Thrombosis

Hull RD, Raskob GE, Pineo GF, Green D, Trowbridge AA, Elliott CG, Lerner RG, Hall J, Sparling T, Brettell HR, Norton J, Carter CJ, George R, Merli G, Ward J, Mayo W, Rosenbloom D, Brant R (Univ of Calgary, Alberta, Canada; Univ of British Columbia, Vancouver, Canada; Lions Gate Hosp, Vancouver, Canada; et al)
N Engl J Med 326:975–982, 1992   3–50

Background.—Compared with conventional unfractionated heparin, low-molecular-weight heparin has a high bioavailability and a prolonged half-life. However, there is little information on the relative efficacy of low-molecular-weight heparin in the treatment of deep venous thrombosis.

Methods.—Fixed-dose subcutaneous low-molecular-weight heparin given once a day was compared with adjusted-dose intravenously administered heparin given by continuous infusion in a multicenter, double-blind clinical trial. It constituted the initial treatment for patients with proximal-vein thrombosis. Objective documentation of clinical outcomes was used.

Findings.—Six of 213 patients given low-molecular-weight heparin and 15 of 219 patients given intravenously administered heparin had new episodes of venous thromboembolism. Major bleeding associated

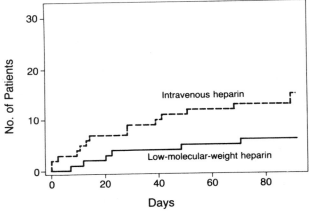

Fig 3–14.—Frequency of objectively documented recurrent venous thromboembolism in the treatment groups. This outcome occurred in 6 of 213 patients receiving low-molecular-weight heparin (2.8%) as compared with 15 of 219 patients receiving intravenously administered heparin (6.9%) (P = .049). (Courtesy of Hull RD, Raskob GE, Pineo GF, et al: N Engl J Med 326:975–982, 1992.)

with the initial treatment was seen in 1 patient in the low-molecular-weight group and in 11 in the intravenously administered heparin group, representing a risk reduction of 91%. However, this apparent protection against major bleeding was lost during long-term treatment. Minor bleeding occurred infrequently. Mortality was 4.7% in the low-molecular-weight heparin group and 9.6% in the intravenously administered heparin group, for a risk reduction of 51% (Fig 3–14). Most events (ac-

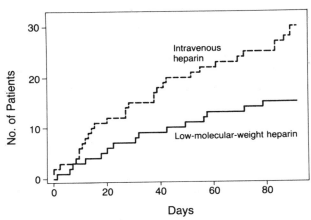

Fig 3–15.—Time-to-event analysis for patients who had recurrent venous thromboembolism or died. Fifteen of 213 patients receiving low-molecular-weight heparin (7%) had objectively documented recurrent venous thromboembolism or died as compared with 30 of 219 patients receiving intravenously administered heparin (13.7%) (P = .024). In each group, most of these events occurred within the first 6 weeks. (Courtesy of Hull RD, Raskob GE, Pineo GF, et al: N Engl J Med 326:975–982, 1992.)

cording to which effectiveness was determined) occurred during the first 6 weeks of follow-up (Fig 3–15).

Conclusion.—Low-molecular-weight heparin is at least as safe and effective as intravenously administered heparin treatment. In addition, it is easier to give. Such treatment may enable patients with uncomplicated proximal deep venous thrombosis to be cared for on an outpatient basis.

Comparison of Subcutaneous Low-Molecular-Weight Heparin With Intravenous Standard Heparin in Proximal Deep-Vein Thrombosis

Prandoni P, Lensing AWA, Büller HR, Carta M, Cogo A, Vigo M, Casara D, Ruol A, ten Cate JW (Univ Hosp of Padua, Italy; Academic Med Ctr, Amsterdam)
Lancet 339:441–445, 1992

3–51

Objective.—Fixed-dose subcutaneous low-molecular-weight heparin (LMWH) therapy was compared with standard adjusted-dose intravenously administered heparin.

Methods.—Half of the 170 consecutive symptomatic patients who had venographically confirmed proximal deep venous thrombosis received standard heparin therapy to prolong the activated partial thromboplastin time to 1.5–2 times the baseline value. The other patients received LMWH in doses adjusted for body weight for 10 days. Orally administered coumarin therapy began after 1 week and continued for at least 3 months. Perfusion lung scanning was done at baseline and on day 10, or earlier if clinically indicated.

Results.—Recurrent venous thromboembolism did not differ significantly in the 2 treatment groups, but venographic scores favored the LMWH group (table). Clinically significant bleeding was infrequent in both groups.

Conclusion.—Fixed-dose subcutaneous LMWH is at least as effective and safe as standard adjusted-dose intravenously administered heparin

Changes in Venographic Score		
	No *(%)* of patients	
—	Standard heparin (n=85)	LMWH (n=83)
Improvement ≥20%	20 *(24%)*	25 *(30%)*
Improvement <20%	16 *(19%)*	25 *(30%)*
Unchanged	35 *(41%)*	28 *(35%)*
Worsening <20%	6 *(7%)*	3 *(3%)*
Worsening ≥20%	8 *(9%)*	2 *(2%)*

(Courtesy of Prandoni P, Lensing AWA, Büller HR, et al: *Lancet* 339:441–445, 1992.)

treatment for symptomatic proximal vein thrombosis. Patients may be treated at home because laboratory monitoring is not necessary.

▶ This comment is for both Abstract 3–50 and Abstract 3–51. A number of studies have been completed recently that compared subcutaneous LMWH with standard unfractionated heparin given intravenously in the standard manner. These 2 studies concluded that the low-molecular-weight subcutaneous material is as effective as standard-dose heparin given intravenously. From these studies, it is apparent that the subcutaneous LMWH is easier to administer and does not require as rigorous monitoring as does intravenous standard heparin. No study yet published has claimed that the low-molecular-weight material is better or more effective than standard-dose intravenous heparin. A recent meta-analysis (Abstract 3–49) of LMWH vs. standard heparin in general concluded that there is now no convincing evidence that LMWH compared with standard heparin generates a clinically important improvement in the benefit-risk ratio. The price of the LMWH preparations is considerably greater than the standard unfractionated heparin. In certain situations, however, it may be more convenient to use the low-molecular-weight preparations knowing that the efficacy is equal to that of unfractionated heparin. Presently, there appears to be no reason for automatically discontinuing the use of standard-dose intravenous unfractionated heparin.—W.R. Bell, M.D.

Optimal Therapeutic Level of Heparin Therapy in Patients With Venous Thrombosis

Hull RD, Raskob GE, Rosenbloom D, Lemaire J, Pineo GF, Baylis B, Ginsberg JS, Panju AA, Brill-Edwards P, Brant R (Univ of Calgary, Alberta, Canada; McMaster Univ, Hamilton, Ont, Canada)
Arch Intern Med 152:1589–1595, 1992   3–52

Purpose.—Heparin administration poses difficult problems. It is currently ordered on an intuitive basis, which, because of fear of bleeding, leads to inadequate therapy. Prospective trials point out the importance of exceeding the lower limit of the therapeutic range; failure to do so carries high rates of recurrent venous thromboembolism. An approach to minimize subtherapeutic heparin dosing and to assess activated partial thromboplastin time (APTT) as a basis for decreasing heparin dosage was evaluated.

Methods.—The double-blind study included 199 consecutive patients with proximal deep venous thrombosis who were randomized to receive initial heparin therapy alone vs. heparin with simultaneous warfarin sodium, and to receive 5 vs. 10 days of intravenous heparin treatment. The regimen began with an intravenous bolus of 5,000 units of heparin sodium followed by continuous infusion of 40,000 units/day for patients at low risk of bleeding and 30,000 units/day for those at high risk. The heparin and warfarin treatments were monitored by laboratory testing, with the heparin dose adjusted by means of APTT according to a nomogram. The outcome was assessed by documentation of thromboembolic and bleeding complications.

Results.—The heparin levels were subtherapeutic for 24 hours or more in only 1% of patients receiving heparin only and in 2% of those receiving heparin and warfarin. Both groups had a 7% incidence of recurrent venous thromboembolism. Supratherapeutic values were present in 69% of patients receiving combined therapy vs. in 24% of those receiving heparin. Rates of bleeding complications were 9% and 12%, respectively.

Conclusion.—No association was found between supratherapeutic APTT responses and bleeding. This is in contrast to the relationship observed between subtherapeutic APTT and recurrent venous thromboembolism. For patients with deep venous thrombosis, a 5-day course of heparin appears to be as effective as a 10-day course.

▶ The authors have clearly demonstrated that subtherapeutic APTT values in the management of patients with venous thrombosis are highly undesirable and clearly predispose to recurrence of venous thromboembolic disease. Another feature of this excellent report is the wide-ranging scatter of APTT times while receiving heparin anticoagulation. The authors stated that there is no association between supratherapeutic APTT responses and hemorrhage. This must be very cautiously interpreted. A definition of a supratherapeutic APTT value was greater than 85 seconds. Although there may be little to no bleeding at a value of greater than 85 but less than 100 seconds, in patients whose APTT value is greater than several hundred seconds, the frequency of bleeding will be extremely high and very close to 100%. Thus, the reader must not come to the conclusion, based on the statement by the authors in this report, that there is no danger to supratherapeutic APTT values. The authors really mean that there is no danger to supratherapeutic APTT values within the range that they examined.—W.R. Bell, M.D.

Heparin Binding to Plasma Proteins, an Important Mechanism for Heparin Resistance
Young E, Prins M, Levine MN, Hirsh J (McMaster Univ, Hamilton, Ont, Canada)
Thromb Haemost 67:639–643, 1992   3–53

Objective.—Heparin dose requirements vary widely in patients treated for venous thromboembolism. To determine whether binding of heparin to plasma proteins other than antithrombin III is a factor in increased heparin needs, an assay was developed to determine the proportion of heparin that is reversibly neutralized by such protein binding.

Patients and Methods.—Thirty-two patients with confirmed deep venous thrombosis and 3 with pulmonary embolism were studied. Pretreatment and 6-hour post-treatment samples were available from 19 of them. The assay is based on low-affinity heparin, which does not bind to antithrombin III and has practically no anti–factor Xa activity. Heparin levels, measured as anti–factor Xa activity, were estimated before and after adding the low-affinity heparin.

Results.—Reversible heparin neutralization caused by binding to plasma proteins is a major factor in the anticoagulant response to standard heparin 6 hours after administration. Reversible heparin neutralization in 6-hour post-treatment samples was higher in heparin-resistant patients than in others, although not to a significant extent.

Conclusion.—Reversible heparin neutralization secondary to plasma protein binding is a factor in the response to a fixed dose of heparin, but it is not the only cause of a reduced anticoagulant response in vivo. Other possible factors are heparin binding to endothelium, binding to extracellular matrix, and factors altering heparin clearance.

▶ Data in this article identify that apparent heparin resistance may be caused by excessive quantities of heparin that can be bound by various plasma proteins in some patients. Whether these various proteins are abnormal proteins or whether they are present in abnormal or excessive quantities remains to be established. These proteins that bind heparin do not contain tissue thromboplastin.—W.R. Bell, M.D.

Sustained Antithrombotic Activity of Hirudin After its Plasma Clearance: Comparison With Heparin

Agnelli G, Renga C, Weitz JI, Nenci GG, Hirsh J (Università di Perugia, Italy; Hamilton Civic Hosp Research Ctr, Ont, Canada)
Blood 80:960–965, 1992   3–54

Background.—Recurrent thrombosis often develops when heparin therapy is withdrawn prematurely, presumably because of the accretion of fibrin onto existing thrombi after conversion of fibrinogen to fibrin by both circulating and thrombus-bound thrombin. Heparin effectively inhibits fluid-phase thrombin, but it is much less effective in inhibiting thrombus-bound thrombin.

Hypothesis.—Hirudin, in contrast to heparin, inactivates both free and thrombus-bound thrombin and, therefore, has the potential of preventing thrombotic extension even after being cleared from the circulation.

Methods.—The time course of fibrin accretion onto preexisting thrombi was examined in the rabbit jugular vein after 3-hour infusions of saline, heparin, and hirudin. Both heparin and recombinant hirudin were infused at a level that doubled the activated partial thromboplastin time.

Results.—Infusion of .75 mg of heparin per kg lowered the accretion of iodine-125–labeled fibrinogen from 59 to 34 µg, compared with saline. Infusion of 1.25 mg of recombinant hirudin per kg further reduced accretion to 21 µg. Accretion was much lower in the hirudin-treated animals 9 hours after the end of infusion. In vitro studies demonstrated persistent inhibition of fibrinopeptide A generation after the incubation of human fibrin clots with plasma containing recombinant hirudin. Such inhibition was not noted after incubating clots in plasma preincubated with heparin.

Conclusion.—The antithrombotic action of hirudin persists after it is cleared from the plasma, presumably because it inactivates thrombus-bound thrombin. It is possible that shorter anticoagulation would be feasible by replacing heparin with hirudin.

▶ The data in this study support the contention that hirudin remains effective even after it is cleared from the plasma. This lends further support to the view that hirudin can, once it is bound to the tissue phase of thrombin generation, continue to exert an antithrombotic activity. However, how will the effect of hirudin be monitored? It continues to be effective for some time (how long?) after it has disappeared from detection in the plasma.—W.R. Bell, M.D.

Efficacy and Safety of Early Versus Late Initiation of Warfarin During Heparin Therapy in Acute Thromboembolism
Mohiuddin SM, Hilleman DE, Destache CJ, Stoysich AM, Gannon JM, Sketch MH Sr (Creighton Univ, Omaha, Neb)
Am Heart J 123:729–732, 1992   3–55

Objective.—Because there is no universally agreed on approach to starting systemic anticoagulant therapy, 2 regimens differing in the timing of warfarin administration were compared.

Methods.—Sixty-three patients with acute thromboembolism received warfarin within 48 hours of the start of heparin therapy, whereas 56 others received warfarin after at least 96 hours of heparin therapy. Heparin was given by infusion to maintain an activated partial thromboplastin time 1.5–2 times control values. The warfarin therapy began at 10 mg daily for 3 days, and the dose then was titrated to maintain a prothrombin time of 1.2–1.5 times the control value.

Results.—The mean time to the start of warfarin therapy was 31 hours in the early group and 108 hours in the late group. Early-treated patients were hospitalized for a significantly shorter time, and heparin-related infusion phlebitis and thrombocytopenia were less frequent in this group. There were no significant group differences in the frequency of bleeding, recurrent thromboembolism, or mortality (table).

Outcome Criteria in the Study Group

Variable	Early group (n = 63)	Late group (n = 56)	p Value
Length of hospital stay (days)	8.62 ± 2.50	13.0 ± 4.31	<0.01
Cost of hospitalization ($)	10,485 ± 6713	14,987 ± 7340	<0.05
Bleeding events (n/%)			
Minor	8/13	6/11	NS
Major	1/2	1/2	NS
Intracranial hemorrhage	0/0	2/4	NS
Recurrent thromboembolic events (n/%)	1/2	2/4	NS
Infusion phlebitis (n/%)	1/2	10/18	<0.05
Thrombocytopenia (n/%)	0/0	8/14	<0.05
Mortality (n/%)	0/0	3/5	NS

(Courtesy of Mohiuddin SM, Hilleman DE, Destache CJ, et al: *Am Heart J* 123:729–732, 1992.)

Conclusion.—Early addition of warfarin to heparin therapy in patients with acute thromboembolism is safer and less expensive than later treatment, and it is equally effective.

► Frequently, after the initiation of heparin anticoagulation, the question is asked, When should warfarin anticoagulation be initiated? This study in a relatively small number of patients suggests that these 2 agents should be started concomitantly, if possible, and that as soon as warfarin anticoagulation is in the therapeutic range, anticoagulation with heparin should be discontinued. This study suggests that waiting for several days while on heparin anticoagulation before starting warfarin anticoagulation does not improve the outcome with respect to recurrence of thrombotic disease. Thus, treatment with heparin alone for several days before the initiation of warfarin anticoagulation apparently has no beneficial effect. If the 2 agents are started concomitantly, the length of hospitalization, the frequency of heparin-associated bleeding and thrombocytopenia, and other untoward side effects are significantly reduced.—W.R. Bell, M.D.

Factors Affecting the Precision of Warfarin Treatment

Britt RP, James AH, Raskino CL, Thompson SG (Hillingdon Hosp, Uxbridge, Middlesex, England; London School of Hygiene & Tropical Medicine, London)
J Clin Pathol 45:1003–1006, 1992   3–56

Objective.—Factors determining the precision of anticoagulant control were sought by examining the records of 2,207 warfarin-treated patients at 7 district hospitals.

Method.—Precision of control was taken as the deviation of the observed International Normalized Ratio (INR) from a target INR.

Extent of Under- or Overtreatment by Hospital and Diagnostic Group:
Percentage of Patients With Observed INR More Than .5 From Target, and
Mean Absolute Deviation of Observed INRs From Target

	Numbers of patients	*Percentage of patients*		*Mean absolute deviation ‡*
		undertreated	*overtreated*	
Observed minus target INR		< -0.5	$> +0.5$	
Hospital: *				
6	114	12%	21%	0·44
1	658	13%	17%	0·45
5	334	15%	16%	0·48
7	403	22%	21%	0·56
4	304	19%	17%	0·57
0	159	23%	24%	0·65
3	235	31%	14%	0·77
Diagnostic group: *				
Coronary disease	78	13%	18%	0·43
Deep vein thrombosis	377	20%	17%	0·48
Heart disease ± AF †	505	15%	18%	0·50
Pulmonary embolism	297	13%	19%	0·55
Prosthetic heart valve	461	25%	17%	0·59
Arterial disease	247	23%	17%	0·61
Prophylaxis	20	10%	30%	0·61

* Hospitals (and diagnostic groups) in order of increasing mean absolute deviation of observed INR from target: 222 patients had missing or unclassified diagnostic information.
† *Abbreviation:* AF, atrial fibrillation.
‡ $P < .0001$ for differences between hospitals; $P = .001$ for differences between diagnostic groups.
(Courtesy of Britt RP, James AH, Raskino CL, et al: *J Clin Pathol* 45:1003–1006, 1992.)

Findings.—Although observed INRs were, on the average, on target, 36% of the patients had a value more than .5 from target, and 12% had INRs more than 1 from target. After adjusting for the target INR in a multiple regression analysis, higher doses for a given target ratio were significantly related to overtreatment. Patients with a high-target INR were more likely to be undertreated. There were interhospital differences in the degree of anticoagulant control (table). Differences in control in different diagnostic groups were not significant after adjusting for hospital and other factors.

Conclusion.—Anticoagulant therapy requires especially close scrutiny in patients with a history of overtreatment or undertreatment. Further attention to interhospital differences in anticoagulant control may allow more uniform treatment.

▶ The anticoagulant warfarin is known to have an inherent appreciable risk of bleeding, anywhere between 5% to 13% of patients taking this medication. The frequency of bleeding does not seem to be preventable through regulation of the prothrombin time. The points emphasized by these authors are potentially of considerable importance. For additional information on this topic, please see reference 1.—W.R. Bell, M.D.

Reference

1. Bianco TM, et al: *Pharmacol Ther* 12:435–439, 1992.

Aging and the Anticoagulant Response to Warfarin Therapy

Gurwitz JH, Avorn J, Ross-Degnan D, Choodnovskiy I, Ansell J (Beth Israel Hosp, Boston; Brigham and Women's Hosp, Boston; Hebrew Rehabilitation Ctr for Aged, Boston; et al)
Ann Intern Med 116:901–904, 1992   3–57

Background.—Thromboembolic and vascular disorders requiring long-term oral anticoagulant therapy with warfarin are relatively prevalent in elderly persons, but there is particular concern about the risk of bleeding in these patients. An age-related increase in sensitivity has been proposed for oral anticoagulants. A cumulative 5% incidence of major bleeding has been found during 1 year of treatment, with minor bleeding complications exceeding 20%.

Patients and Methods.—A total of 530 patients was followed in an anticoagulation clinic from 1980 to 1990. The series included 149 patients, aged 60–69 years, and 177 patients aged 70 years and older.

Results.—The older patients had more medical problems, took more medication, and weighed less than the younger ones. The prothrombin time ratio adjusted for the warfarin dose was significantly increased in older patients (Fig 3–16), even after controlling for relevant clinical and demographic variables. Women and patients using more medications

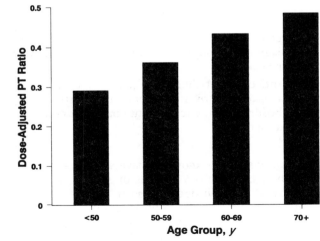

Fig 3–16.—Relationship between the dose-adjusted prothrombin time (PT) ratio and age group (P < .001). (Courtesy of Gurwitz JH, Avorn J, Ross-Degnan D, et al: *Ann Intern Med* 116:901–904, 1992.)

were more sensitive to warfarin. Heavier patients and those using warfarin longer than 6 months were less sensitive.

Conclusion.—Older patients are more sensitive to warfarin and, therefore, require close monitoring because the intensity of anticoagulant effect is the chief predictor of bleeding in warfarin-treated patients. Age appears to be an independent risk factor for bleeding complications from warfarin.

▶ The authors studied a very reasonable sample size of 530 patients undergoing warfarin anticoagulation. They were clearly able to show that as age increases, the dose of warfarin required to maintain a therapeutic prothrombin time is progressively lower in quantity. The practicing physician must be aware of this and consider the age of a patient when warfarin is prescribed.—W.R. Bell, M.D.

Monitoring "Mini-Intensity" Anticoagulation With Warfarin: Comparison of the Prothrombin Time Using a Sensitive Thromboplastin With Prothrombin Fragment F_{1+2} Levels
Millenson MM, Bauer KA, Kistler JP, Barzegar S, Tulin L, Rosenberg RD (Beth Israel Hosp, Boston; Brockton-West Roxbury VA Med Ctr, Boston; Massachusetts Gen Hosp, Boston; et al)
Blood 79:2034–2038, 1992   3–58

Background.—Warfarin therapy based on a target International Normalized Ratio (INR) range of 1.7–2.5 is effective in many clinical settings. However, the minimal degree of anticoagulation needed to prevent thrombosis is uncertain.

Objective and Methods.—To determine whether a less intensive regimen is feasible, patients with a history of cerebral embolism and those with acute carotid occlusion causing either transient ischemia or stroke were given warfarin for several months by using a target INR range of 1.3–1.6. In the determination of prothrombin time (PT), a sensitive thromboplastin was used. Plasma values of F_{1+2} were obtained as a marker of factor Xa action on prothrombin in vivo.

Results.—All but 1 of 21 patients could be reliably regulated with warfarin in the target INR range. The level of F_{1+2} was significantly lowered from baseline in all cases; the mean reduction was 49%. The degree of suppression of prothrombin activation correlated closely with baseline values. When less sensitive thromboplastins were used, far fewer prothrombin time estimates were within the target range. When the sensitive product was used, 68% of all plasma samples taken during stable anticoagulation were within the target range.

Conclusion. — "Mini-intensity" warfarin anticoagulation is an appropriate way of using the drug for antithrombotic purposes.

▶ Using a sensitive technique, namely, the measurement of prothrombin fragment F_{1+2} concentrations in the blood, these authors established that a dose of between 3 and 4 mg of warfarin per day was adequate to achieve this therapeutic range. This suggests that warfarin may be used in lower doses than is currently the standard acceptable practice. This translates into a prothrombin time in the range of 14–18 seconds being as therapeutically efficacious as extending the range up to a prothrombin time of 25 seconds. However, no data are supplied on how well protected a patient is who has a considerable reduction in his or her prothrombin F_{1+2} level. Another concern is that the patient population size (20) was exceedingly small. Thus, clearly additional studies must be performed before a universal recommendation can be made.—W.R. Bell, M.D.

Fibrinolysis

Urgent Therapy for Stroke: Part I. Pilot Study of Tissue Plasminogen Activator Administered Within 90 Minutes

Brott TG, Haley EC Jr, Levy DE, Barsan W, Broderick J, Sheppard GL, Spilker J, Kongable GL, Massey S, Reed R, Marler JR (Univ of Cincinnati, Ohio; Univ of Virginia, Charlottesville; Cornell Univ, New York; et al)

Stroke 23:632–640, 1992   3–59

Post-Treatment Arteriography and Major Neurologic Improvement at 2 Hours		
Angiographic lesion*	Early improvement	No early improvement
No. with arteriography	18	36
No. with complete occlusion*	6 (33%)	21 (58%)
ICA occlusion	1	3
ICA occlusion with distal intracranial MCA occlusion(s)	0	6
MCA trunk occlusion	1	3
MCA trunk occlusion with distal branch occlusion(s)	0	3
MCA branch occlusion(s) only	3	6
Other occlusions	1†	0
No. without complete occlusion	12	15

Abbreviations: ICA, internal carotid artery; *MCA,* middle cerebral artery.
Note: Major neurologic improvement measured by improvement of ≥ 4 points in the NIH Stroke Scale score.
* Only lesions in the vascular distribution of the clinical deficit are indicated.
† Left vertebral artery occlusion.
(Courtesy of Brott TG, Haley EC Jr, Levy DE, et al: *Stroke* 23:632–640, 1992.)

Background.—Acute thrombus formation and arterial occlusion are the critical pathologic events in at least 70% of strokes. In animals, ischemic brain injury probably takes place when occlusion exceeds 2–3 hours. Recombinant tissue plasminogen activator (rt-PA) was assessed as urgent treatment for acute cerebral infarction.

Methods.—Seventy-four patients received .35–1.08 mg of rt-PA per kg starting within 90 minutes of the onset of symptoms of acute ischemic stroke, using a dose-escalation design.

Results.—Three patients given higher doses of rt-PA had intracranial hematoma and deteriorated neurologically. None of 58 patients given a maximum of .85 mg/kg had hematoma. One or more complete arterial occlusions were identified in 27 patients (50%) (table). Thirty percent of patients had major neurologic improvement 2 hours after the start of treatment, and 46% had improvement at 24 hours. Significant improvement did not correlate with either increasing doses or the type of stroke.

Conclusion.—The potential clinical benefit from early administration of rt-PA warrants a randomized trial in patients with acute stroke.

Urgent Therapy for Stroke: Part II. Pilot Study of Tissue Plasminogen Activator Administered 91–180 Minutes From Onset
Haley EC Jr, Levy DE, Brott TG, Sheppard GL, Wong MCW, Kongable GL, Torner JC, Marler JR (Univ of Virginia, Charlottesville; Cornell Univ, New York; Univ of Cincinnati, Ohio; et al)
Stroke 23:641–645, 1992   3–60

Background.—There has been renewed interest in thrombolytic therapy as potential treatment for patients with acute ischemic stroke. Recently, the safety of dose escalation of tissue plasminogen activator in patients with very early neurologic symptoms was examined. Whether this stringent entry window may be safely lengthened was determined.

Methods.—Tissue plasminogen activator was tested in patients with symptoms of 91–180 minutes' duration before treatment. An open-label, dose-escalation study design was used. Twenty patients at 3 hospitals were treated in 13 months. End points included the incidence of symptomatic and asymptomatic intracranial hemorrhage, other bleeding, and clinical outcome at different periods.

Results.—Eight patients received .6 mg/kg, 6 patients received .85 mg/kg, and 6 received .95 mg/kg of tissue plasminogen activator. One patient in the highest and 1 in the second highest dose group had fatal intracerebral hemorrhages. Three patients, or 15%, improved by 4 points or more on the NIH Stroke Scale by 24 hours. Table 1 summarizes the dose, baseline NIH Stroke Scale scores, and all bleeding complications

TABLE 1.—Dose, Baseline Scores, and Bleeding

Dose tier	Patient No.	Total rt-PA dose (mg)	Baseline score*	Bleeding complications
II	1	37.4	16	Oozing at venipuncture
	2	44.0	14	Hematuria
	3	43.4	24	ASX hemorrhagic conversion
	4	35.0	15	Hematuria
	5	40.2	17	None
	6	37.2	10	None
	7	47.0	4	None
	8	44.0	9	None
IV	9	69.0	23	Gingival bleeding
	10	50.0	21	Intracerebral hemorrhage
	11	50.0	6	None
	12	60.0	24	Gingival bleeding
	13	67.0	27	None
	14	51.2	24	Hematuria, ASX hemorrhagic conversion
IV-E	15	60.0	22	Hematoma at venipuncture
	16	56.4	12	ASX hemorrhagic conversion
	17	70.0	18	Intracerebral hemorrhage
	18	78.0	18	ASX hemorrhagic conversion
	19	71.2	5	None
	20	75.0	24	Guaiac positive stool

Abbreviations: rt-PA, recombinant tissue plasminogen activator; ASX, asymptomatic.
* NIH Stroke Scale scores.
(Courtesy of Haley EC Jr, Levy DE, Brott TG, et al: *Stroke* 23:641–645, 1992.)

noted. The clinical outcomes of the patients by dose tier are summarized in Table 2.

Conclusion.—Tissue plasminogen activator treatment of acute ischemic stroke 91–180 minutes from onset in doses of .85 mg/kg or greater appears to be accompanied by a risk of intracerebral bleeding of about 17%. In this series, the rate of early neurologic improvement was small, but this does not exclude the possibility of improving on the natural history. Further research with placebo and stratification by time to therapy is merited.

▶ Although there has been a progressive increase in the number of studies performed using thrombolytic therapy in the treatment of stroke, this treatment is being performed only at a few centers. In these studies (Abstracts 3–59 and 3–60), when tissue plasminogen activator has been used, no apparent benefits have been detectable when one considers the hemorrhagic risk vs. neurologic improvement. The problem of hemorrhage could perhaps be improved if treatment is initiated earlier. In addition, if the thrombolytic agent urokinase, which is known to have a considerably lower frequency of CNS hemorrhagic problems, is used, a greater degree of neurologic benefit and a lower frequency of hemorrhage in patients with ischemic stroke may

TABLE 2.—Clinical Outcome

Dose tier	No. of patients	No. with MNI at 2 hours	No. with MNI at 24 hours	Outcome at 3 months
II	8	3	2	2 D, 4 NL or Mild L, 2 Mod L
IV	6	1	1	3 D, 2 Mod L, 1 LTF
IV-E	6	1	0	1 D, 1 NL, 4 Mod L
Total	20	5 (25%)	3 (15%)	

Abbreviations: MNI, major neurologic improvement (improvement of ≥ 4 points in NIH Stroke Scale score); *D*, dead; *NL*, no limitation in activities of daily living; *Mild L*, mild limitation; *Mod L*, moderate limitation; *LTF*, lost to follow-up. (Courtesy of Haley EC Jr, Levy DE, Brott TG, et al: *Stroke* 23:641–645, 1992.)

result. We must await the conclusion of such studies before firmly stating that thrombolytic therapy is not beneficial in this disease situation.—W.R. Bell, M.D.

Effect of Ultrasound on Tissue-Type Plasminogen Activator-Induced Thrombolysis

Lauer CG, Burge R, Tang DB, Bass BG, Gomez ER, Alving BM (Walter Reed Army Inst of Research, Washington, DC; Walter Reed Army Med Ctr, Washington, DC)
Circulation 86:1257–1264, 1992   3–61

Introduction.—The efficacy of fibrinolytic treatment is limited by the surface area of the clot available to bind the thrombolytic agent, such as tissue-type plasminogen activator (t-PA). It was hypothesized that exposure of the clot to ultrasound during thrombolytic treatment might enhance lysis by exposing additional fibrin binding sites for t-PA.

Methods.—Clots of whole human blood containing radiolabeled fibrinogen were incubated for 200 minutes with Tris-albumin buffer containing t-PA in concentrations of 3–3,000 IU/mL. In paired experiments, one of the clots was also exposed to intermittent ultrasound at 1 MHz and 1.75 W/cm² (Fig 3–17). Two-second exposures were followed by 2-second rest intervals. In addition, paired studies were done in a rabbit model of jugular vein thrombosis.

Results.—Clot lysis was significantly greater after ultrasound exposure at all concentrations of t-PA (Fig 3–18). For clots incubated with t-PA, 300 IU/mL, ultrasound exposure increased lysis from a mean of 42% to

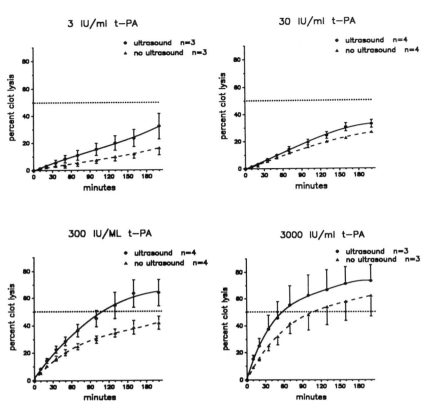

Fig 3–17.—Graphs showing effect of intermittent ultrasound (1 MHz, 1.75 W/cm²) on whole blood clot lysis induced by different concentrations of t-PA in Tris-albumin buffer. Ultrasound was delivered during 2 seconds with a 2-second rest interval. (Courtesy of Lauer CG, Burge R, Tang DB, et al: *Circulation* 86:1257–1264, 1992.)

a mean of 64% at 200 minutes. Similar results were obtained in the rabbit model. Ultrasound exposure alone produced minimal lysis.

Conclusion.—Intermittent ultrasound exposure significantly enhances t-PA–induced thrombolysis both in vitro and in vivo. Possibly acoustic microstreaming gently perturbs the clot, allowing increased binding of t-PA to fibrin. Whether the risk of pulmonary embolism is increased remains to be seen.

▶ The authors have shown the usefulness of ultrasound in enhancing the ability of the plasminogen/plasmin proteolytic enzyme system to bring about the dissolution of in vitro–formed clots. This observation, which was recognized years ago by our group, should be extended further by perhaps placing ultrasonic devices in catheters that can be imbedded in thrombi or placed adjacent to an in vivo thrombus formation. This may aid in the dissolution

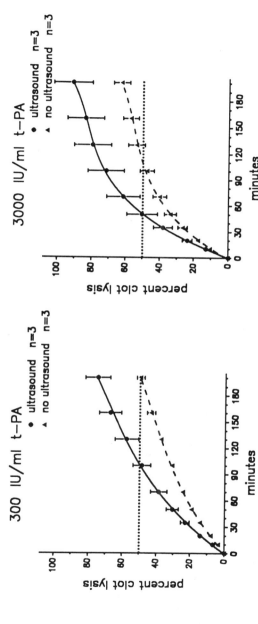

Fig 3-18.—Graphs showing effect of intermittent ultrasound (1 MHz, 1.75 W/cm²) on whole blood clot lysis induced by t-PA in plasma. (Courtesy of Lauer CG, Burge R, Tang DB, et al: *Circulation* 86:1257–1264, 1992.)

and restoration of blood flow in thrombus-obstructed vessels.—W.R. Bell, M.D.

Choice of Agent for Peripheral Thrombolysis

Earnshaw JJ, Scott DJA, Horrocks M, Baird RN (Bristol Royal Infirmary, England)
Br J Surg 80:25–27, 1993   3–62

Background.—Accumulating evidence suggests that tissue plasminogen activator (t-PA) may be a quicker and more effective agent than streptokinase for peripheral thrombolysis. However, when compared with streptokinase, 24 hours of t-PA treatment is 10 times more expensive. Peripheral thrombolysis clinical results of both t-PA and streptokinase were compared to determine whether the additional expense of t-PA is justified.

Patients and Methods.—During a 15-month period, 23 patients with acute limb-threatening ischemia were treated with .5 mg h^{-1} t-PA. This group was compared with 20 consecutive patients who had previously received 5,000 (10 patients) or 10,000 (10 patients) units h^{-1} streptokinase during a similar 15-month period.

Results.—The median duration of lysis was 18 and 22 hours for streptokinase and t-PA, respectively. No significant differences in successful complete and partial lysis rates were noted between groups (t-PA = 61%; streptokinase = 65%). Additionally, no major between-group limb salvage differences were found (t-PA = 65%; streptokinase = 55%). Rates of complications, including catheter-related, minor and major hemorrhage, early rethrombosis, and major vascular reconstruction, were also comparable between groups.

Conclusion.—Study results indicated that there was no advantage in using t-PA rather than streptokinase for peripheral thrombolysis, particularly when considering the added cost. Perhaps peripheral thrombolysis research should concentrate on developing safe and effective low-dose streptokinase regimens and new physical modes of speeding clot lysis, including lacing, mechanical disruption, and pulse-spray lysis.

▶ The authors of this thorough study clearly demonstrated that there is absolutely no statistical significant difference between streptokinase and recombinant t-PA in the results of thrombus dissolution in the peripheral arterial circulation. The authors pointed out that the complications with the recombinant t-PA are actually slightly higher than those seen with streptokinase. It has been repeatedly shown with respect to coronary artery thrombosis that there is no statistically significant difference in the success rate with these 2 agents, and now this study had a similar conclusion for the peripheral arterial circulation. Once again the question must be posed, Is an agent that costs 10–20 times more than streptokinase without producing any significantly greater benefit a reasonable choice?—W.R. Bell, M.D.

Coagulation, Fibrinolytic, and Inhibitory Proteins in Acute Myocardial Infarction and Angina Pectoris
Vaziri ND, Kennedy SC, Kennedy D, Gonzales E (Univ of California, Irvine)
Am J Med 93:651–657, 1992   3–63

Introduction.—Although a role for thrombus formation in the development of acute myocardial infarction and unstable angina is established, coagulation and fibrinolysis have not been systematically examined. Coagulation, fibrinolytic, and inhibitory proteins in 14 patients with acute infarction, 10 patients with clinical and ECG evidence of myocardial ischemia, and 32 normal subjects were analyzed.

Findings.—Levels of factor XII were significantly lower in patients with infarction than in normal control subjects, but there was no significant difference in factor XII antigen levels. Plasma levels of high-molecular-weight kininogen were significantly reduced in patients with acute infarction and also those with angina. Factor XI activity was higher in these groups than in normal subjects, and factor IX coagulant activity also was increased. Factor VIII coagulant activity was elevated in patients with angina, and both patient groups had markedly higher levels of vWF antigen than did normal subjects. Factor V levels were reduced in patients with acute infarction. Both patient groups had relatively low factor II coagulant activity and antigen concentrations. Fibrinogen levels were significantly elevated in both groups. Only patients with infarction had significantly increased plasma levels of tissue plasminogen activator. Levels of D-dimer were higher in both patient groups than in control subjects.

Conclusion.—Activation of the intrinsic pathway, thrombin generation, fibrin formation, and fibrin degradation may be present in patients with acute myocardial infarction. A prothrombotic state also is present in patients with myocardial ischemia.

▶ The authors identified alterations in certain coagulation glycoproteins that apparently are associated with myocardial infarction and angina pectoris. However, these changes should also be examined in other patients who are not experiencing myocardial infarction but may have an acute, systemic illness of any variety. The reader comes away with the impression that if these measurements are made, the presence of acute myocardial infarction can actually be identified or diagnosed. This, indeed, may not be true. These studies need to be repeated using the appropriate control populations of patients with acute illnesses not experiencing myocardial infarction.—W.R. Bell, M.D.

Plasma Crosslinked Fibrin Polymers: Quantitation Based on Tissue Plasminogen Activator Conversion to D-Dimer and Measurement in Normals and Patients with Acute Thrombotic Disorders

Kornberg A, Francis CW, Marder VJ (Univ of Rochester, NY)
Blood 80:709–717, 1992   3–64

Introduction.—Soluble fibrin is found in low concentrations in normal plasma and in increased concentrations in patients with thrombotic disease. Evaluation of plasma-soluble fibrin can be based on the identification of covalently cross-linked fibrin polymers (XLFPs) formed as a result of in vivo hemostatic activation. The plasmic degradation of XLFPs in vitro was investigated to determine the pattern of cross-linking and the composition of the degradation products.

Methods.—Blood samples obtained from normal persons and patients were prepared for electrophoresis or plasmic digestion. Plasma XLFPs were identified by sodium dodecylsulfate-agarose electrophoresis and Western blotting and were quantitated by gel scanning. Enzyme-linked immunosorbent assay was used to measure D-dimer, the primary plasmic

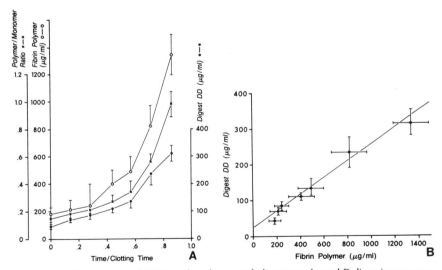

Fig 3–19.—Measurement of XLFPs in thrombin-treated plasma samples and D-dimer immunoreactivity of plasmic digests. **A,** thrombin (.01 unit/mL) and calcium chloride (10 mmol/L) were added to stored, pooled normal plasma, incubated at 37°C, and aliquots were withdrawn. Samples were subjected to sodium dodecylsulfate 2% agarose electrophoresis and Western blotting with antifibrinogen antiserum, and the concentration of plasma fibrin polymer (*open circles*) was determined by gel scanning and comparison with a standard curve of purified fibrinogen at known concentrations. The ratio of polymer/monomer (*x's*) was determined directly from the gel scan tracing. Plasmic digests of the same plasma aliquots were prepared and D-dimer immunoreactivity (*filled circles*) of the digests was measured by enzyme-linked immunosorbent assay. The values represent mean ± SD of 3 experiments. **B,** correlation between plasma concentration of XLFPs and D-dimer immunoreactivity in plasmic digests. As determined by linear regression, the equation for the line is $y = .23X + 23$ ($r = .98$). (Courtesy of Kornberg A, Francis CW, Marder VJ: *Blood* 80:709–717, 1992.)

derivation of XLFPs. Results were confirmed by sodium dodecylsulfate-polyacrylamide gel electrophoresis and Western blotting of the digests.

Results.—Supplementation of plasma with plasminogen (5 units/mL) and incubation with recombinant tissue plasminogen activator were required for complete degradation of XLFPs, suggesting that normal plasma plasminogen concentration limits plasmic degradation in vitro. The principal terminal degradation products of XLDPs were fragments D, DD, and E. Cross-linked fibrin polymers increased progressively before clotting with the addition of a low concentration of thrombin to plasma in vitro (Fig 3–19). Compared with normals, patients with stroke, myocardial infarction, and venous thrombosis had significantly elevated plasma XLFPs and D-dimer concentrations in plasmic digests. The plasma concentration of XLFPs and the D-dimer immunoreactivity of plasma after plasmic degradation exhibited a strong correlation ($r = .87$).

Conclusion.—Cross-linked fibrin polymers in plasma are cross-linked primarily through gamma-chains and degrade to fragment DD with plasminogen activation. In addition, the immunoreactivity of in vitro plasmic digests of plasma reflects the concentration of XLFPs. Such concentrations may be a useful means of indirectly measuring in vivo hemostatic activation in patients with thrombotic disease.

▶ This report of very small numbers of patients with different thrombotic disorders suggests that identification of XLFPs may be helpful in identifying the presence of a hypercoagulable state.—W.R. Bell, M.D.

---

von Willebrand Factor, Plasminogen Activator Inhibitor-1 and C-Reactive Protein Are Markers of Thrombolytic Efficacy in Acute Myocardial Infarction
Andreotti F, Hackett DR, Haider AW, Roncaglioni MC, Davies GJ, Beacham JL, Kluft C, Maseri A (Hammersmith Hosp, London; Gaubius Lab, Leiden, The Netherlands)
Thromb Haemost 68:678–682, 1992   3–65

Background.—Effective thrombolysis in patients with evolving myocardial infarction limits the elevations of C-reactive protein, vWF, and plasminogen activator, but it is unclear whether estimating these factors will detect myocardial reperfusion.

Study Plan.—Plasma levels of these factors were monitored in 30 patients with acute myocardial infarction who received tissue-type plasminogen activator (t-PA). Blood was sampled before treatment, every 4 hours for 24 hours, and then daily for as long as 3 days. Double-chain recombinant t-PA was given either by continuous infusion or in bolus form, and coronary angiography was done 90 minutes and 24 hours after treatment began.

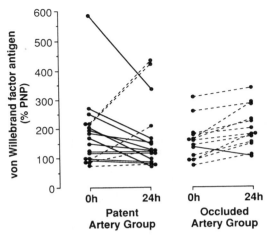

Fig 3–20.—*Abbreviation:* PNP, pooled normal plasma. The plasma vWF at time 0 hours and 24 hours in the patients with patent and occluded artery. (Courtesy of Andreotti F, Hackett DR, Haider AW, et al: *Thromb Haemost* 68:678–682, 1992.)

Findings.—Nineteen patients had a patent infarct vessel after 90 minutes of t-PA treatment. In 17 patients, the vessel remained patent at 24 hours. Levels of plasma vWF antigen remained unchanged or decreased in 12 of 17 patients with a patent infarct artery but in only 1 of those

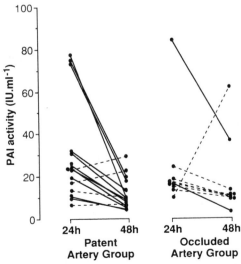

Fig 3–21.—Plasminogen activator inhibitor (PAI) activity at 24 hours and 48 hours in the patients with patent and occluded artery. A 24- to 48-hour PAI > 2 was used as a marker of coronary recanalization (*continuous lines*). The *dashed lines* represent a ratio ≤ 2. (Courtesy of Andreotti F, Hackett DR, Haider AW, et al: *Thromb Haemost* 68:678–682, 1992.)

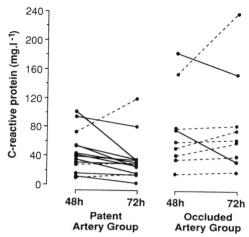

Fig 3–22.—C-reactive protein at 48 hours and 72 hours in the patients with patent and occluded artery. A 48- to 72-hour C-reactive protein > 1 was the index of reperfusion (*continuous lines*). The *dashed lines* indicate a ratio ≤ 1. (Courtesy of Andreotti F, Hackett DR, Haider AW, et al: *Thromb Haemost* 68:678–682, 1992.)

with persistent occlusion (Fig 3–20). Plasminogen activator inhibitor activity declined significantly faster in patients with a patent vessel (Fig 3–21). A decline in C-reactive protein was much more frequent when thrombolysis succeeded (Fig 3–22).

Conclusion.—Changes in levels of vWF, plasminogen activator inhibitor, and C-reactive protein in the first 3 days of myocardial infarction can serve as markers of the effectiveness of thrombolysis with t-PA.

▶ This article suggested that measurement of plasma levels of certain components perhaps may reliably predict myocardial reperfusion. The mechanism whereby these changes occur needs to be defined. This finding also should be confirmed in a much, much larger series of patients before there is complete implementation of these diagnostic techniques. Although these techniques may be helpful, they are difficult and require considerable time to assay in the coagulation laboratory.—W.R. Bell, M.D.

Glycoproteins IIb and IIIa: Insights into Platelet Aggregation Derived from the Study of Glanzmann's Thrombasthenia

PAUL F. BRAY, M.D.

Johns Hopkins University School of Medicine, Baltimore, Maryland

Introduction

Blood platelets are crucial in the maintenance of normal hemostasis and vascular integrity, and they have a central role in the acute development of unstable angina, myocardial infarction, and other thrombotic diseases. When a blood vessel is injured, platelets aggregate at the injury site and form a platelet plug that acts as a barrier to stop hemorrhage. Platelet aggregation occurs when fibrinogen binds to the surface of activated platelets, thereby linking platelets to one another. The fibrinogen receptor is a complex of 2 distinct glycoproteins, IIb and IIIa (GPIIb and GPIIIa). A model for platelet aggregation is shown in Figure 1.

Glanzmann's thrombasthenia (GT) is an inherited bleeding disorder caused by quantitative or qualitative defects in GPIIb of GPIIIa (1). Platelets from these patients are normal in number but are unable to bind fibrinogen and, hence, to aggregate. Recent studies characterizing the genetic defects implicated in GT have provided valuable insights into critical functional domains of GPIIb and GPIIIa. This special article reviews the biochemistry and molecular and cellular biology of GPIIb-IIIa, and emphasizes how characterization of molecular defects in GT has greatly contributed to the current understanding of receptor function.

GPIIb and GPIIIa

The initial evidence implicating GPIIb and GPIIIa in platelet aggregation came from studies of patients with GT. Platelets from these patients fail to aggregate normally in response to physiologic agonists (2). Thrombasthenic platelets, when analyzed on SDS polyacrylamide gels, have absent or markedly reduced quantities of GPIIb and GPIIIa (3, 4) and are unable to bind fibrinogen (2, 5). In addition to this genetic evidence, abundant biochemical and immunologic data demonstrate that GPIIb-IIIa serves as the fibrinogen receptor (for review, see reference 6).

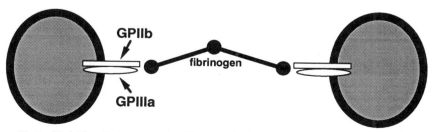

Fig 1.—Model for platelet aggregation. Fibrinogen binds to the GPIIb-IIIa receptor on the surface of activated platelets. (Courtesy of P.F. Bray, M.D.)

BIOCHEMISTRY

The GPIIb-IIIa complex is a calcium-dependent heterodimer present at about 40,000–50,000 copies per cell (7), representing about 1.5% of the total platelet proteins. The GPIIb is a glycoprotein of Mr~140,000 daltons composed of a larger alpha-subunit (Mr~120,000 daltons) disulfide linked to a smaller beta-subunit (Mr~20,000 daltons). The GPIIb$_\alpha$ and GPIIb$_\beta$ are derived from a single-chain precursor (8) and are cleaved post-translationally. The GPIIIa is a single-chain glycoprotein with numerous intrachain disulfide bonds that cause it to migrate differently during reduced (Mr~105,000 daltons) or nonreduced (Mr~90,000) SDS-polyacrylamide gel electrophoresis. Structural studies suggest that the 2 polypeptides form a calcium-dependent complex when analyzed by crossed immunoelectrophoresis (9).

MOLECULAR BIOLOGY

The complementary DNA (cDNA) cloning of GPIIb and GPIIIa proved both important and interesting. Because standard cDNA cloning requires a source of messenger RNA (mRNA), which is absent in platelets, platelets could not be used as a source for the starting material. The discovery of a human erythroleukemia (HEL) cell line with megakaryocytic properties proved useful for these and many subsequent molecular and cellular biology studies on platelets (8). The isolation and sequencing of the cDNAs for GPIIb and GPIIIa from HEL cell cDNA libraries confirmed much of the biochemical data (10–13). The GPIIb cDNA codes for 1,039 amino acids: 137 for GPIIb$_\beta$, 871 for GPIIb$_\alpha$, and a 31–amino acid signal peptide (11). The GPIIb$_\beta$ has a hydrophobic sequence of 26 amino acids near the carboxyl-terminus representing a short transmembrane domain (10). Four domains of 12 amino acids each are present in GPIIb$_\alpha$ that are homologous to calcium-binding regions of calmodulin and troponin C. A 3.4-kilobase (kb) mRNA was identified by Northern blotting of HEL-cell mRNA. An alternately spliced mRNA for GPIIb that has a 34–amino acid deletion in the extracellular domain of GPIIb$_\beta$ has also been identified (14). The GPIIIa cDNA encodes a 788–amino acid protein containing a long amino-terminal extracellular domain with several potential N-linked glycosylation sites and 4 cysteine-rich tandem repeats (12–13). A 29-residue hydrophobic transmembrane segment is followed by a short carboxyl-terminal cytoplasmic domain.

The genes for GPIIb and GPIIIa are quite large, approximately 20 kb and 40 kb, respectively. The majority of both genes have been cloned. The intron-exon structure has been completely determined for GPIIb (15). It spans approximately 17.2 kb, has 30 exons, and is transcribed into a 3.4-kb mRNA. The full size for the GPIIIa gene has yet to be determined but is at least 40 kb. The mature GPIIIa protein is derived from 14 exons (16). The region of the gene upstream and including the signal peptide has only been isolated recently (17). The genes for GPIIb and GPIIIa are physically linked within 260 kb of one another on chromosome 17q21.23 (18).

Moving?

I'd like to receive my *Year Book of Hematology* without interruption.
Please not the following change of address, effective:

Name: _____

New Address: _____

_____

City: _____ State: _____ Zip: _____

Old Address: _____

_____

City: _____ State: _____ Zip: _____

Reservation Card

Yes, I would like my own copy of *Year Book of Hematology*. Please begin my subscription with the current edition according to the terms described below.* I understand that I will have 30 days to examine each annual edition. If satisfied, I will pay just $64.95 plus sales tax, postage and handling (price subject to change without notice).

Name: _____

Address: _____

City: _____ State: _____ Zip: _____

Method of Payment
○ Visa ○ Mastercard ○ AmEx ○ Bill me ○ Check (in US dollars, payable to Mosby, Inc.)

Card number: _____ Exp date: _____

Signature: _____

LS-0908

*Your *Year Book* Service Guarantee:

When you subscribe to the *Year Book*, we'll send you an advance notice of future volumes about two months before they publish. This automatic notice system is designed to take up as little of your time as possible. If you do not want the *Year Book*, the advance notice makes it quick and easy for you to let us know your decision, and you will always have at least 20 days to decide. If we don't hear from you, we'll send you the new volume as soon as it's available. And, of course, the *Year Book* is yours to examine free of charge for 30 days (postage, handling and applicable sales tax are added to each shipment.).

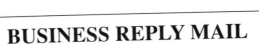

BUSINESS REPLY MAIL
FIRST CLASS MAIL   PERMIT No. 762   CHICAGO, IL

POSTAGE WILL BE PAID BY ADDRESSEE

Chris Hughes
Mosby-Year Book, Inc.
200 N. LaSalle Street
Suite 2600
Chicago, IL 60601-9981

NO POSTAGE
NECESSARY
IF MAILED
IN THE
UNITED STATES

BUSINESS REPLY MAIL
FIRST CLASS MAIL   PERMIT No. 762   CHICAGO, IL

POSTAGE WILL BE PAID BY ADDRESSEE

Chris Hughes
Mosby-Year Book, Inc.
200 N. LaSalle Street
Suite 2600
Chicago, IL 60601-9981

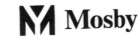 Mosby

Dedicated to publishing excellence

INTEGRINS

The amino acid sequences of GPIIb and GPIIIa helped define the integrin family of adhesion molecules. Integrins are structurally related molecules that bind adhesive glycoproteins (for review, see reference 19). Integrins consist of a large alpha-subunit and a smaller beta-subunit (not to be confused with $GPIIb_\alpha$ and $GPIIb_\beta$). The term integrin was coined to refer to an integral membrane protein that served as a bridge between the extracellular matrix and the cytoskeleton of the cell. Adhesive reactions are crucial to many diverse biological systems, including embryogenesis, inflammation, cell differentiation, tumor metastasis, wound repair, as well as hemostasis, and it is not surprising that all cells have integrins. Using the terminology of the integrins, platelets contain α_{IIb} and β_3. Figure 2 illustrates how GPIIb-IIIa, and most integrins, reside in the membrane.

The GPIIb gene is only expressed in the megakaryocyte/platelet lineage. The GPIIIa, or integrin β_3, also pairs with the integrin α_v, to form the vitronectin receptor, or $\alpha_v\beta_3$ (20–21). The GPIIIa expression is less restricted than GPIIb and has been identified in endothelial cells, human

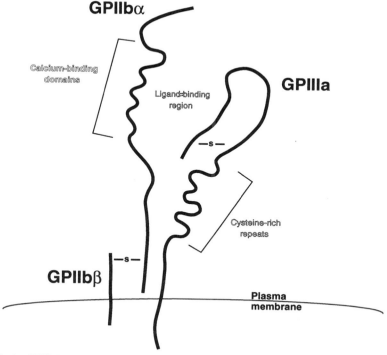

GPIIbα

Calcium-binding domains

Ligand-binding region

GPIIIa

—s—

Cysteine-rich repeats

—s—

GPIIbβ

Plasma membrane

Fig 2.—GPIIb-IIIa as a prototypic integrin. A model for the fibrinogen receptor in the platelet plasma membrane. $GPIIb_\alpha$ contains 4 calcium-binding domains and GPIIIa has 4 cysteine-rich domains. (Courtesy of P.F. Bray, M.D.)

placental syncytiotrophoblast brush border, and human osteoclasts as $\alpha_v\beta_3$. Less convincing data suggest that monocyte-derived macrophages and cultured human embryonic fibroblasts may express $\alpha_v\beta_3$. Several melanoma and osteosarcoma cell lines and a variety of nonhuman tissues have been reported to express β_3.

The GPIIb-IIIa belongs to a subclass of integrins characterized by their ability to bind ligands containing the Arg-Gly-Asp-Ser, or RGDS, sequence (22). This sequence, which was originally identified as the binding domain on the adhesive molecule fibronectin, was present in many other adhesive molecules, including fibrinogen (23). There is an additional region on fibrinogen that binds to GPIIb-IIIa: the gamma-chain dodecapeptide, HHLGGAKQAGDV (24). Biochemical cross-linking studies have provided a gross picture of the sites on the GPIIb-IIIa receptor that bind fibrinogen. Three regions have been identified: (1) amino acids 109–171 of GPIIIa (25); (2) amino acids 294–314 on GPIIb (26); and (3) amino acids 211–222 on GPIIIa (27). Localization of functionally critical residues is being further refined by the genetic analysis of mutations in the genes for GPIIb and GPIIIa (next section). Figure 2 shows how a pocket is formed by GPIIb and GPIIIa. This pocket is mutually exclusive, i.e., it can bind 1 or the other, but not both RGDS and the dodecapeptide.

Glanzmann's thrombasthenia

Dr. Glanzmann, a German pediatrician, originally described a bleeding diathesis in children that was characterized by diminished clot retraction. He thought this disorder was caused by abnormal blood platelets. The bleeding is of moderate severity and is usually present in the neonatal period (for review, see reference 1). This disorder, inherited in a classic mendelian autosomal recessive fashion, is the most common inherited abnormality of platelets. Glanzmann's thrombasthenia most often occurs in areas with a high incidence of consanguinity, and sporadic cases are unusual. It is characterized by mucocutaneous bleeding of mild to moderate severity. Platelets are normal in appearance and number, the bleeding time is prolonged, and there is absent platelet aggregation to all physiologic stimuli. Electrophoretic analysis of platelet proteins from the vast majority of patients with this disorder demonstrates a lack of GPIIb and GPIIIa (3). A handful of qualitative defects in GPIIb or GPIIIa have been described. Bleeding occurs in individuals with GT because their platelets are unable to bind fibrinogen and aggregate. For many years, investigators have been puzzled as to why 2 proteins should be missing in 1 disease.

At the protein level, GT has been well studied and has traditionally been classified according to the amount of residual GPIIb and GPIIIa in patient's platelets (columns 5 and 6 of Table 1). Originally, patients with thrombasthenia were divided into 2 groups: type I platelets completely lacked intracellular fibrinogen and did not support clot retraction, whereas type II platelets had decreased but detectable platelet fibrinogen

TABLE 1.—"Classic" Classification of GT

Type	GPIIb-IIIa Level	Platelet Aggregation	FGN Binding	Clot Retraction	FGN Deficiency in α Granules	Western Blot	
						IIb	IIIa
I	None to barely detectable	None	None	None	Moderate to severe	Occl Trace	Occl Trace
II	Low (5% to 20%)	Minimal	Minimal	Retarded	30% to 50%	Low	Low
III (Variants)	Normal	None to minimal	None to minimal	?	Variable	nl	nl

Abbreviation: FGN, fibrinogen.
(Courtesy of P.F. Bray, M.D.)

and clot retraction (28). Estimates of the amount of surface GPIIb-IIIa on the platelets of type I patients are 0% to 5%; platelets from type II patients have 5% to 20% GPIIb-IIIa (1). According to this classification, 78% of patients have type I disease, 14% are type II, and 8% are type III. Type III patients, or variant GT, have normal levels of immunologically detectable GPIIb-IIIa, but it is functionally abnormal. With the advent of more sophisticated laboratory techniques, characteristic abnormalities of protein content, platelet aggregation, and fibrinogen binding were identified (columns 2–4 of Table 1). Although GPIIb and GPIIIa are generally undetectable by conventional techniques in type I platelets, trace amounts (< 5% normal) can be demonstrated by sensitive iodine-125 Western immunoblotting (29).

GENETICS

From the genetic point of view, the protein classification system in Table 1 is not an accurate way to convey information regarding the molec-

TABLE 2.—Mutant Alleles Causing GT With Decreased Amounts of GPIIb-IIIa

Gene	Description	Reference
GPIIIa	15-kb Inversion/1-kb deletion from break points in 3 Alu sequences	30, 32
GPIIIa	11-bp Deletion in exon 12 → premature termination	33
GPIIIa	86-bp Deletion of exon 1 → premature termination; 3-point mutations at exon i-intron i	34
GPIIIa	Point mutation exon 4: ATgt → ATat, abnormal RNA splicing	35
GPIIIa	Point mutation exon 8: GGTGAgt → AGTGAgt, abnormal RNA splicing	35
GPIIb	4.5-kb Deletion of exons 2-9	36
GPIIb	13-bp Deletion in exon 4 → abnormal RNA splicing	33
GPIIb	Point mutation: CGA → TGA, Arg^{584} → stop	37
GPIIb	Point mutation exon 26: CAG → GAG; abnormal RNA splicing	37
GPIIb	Point mutation: Gly^{418} → Asp^{418}; GPIIb is 45 kD and presumably nonfunctional	38
GPIIb	Point mutation: Gly^{273} → Asp^{273}	39

(Courtesy of P.F. Bray, M.D.)

TABLE 3.—Mutations Causing Variant GT

Gene	Description	Reference
GPIIIa	Asp^{119} → Tyr^{119} point mutation	40
GPIIIa	Arg^{214} → Gln^{214} point mutation	41
GPIIIa	Arg^{214} → Trp^{214} point mutation unusually sensitive to EDTA dissociation at 22°C	42
GPIIIa	Ser^{752} → Pro^{752} point mutation in cytoplasmic domain; half normal numbers on platelet surface, nl internal pool	43

Abbreviation: EDTA, ethylenediamine tetraacetic acid.
(Courtesy of P.F. Bray, M.D.)

ular defect causing the disease. At the DNA level, it makes more sense to refer to "GPIIb mutations" or "GPIIIa mutations." This became clear once it was shown that the disease could be caused by mutations in only 1 gene (30), with the other being structurally normal. This experiment of nature was confirmed in the laboratory when O'Toole et al. (31) showed that both the GPIIb and GPIIIa subunits are needed for efficient surface expression of the complex in transfected COS cells. It is likely that an unpaired GPIIb or GPIIIa is degraded after synthesis in the endoplasmic reticulum. Using thalassemia as an example, a much more precise definition of the molecular pathogenesis is made when describing a patient as having a "β39 mutation" rather than a "low hemoglobin." Likewise, the distinction between type I and type II patients is artificial. Already, mutations have been described at the level of the gene for GPIIb and GPIIIa, which makes any attempt to classify according to a rigid definition of the amount of protein misleading. Thus, I will arbitrarily group all mutations according to whether or not there is immunologically detectable protein.

Table 2 summarizes the molecular defects causing nonvariant GT according to which gene is defective. Similar numbers of mutations have been described in both the genes for GPIIb and GPIIIa, which eventually lead to the production of reduced protein. No particular abnormal allele predominates. Large gene rearrangements as well as point mutations that result in abnormal mRNA splicing have yielded the thrombasthenic phenotype.

The especially interesting mutations have been the variants, which are listed in Table 3. In all cases, these are caused by point mutations affecting amino acids critical to receptor function, but not to receptor synthesis. The first 3 abnormal alleles contain nucleotide substitutions that change amino acids in the region of GPIIIa that had been previously shown to cross-link to the RGDs peptide, amino acids 109–171 and

211–222 (25, 27). The fourth variant is particularly important because it provides the first evidence for linkage between platelet cytoplasmic events and receptor activation. Chen et al. (43) found no defect in the intrinsic ability of the platelets from the kindred they studied to bind to fibrinogen. This suggests that in normal platelets, the cytoplasmic domain of GPIIIa responds to signals generated when platelets are stimulated by agonists, with subsequent conversion of an inactive receptor to one that is able to bind fibrinogen. The lack of identified mutations in the GPIIb gene that result in the variant type of GT is most likely coincidence caused by the small number of patients characterized. Thus, the characterization of amino acid substitutions that disrupt function of the GPIIb-IIIa receptor has confirmed the biochemical studies and greatly refined our understanding of the crucial residues involved in fibrinogen binding and receptor activation.

Clinical Significance

Initially, clinical studies on GPIIb-IIIa function addressed the role of the fibrinogen receptor in bleeding disorders and confirmed the essential role of GPIIb-IIIa in normal platelet function. More recently, a putative hyper-responsiveness of platelets has been incriminated in specific thrombotic syndromes. For example, in patients after myocardial infarction, spontaneous platelet aggregation appears to be a powerful predictor for the incidence of death (44). Aspirin and heparin have clinical usefulness in the treatment of patients who have had myocardial infarction, but both have limitations (45–49).

New therapies for cardiovascular disease have been developed that specifically interrupt fibrinogen binding to GPIIb-IIIa. Clinical trials in unstable coronary situations (unstable angina, high-risk angioplasty) have used the human/mouse chimeric c7E3-Fab (an anti-GPIIb-IIIa monoclonal antibody). This reagent was shown to prevent platelet aggregation induced by 20 μM of adenosine diphosphate and to be safe in terms of bleeding complications (50). Immune responses were not detectable when the chimeric antibody was used in phase I trials. In addition, this treatment was successful in preventing reocclusion in a canine model of coronary angioplasty (51).

A growing number of peptides derived from snake venoms have been found that inhibit platelet aggregation and contain an RGDS or RGDS-like sequence (52). Integrelin, a cyclic heptapeptide derived from the southeastern pygmy rattlesnake, has a lysine instead of an arginine (KGD vs. RGD) that dramatically increases the specificity of this heptapeptide for GPIIb-IIIa. Integrelin is about 5,000 times more potent than other RGD-containing peptides at specifically blocking GPIIb-IIIa and platelet aggregation. The off-rate of Integrelin from the receptor is about 1 order of magnitude faster than the off-rate of the antibodies (unpublished data), allowing a more rapid reversal of the effect of the peptide. This property may be useful in case of severe hemorrhage, or if emergent cardiac surgery becomes necessary.

Future

Despite the presence of GPIIb-IIIa on the surface of the platelet and the presence of fibrinogen in the circulation, platelets must be activated by an agonist before GPIIb-IIIa becomes competent to bind its ligand. The changes that these molecules undergo are not understood, and elucidating these changes is a very active area of investigation.

To study the mechanism of receptor activation, investigators began expressing recombinant GPIIb-IIIa in heterologous cell lines. Bodary et al. (63) expressed GPIIb-IIIa in the human embryonal kidney cell line, 293, and demonstrated levels of expression comparable with that in platelets. The transfected cells were able to bind to fibrinogen-coated plates. However, when these cells were stimulated with adenosine diphosphate, no binding of fibrinogen *in solution* occurred. This has been the experience of other investigators (54) and is important because platelets respond differently to fibrinogen in solution than to fibrinogen on a substrate (55). Although the nonactivated conformation of GPIIb-IIIa can bind insoluble fibrinogen, only the activated conformation binds to soluble fibrinogen. It is, therefore, essential that we acquire a greater understanding of *soluble* fibrinogen binding.

Expression of a GPIIb-IIIa receptor in CHO cells in which the cytoplasmic domain of GPIIb had been truncated resulted in an increased affinity of ligand for receptor in a complex assay assessing fibrinogen binding (56). These data suggested a possible negative regulatory role for the cytoplasmic domain of GPIIb in receptor activation. As mentioned, evidence from the analysis of a patient with GT suggests a *positive* role for the cytoplasmic domain of GPIIIa in receptor activation (43). Smyth and colleagues (57) have shown that phosphatidic acid increases fibrinogen binding in vitro to antibody "captured" GPIIb-IIIa but does not affect binding in intact platelets (57). These observations bear further investigation.

In summary, the molecular biology and genetics of the platelet fibrinogen receptor have moved at a very rapid pace during the past few years. The "bedside" study of a rare inherited disease has led to the "benchside" laboratory discovery and development of new reagents with which to combat vascular thrombotic disease.

References

1. George JN, Caen JP, Nurden AT: Glanzmann's thrombasthenia: the spectrum of clinical disease. *Blood* 75:1383–1395, 1990.
2. Bennett JS, Vilaire G: Exposure of platelet fibrinogen receptors by ADP and epinephrine. *J Clin Invest* 64:1393–1401, 1979.
3. Nurden AT, Caen JP: An abnormal platelet glycoprotein pattern in three cases of Glanzmann's thrombasthenia. *Br J Haematol* 28: 253–260, 1974.
4. Phillips DR, Agin PP: Platelet plasma membrane glycoproteins. *J Biol Chem* 252:2121–2126, 1977.
5. Peerschke E, Zucker MB, Grant RA, et al: Correlation between fibrinogen binding to human platelets and platelet aggregability. *Blood* 55:841–847, 1980.

6. Phillips DR, Charo IF, Parise LV, et al: The platelet membrane glycoprotein IIb-IIIa complex. *Blood* 71:831–843, 1988.
7. McEver RP, Baenziger NL, Majerus P: Isolation and quantitation of the platelet membrane deficiency in thrombasthenia using a monoclonal hybridoma antibody. *J Clin Invest* 66:1311–1318, 1980.
8. Bray PF, Rosa J-P, Lingappa VR, et al: Biogenesis of the platelet receptor for fibrinogen: evidence for separate precursors for glycoproteins IIb and IIIa. *Proc Natl Acad Sci USA* 83:1480–1484, 1986.
9. Kunicki TJ, Pidard D, Rosa JP, et al: The formation of calcium-dependent complexes of platelet membrane glycoproteins IIb and IIIa in solution as determined by crossed immunoelectrophoresis. *Blood* 58:268–278, 1981.
10. Bray PF, Rosa J-P, Johnston GI, et al: Platelet glycoprotein IIb: chromosomal location and tissue expression. *J Clin Invest* 80:1812–1817, 1987.
11. Poncz M, Eisman R, Heidenreich R, et al: Structure of the platelet membrane glycoprotein IIb. *J Biol Chem* 262:8476–8482, 1987.
12. Rosa J-P, Bray PF, Gayet O, et al: Cloning of glycoprotein IIIa cDNA from human erythroleukemia cells and localization of the gene to chromosome 17. *Blood* 72:593–600, 1988.
13. Fitzgerald LA, Steiner B, Rall SC Jr, et al: Protein sequence of endothelial glycoprotein IIIa derived from a cDNA clone. *J Biol Chem* 262:3936–3939, 1987.
14. Bray PF, Leung S-I, Shuman MA: Human platelets and megakaryocytes contain alternately spliced glycoprotein IIb mRNAs. *J Biol Chem* 265:9587–9590, 1990.
15. Heidenreich R, Eisman R, Surrey S, et al: Organization of the gene for platelet glycoprotein IIb. *Biochemistry* 29:1232–1244, 1990.
16. Zimrin AB, Gidwitz S, Lord S, et al: The genomic organization of platelet glycoprotein IIIa. *J Biol Chem* 265:8590–8595, 1990.
17. Villa-Garcia M, Li L, Reily G, et al: Characterization of the 5′ region of the gene for platelet glycoprotein IIIa. *Blood* 80:164a, 1992.
18. Bray PF, Barsh G, Rosa J-P, et al: Physical linkage of the genes for platelet membrane glycoproteins IIb and IIIa. *Proc Natl Acad Sci USA* 85:8683–8687, 1988.
19. Hynes RO: Integrins: modulation, and signalling in cell adhesion. *Cell* 69:11–25, 1992.
20. Ginsberg MH, Loftus J, Ryckwaert J-J, et al: Immunochemical and amino-terminal sequence comparison of two cytoadhesions indicates they contain similar or identical β subunits and distinct α subunits. *J Biol Chem* 262:5437–5440, 1987.
21. Giltay JC, Leeksma OC, von dem Borne AEG Jr, et al: Alloantigenic composition of the endothelial vitronectin receptor. *Blood* 72:230–233, 1988.
22. Pytela R, Pierschbacher MD, Ginsberg MH, et al: Platelet membrane glycoprotein IIb/IIIa: member of a family of Arg-Gly-Asp–specific adhesion receptors. *Science* 231:1559–1562, 1986.
23. Pierschbacher MD, Ruoslahti E: Cell attachment activity of fibronectin can be duplicated by small synthetic fragments of the molecule. *Nature* 309:30–33, 1984.
24. Kloczewiak M, Timmons S, Lukas TJ, et al: Platelet receptor recognition site on human fibrinogen. Synthesis and structure-function relationship of peptides corresponding to the carboxy-terminal segment of the γ chain. *Biochemistry* 23:1767–1774, 1984.
25. D'Souza SE, Ginsberg MH, Burke TA, et al: Localization of an Arg-Gly-Asp recognition site within an integrin adhesion receptor. *Science* 242:91–93, 1988.
26. D'Souza SE, Ginsberg MH, Burke TA, et al: The ligand binding site of the platelet integrin receptor GPIIb-IIIa is proximal to the second calcium binding domain of its α subunit. *J Biol Chem* 265:3440–3446, 1990.
27. Charo IF, Nanizzi L, Phillips DR, et al: Inhibition of fibrinogen binding to GPIIb-IIIa by a GPIIIa peptide. *J Biol Chem* 266:1415–1421, 1991.
28. Caen JP: Glanzmann's thrombasthenia. *Clin Haematol* 1:383–392, 1972.
29. Nurden AT, Didry D, Kieffer N, et al: Residual amounts of glycoproteins IIb and IIIa may be present in the platelets of most patients with Glanzmann's thrombasthenia. *Blood* 65:1021–1024, 1985.

30. Bray PF, Shuman MA: Identification of an abnormal gene for the GPIIIa subunit of the platelet fibrinogen receptor resulting in Glanzmann's thrombasthenia. *Blood* 75:881–888, 1990.

31. O'Toole TE, Loftus JC, Plow EF, et al: Efficient surface expression of platelet GPIIb-IIIa requires both subunits. *Blood* 74:14–18, 1989.

32. Li L, Bray PF: Homologous recombination among 3 intragene Alu sequences causes an inversion-deletion resulting in the hereditary bleeding disorder Glanzmann thrombasthenia. *Am J Hum Genet* (in press).

33. Newman PJ, Seligsohn U, Lyman S, et al: The molecular genetic basis of Glanzmann thrombasthenia in the Iraqi-Jewish and Arab populations in Israel. *Proc Natl Acad Sci USA* 88:3160–3164, 1991.

34. Simsek S, Heyboer H, de Bruihne LG, et al: Glanzmann's thrombasthenia caused by homozygosity for a splice defect that leads to deletion of the first coding exon of the glycoprotein IIIa mRNA. *Blood* 81:2044–2049, 1993.

35. Jin Y, Bray PF: The single strand chain polymorphism (SSCP) technique identifies two mutations in Glanzmann thrombasthenia and platelet-specific alloantigens. (In preparation.)

36. Burk CD, Newman PJ, Lyman S, et al: A deletion in the gene for glycoprotein IIb associated with Glanzmann's thrombasthenia. *J Clin Invest* 87:270–276, 1991.

37. Kato A, Yamamoto K, Miyazaki S, et al: Molecular basis for Glanzmann's thrombasthenia (GT) in a compound heterozygote with the GPIIb gene: a proposal for the classification of GT based on the biosynthetic pathway of glycoprotein IIb-IIIa complex. *Blood* 79:3212–3218, 1992.

38. Wilcox DA, Wautier J-L, Pidard D, et al: An amino acid substitution within the fourth calcium binding region of GPIIb results in degradation of the integrin GPIIb-IIIa and type I Glanzmann thrombasthenia. *Circulation* 86:I-682, 1992.

39. Bennett JS, Vilaire G, Rifat S, et al: Effect of a Gly$\rightarrow$Asp mutation in the first calcium binding domain of platelet glycoprotein IIb on the expression of the glycoprotein IIb-IIIa complex. *Blood* 80:73a, 1992.

40. Loftus JC, O'Toole TE, Plow EF, et al: A β_3 integrin mutation abolishes ligand binding and alters divalent cation-dependent conformation. *Science* 249:915–918, 1990.

41. Bajt ML, Ginsberg MH, Frelinger AL III, et al: A spontaneous mutation of integrin $\alpha_{IIb}\beta_3$ (platelet glycoprotein IIb-IIIa) helps define a ligand binding site. *J Biol Chem* 267:3789–3794, 1992.

42. Lanza F, Stierlé A, Fournier D, et al: A new variant of Glanzmann's thrombasthenia (Strasbourg I). Platelets with functionally defective glycoprotein IIb-IIIa complexes and a glycoprotein III ^{214}Arg$\rightarrow^{214}$Trp mutation. *J Clin Invest* 89:1995–2004, 1992.

43. Chen Y-P, Djaffar I, Pidard D, et al: Ser$^{752}\rightarrow$Pro mutation in the cytoplasmic domain of integrin β_3 subunit and defective activation of platelet integrin $\alpha_{IIb}\beta_3$ (glycoprotein IIb-IIIa) in a variant of Glanzmann thrombasthenia. *Proc Natl Acad Sci USA* 89:10169–10173, 1992.

44. Trip MD, Cats VM, van Capelle FJL, et al: Platelet hyperreactivity and prognosis in survivors of myocardial infarction. *N Engl J Med* 322:1549–1554, 1990.

45. ISIS-1 (Second International Study of Infarct Survival) Collaborative Group: Randomized trial of intravenous streptokinase, oral aspirin, both, or neither among 17,187 cases of suspected acute myocardial infarction. ISIS-2. *Lancet* 13:349–360, 1988.

46. Lewis HD, Davis JW, Archibald DG, et al: Protective effects of aspirin against acute myocardial infarction and death in men with unstable angina. *N Engl J Med* 309:396–403, 1983.

47. Steering Committee of the Physicians' Health Study Research Group: Final report on the aspirin component of the ongoing physicians' health study. *N Engl J Med* 321:129–135, 1989.

48. Theroux P, Oiumet H, McCans J, et al: Aspirin, heparin, or both to treat acute unstable angina. *N Engl J Med* 319:1105–1111, 1988.

49. Theroux P, Waters D, Lam J, et al: Reactivation of unstable angina after the discontinuation of heparin. N Engl J Med 327:141–145, 1992.
50. Bernardi MM, Califf RM, Kleiman N, et al: Prolonged bleeding times do not predict hemorrhagic events in patients receiving the 7E3 glycoprotein IIB/IIIa platelet antibody. Circulation 86:260a, 1992.
51. Bates ER, McGillem MJ, Mickelson JK, et al: A monoclonal antibody against the platelet glycoprotein IIb/IIIa receptor complex prevents platelet aggregation and thrombosis in a canine model of coronary angioplasty. Circulation 84:2463–2469, 1991.
52. Dennis MS, Henzel WJ, Pitti RM, et al: Platelet glycoprotein IIb-IIIa protein antagonists from snake venoms: evidence for a family of platelet-aggregation inhibitors. Proc Natl Acad Sci USA 87:2471–2475, 1989.
53. Bodary SC, Napier MA, McLean JW: Expression of recombinant platelet glycoprotein IIbIIIa results in a functional fibrinogen-binding complex. J Biol Chem 264:18859–18862, 1989.
54. O'Toole TE, Loftus JC, Du X, et al: Affinity modulation of the $\alpha_{IIb} \beta_3$ integrin (platelet GPIIb-IIIa) is an intrinsic property of the receptor. Cell Regula 1:883–893, 1990.
55. Savage B, Ruggeri ZM: Selective recognition of adhesive sites in surface-bound fibrinogen by glycoprotein IIb-IIIa on nonactivated platelets. J Biol Chem 266:11227–11233, 1991.
56. O'Toole TE, Mandleman D, Forsyth J, et al: Modulation of the affinity of the integrin $\alpha_{IIb} \beta_3$ (GPIIb-IIIa) by the cytoplasmic domain of α_{IIb}. Science 254:845–847, 1991.
57. Smyth SS, Hillery CA, Parise LV: Phosphatidic and lysophosphatidic acid modulate the fibrinogen binding activity of purified platelet glycoprotein IIb-IIIa. Blood 78:278a, 1991.

4 Hematologic Malignancies

Introduction

A significant number of new diagnostic and therapeutic advances have been reported since the 1994 YEAR BOOK was compiled. The number of true advances that continue to be reported each year is truly amazing, especially when considering the unfavorable research climate in which we continue to function. These advances are the product of the intellect and perseverance of laboratory and clinical investigators around the world and are, indeed, a tribute to them. I attempt to briefly summarize some of the most important of these advances that are described in greater detail in the following pages.

Hodgkin's Disease

Ferry et al. (Abstract 4–4) demonstrate the value in the histologic subclassification of nodular sclerosis according to the criteria of the British National Lymphoma Investigation. With this scheme, relapsed patients with nodular sclerosis who have a significantly better prognosis than others can be identified. This subclassification should now be required in studies of salvage therapy.

The Cancer and Leukemia Group B report the results of a major study in which mechlorethamine, vincristine, procarbazine, and prednisone (MOPP), doxorubicin, bleomycine, vinblastine, and dacarbazine (ABVD), and MOPP alternating with ABVD were compared in patients with advanced stage disease (Abstract 4–7). Patients who received doxorubicin had a significantly better response rate, although failure-free and overall survival did not differ among the treatment options. The study demonstrates the major activity of doxorubicin in the treatment of Hodgkin's disease, but the results do not support the commonly held notion that treatment with alternating noncross-resistant regimens is superior to single-regimen administration, because results with both doxorubicin-based regimens were essentially identical. The study may leave open the question of whether ABVD is better treatment than MOPP in the minds of some, since MOPP was not given as described by the National Cancer Institute. However, it is clear from the study that unacceptable toxicity would have resulted without attenuation of MOPP doses and that ABVD at full dose is better tolerated than MOPP at full dose. One can conclude from this study that when ABVD or MOPP is given with acceptable acute toxicity, results are better with ABVD. In my view, there is some concern for long-term cardiotoxicity with ABVD, but decades may be required to evaluate the validity of that concern.

The question whether autologous bone marrow transplantation is required for optimal results in refractory Hodgkin's disease is raised by Tourani et al. (Abstract 4–17) who report excellent results with a high-dose salvage regimen without autologous marrow transplantation. Desch et al. (Abstract 4–19) attempted to define the optimal timing of autologous transplantation for Hodgkin's disease and conclude that it should be reserved for second relapse. It seems clear from these and other studies that the prognosis for refractory and relapsed patients has considerably improved recently.

Non-Hodgkin's Lymphoma

DeAngelis et al. (Abstract 4–23) demonstrate that cranial irradiation plus high-dose intravenous cytarabine significantly improved disease-free survival compared with irradiation alone in patients with primary CNS lymphoma. There seems to be an increasing incidence of this still-rare lymphoma, and combined modality therapy may now be the treatment of choice.

Fludarabine has been identified by Redman et al. (Abstract 4–24) as a drug with major activity in follicular lymphoma. Although significant and permanent bone marrow suppression can be observed after multiple courses of this agent, it will unquestionably play a major role in low-grade lymphomas.

The Eastern Cooperative Oncology Group (ECOG) (Abstract 4–25) report that interferon-alfa can significantly prolong the time to treatment failure, complete response duration, and overall survival in patients with progressive low-grade or intermediate-grade lymphoma. Others have reported similar findings, and chemotherapy plus interferon may become standard therapy for these lymphomas. Whether interferon must be given along with induction therapy as in the ECOG study or only during remission as in most other studies is an open question at present.

Myeloma and Waldenström's Disease

A simple and potentially useful staging system for myeloma based on measurements of serum C-reactive protein and beta$_2$-microglobulin is proposed by Bataille et al. (Abstract 4–30). C-reactive protein levels reflect IL-6 activity and beta$_2$-microglobulin levels reflect tumor bulk. The system allowed for segregation of myeloma patients into low-, intermediate-, and high-risk groups with significantly different median survivals.

Jagannath et al. (Abstract 4–32) demonstrate the value of adding peripheral blood stem cell infusions to autologous bone marrow transplantation for support of myeloma patients undergoing intensive therapy. More than 80% of patients had complete hematologic recovery within a month. Peripheral stem cells have been shown by others to hasten marrow recovery after transplantation in a number of diseases now.

2-Chlorodeoxyadenosine is shown by Dimopoulos et al. (Abstract 4–33) to have major activity against Waldenström's macroglobulinemia. Responses were obtained in all of 9 previously untreated patients and in 40% of 20 patients who had failed previous treatment. This represents the discovery of an important new treatment for this disease.

Chronic Lymphocytic and Hairy-Cell Leukemia

Fludarabine has been accepted as an important new drug for chronic lymphocytic leukemia (CLL) and other lymphoid neoplasms as noted previously. Robertson et al. (Abstract 4–36) report that the vast majority of complete clinical responders to fludarabine had no detectable minimal residual disease by marrow biopsy, flow cytometry, and immunoglobulin gene rearrangement studies. Such patients had greater response durations than those with minimal residual disease after treatment. Anaissie et al. (Abstract (4–35) from the same institution remind us that the drug is quite immunosuppressive and report that they observed an increased incidence of listeriosis in fludarabine-treated patients with CLL.

Juliusson et al. (Abstract 4–38) show that 2-chlorodeoxyadenosine can produce complete responses in patients with CLL who fail with fludarabine, and Tallman et al. (Abstract 4–34) confirm the high rate of apparent complete responses in hairy-cell leukemia after a single cycle of that agent. However, there have been several demonstrations lately of the detection of minimal residual disease in patients with hairy-cell leukemia in apparent complete response after 2-chlorodeoxyadenosine treatment. To date, there has been no difference in response duration in patients with or without detectable minimal residual disease, but the work of Robertson et al. noted before suggests that such reports might be expected in the future.

Chronic Myelocytic Leukemia

In a fascinating case report, Drobyski et al. (Abstract 4–45) describe a patient with chronic myeloid leukemia (CML) who failed 2 allogeneic bone marrow transplantations but completely eradicated her leukemic clone after graft-vs.-host disease developed from leukocyte transfusions donated by the second marrow donor. Her complete molecular remission had lasted almost a year when the report was prepared. Leukocyte transfusions were an effective form of adoptive immunotherapy in this patient and should be systematically studied in other patients.

Kantarjian et al. (Abstract 4–40) studied interferon-alpha and low-dose cytarabine in advanced CML and found the combination yielded significantly better results than interferon-alpha alone. They suggest studying the combination in the early chronic phase.

Myelodysplasia

No true therapeutic advances have been reported for myelodysplasia in some time. Several interesting reports on prognostic factors have appeared, however. An example is the report by Sullivan et al. (Abstract 4–48) in which patients were tested for circulating CD34+ cells. They found the absence of such cells to be strongly correlated with the lack of transformation to frank leukemia during observation. It seems reasonable to monitor patients with myelodysplasia for the appearance of circulating CD34+ cells, which may be the harbinger of clinical transformation to acute leukemia.

Acute Myeloid Leukemia

A number of important observations concerning the treatment of acute promyelocytic leukemia with all-*trans* retinoic acid have been made recently. Frankel et al. (Abstract 4–69) describe a potentially lethal syndrome of fever and respiratory distress that is related to treatment. Prompt corticosteroid administration may interrupt the progressive deterioration of pulmonary function, but this is not entirely clear. They observed this problem in 9 of 35 patients, which is a higher incidence than that observed in the current intergroup study. Muindi et al. (Abstract 4–70) report that continuous oral administration of the agent for 2–6 weeks was associated with a significant decrease in both the plasma peak level and the area under the concentration × time curve in most patients. They suggest that rapid disappearance of the agent may explain the early relapse observed in some patients who have responded to it. Fenaux et al. (Abstract 4–71) and Dombret et al. (Abstract 4–72) report that all-*trans* retinoic acid followed by standard acute myeloid leukemia (AML) induction chemotherapy is better than retinoic acid alone for treatment of acute promyelocytic leukemia because response rates may be higher with sequential therapy and response duration may be longer. These observations are consistent with the pharmacokinetic observations of Muindi et al.

The ECOG studied the relative merits of allogeneic bone marrow transplantation, continuous maintenance therapy for 2 years, and a single course of high-dose consolidation therapy for patients with AML in complete remission. The results with allogeneic bone marrow transplantation and with consolidation therapy were significantly better than those with maintenance therapy. However, there was no event-free or overall survival difference between the 2 intensive therapies. This study led to the current intergroup study (Abstract 4–78) in which allogeneic or autologous bone marrow transplantation, or high-dose consolidation therapy are the postremission options.

The Southeastern Cancer Study Group (Abstract 4–58) published the fourth prospective, randomized study in which 1 or more significant advantages for idarubicin compared with daunorubicin for induction therapy of AML was demonstrated. Berman and McBride (Abstract 4–59) report that idarubicin kills leukemia cell lines that express P-glyprotein much more effectively in vitro than does daunorubicin. This observation may be related to the clinical therapeutic advantage for idarubicin rather than daunorubicin.

Significant activity of carboplatin in relapsed and refractory leukemia was confirmed by the ECOG. A 36% complete response rate in AML in the first relapse was observed, which clearly warrants further investigation. The ECOG is now studying the drug in advanced CML.

Bajorin et al. (Abstract 4–66) and Nichols et al. (Abstract 4–67) report a noteworthy incidence of secondary AML in patients with germ cell tumor treated with etoposide-containing regimens. Although of concern, information collected to date does not compel the discontinuation of this important drug in germ cell tumor therapy.

Michel et al. (Abstract 4–97) report that the outcome for children receiving allogeneic bone marrow transplantation for AML in the first remission has improved in France in recent years, primarily because of advances in supportive care. Similar reports have appeared from the United States. Blaise et al. (Abstract 4–99) report that busulfan-cyclophosphamide is a safer and more effective preparation for allogeneic transplantation than total body irradiation–cyclophosphamide for patients with AML in the first remission. Clift et al. (Abstract 4–98) find methotrexate alone to be better prophylaxis for graft-vs.-host disease than when combined with cyclosporin.

Acute Lymphocytic Leukemia

Trisomy 21 as the sole acquired chromosomal abnormality in children with ALL occurred in 1.8% of more than 600 well-studied patients at St. Jude Children's Research Hospital (Memphis), and Raimondi et al. (Abstract 4–84) report that they all readily achieved complete remission. They suggest that this karyotype may confer an excellent prognosis in children with acute lymphoblastic leukemia (ALL). Patients known to have Down syndrome were excluded from the analysis. Interestingly, the Pediatric Oncology Group (Abstract 4–65) report that AML in Down syndrome is highly responsive to treatment.

Lanning et al. (Abstract 4–89) report that treatment results in females with high-risk ALL in childhood are superior to those in males, and Schiller et al. (Abstract 4–77) report the same findings in adults with AML.

Westbrook et al. (Abstract 4–85) suggest that the *bcr-abl* gene may impact on the remission duration in adult ALL but not on the response rate. Therefore, identification of this gene should be required for all patients entering clinical trials for ALL.

Kantarjian et al. (Abstract 4–86) show that beta$_2$-microglobulin elevation in adult ALL is associated with a lower response rate, worse survival, and greater incidence of CNS leukemia. This marker should be required in adult ALL studies as well.

Bone Marrow Transplantation

Hepatic veno-occlusive disease is a major treatment-related complication of bone marrow transplantation and is the third leading cause of death in transplant patients. Attal et al. (Abstract 4–107) found that continuous infusion of low-dose heparin resulted in significantly fewer incidences of veno-occlusive disease in patients undergoing autologous or allogeneic bone marrow transplantation, compared with unheparinized controls.

An increasing number of reports concern the role of IL-2 in the treatment of AML with and without bone marrow transplantation. Sykes et al. (Abstract 4–109) found that IL-2 reduces graft-vs.-host disease while not interfering with a graft-vs.-leukemia effect.

Vogelsang et al. (Abstract 4–110) in a phase II study found that thalidomide was a safe and effective treatment for chronic graft-vs.-host disease, and they suggest that a prospective comparison of that agent with prednisone should be done.

Peter H. Wiernik, M.D.

Hodgkin's Disease

Subtypes of Epstein-Barr Virus (EBV) in Hodgkin's Disease: Association Between B-Type EBV and Immunocompromise
Boyle MJ, Vasak E, Tschuchnigg M, Turner JJ, Sculley T, Penny R, Cooper DA, Tindall B, Sewell WA (St Vincent's Hosp, Sydney, Australia; Queensland Inst of Med Research, Brisbane, Australia; Univ of New South Wales, Sydney, Australia)
Blood 81:468–474, 1993   4–1

Purpose.—As many as half the patients with Hodgkin's disease (HD) have associated Epstein-Barr virus (EBV). The EBV in these patients has been reported to be of the A type exclusively. The role of EBV subtypes in HD among both previously healthy and immunocompromised patients was examined.

Methods.—The subjects were 30 patients with HD; 15 had the nodular sclerosing type, 10 had mixed cellularity HD, and 5 had lymphocyte-depleted HD. Biopsy samples from these patients were assessed for EBV sequences by using both the PCR and in situ hybridization.

Findings.—Samples from 9 patients had EBV localized to malignant Reed-Sternberg cells and their mononuclear variants. Seven of these patients had A-type EBV sequences, and 2 had B-type sequences. The latter 2 patients also had evidence of preexisting immune compromise; 1 had HIV infection and severe CD4+ T-lymphocyte depletion; and the other was a debilitated, elderly patient with dementia.

Conclusion.—Epstein-Barr virus appears to be an important cofactor for the development of HD. This study, along with a previous report of B-type EBV in patients with HIV-associated non-Hodgkin's lymphoma, suggests that B-type EBV may be an important human pathogen in immunocompromised patients. The patients with HD who were EBV-positive were significantly younger than the EBV-negative patients.

Distribution and Phenotype of Epstein-Barr Virus–Harboring Cells in Hodgkin's Disease

Herbst H, Steinbrecher E, Niedobitek G, Young LS, Brooks L, Müller-Lantzsch N, Stein H (Free Univ, Berlin; Univ of Birmingham, England; Univ of Saarland, Homburg/Saar, Germany)
Blood 80:484–491, 1992

4–2

Background.—The significance of Epstein-Barr virus (EBV) genomes in patients with Hodgkin's disease (HD) remains controversial. Though EBV DNA has been found in Hodgkin's and Reed-Sternberg (H-RS) cells, it has been argued that the DNA may have come from non–H-RS cells in the tissue biopsies. These criticisms are further supported by the prevalence (90%) of a latent EBV infection, suggesting that some EBV-infected lymphocytes are likely to be found in any lymphoid biopsies. The significance of EBV infection was assessed by examining the presence of EBER1 and EBER2 (small EBV-encoded nonpolyadenylated RNA transcripts) via in situ hybridization in H-RS cells.

Methods.—Lymph node biopsy samples were obtained from 46 patients with HD. To determine the distribution and phenotype of EPV-harboring cells, in situ hybridization using [^{35}S]-labeled RNA probes geared toward the small EBV-encoded nuclear RNAs (EBER1 and EBER2) was performed. Immunohistology for CD20, CD30, CD45RO, and CD68 antigens; the T-cell receptor beta-chain; and latent membrane antigen (LMP) of EBV preceded in situ hybridization in some cases.

Results.—Of the 46 patients with HD, 23 demonstrated EBER transcripts in all H-RS cells. The expression of LMP was noted exclusively in neoplastic cells in 18 of these patients. The EBER+ small reactive cells were found in 42 patients. Of these, an abundant quantity of cells were noted in 3 patients, whereas low numbers were revealed in 39 patients. Therefore, an unrestricted proliferation of reactive EBER+/LMP− lymphoid cells did not accompany the presence of H-RS cells (with or without LMP expression) in most of the patients with HD. A phenotype of mature B lymphocytes and a polyclonal composition for a large proportion of the EBER+ small cells were noted via coincident in situ hybridization using [^{35}S-] labeled immunoglobulin light-chain gene probes and nonisotopically labeled EBER probes. However, CD20 expression was not detectable in many of these cells (in contrast to noninfected cells). Therefore, downregulation of particular differentiation antigens in latently EBV-infected small lymphoid cells may be indicated in vivo.

Conclusion.—The presence of EBV DNA and LMP expression in H-RS cells is the most frequently observed abnormality in patients with HD. This supports the contention that EBV is at least 1 of possibly several etiologic agents responsible for cellular transformation in a subset of patients with HD. However, more studies are needed before the significance of EBV infection in HD pathogenesis can be conclusively established.

▶ The Boyle et al. article (Abstract 4–1) suggests that if EBV is etiologically related to HD, different types may cause the disease under different circumstances. The Herbst et al. article (Abstract 4–2) described a method by which EBV-infected cells can be identified with light microscopy and demonstrates that EBV is present primarily in Hodgkin's cells rather than reactive cells.—P.H. Wiernik, M.D.

IgE in Reed-Sternberg Cells of Hodgkin's Disease With Eosinophilia
Samoszuk M (Univ of California, Irvine)
Blood 79:1518–1522, 1992   4–3

Introduction.—In Hodgkin's disease (HD) of the nodular sclerosis and mixed cellularity types, tissues often are infiltrated by eosinophils that undergo degranulation. Increased levels of serum IgE also are recognized in patients with HD. A sensitive, specific immunohistochemical procedure was used to determine the distribution of IgE in fixed tissues.

Patients.—The study comprised 1 patient with lymphocyte-predominance HD, 7 patients with nodular sclerosing HD, and 6 patients with mixed-cellularity HD. Five patients with benign hyperplastic lymphoid hyperplasia and 5 with B-cell lymphoma lacking eosinophilia also were examined.

Results.—Eleven of 14 patients with HD exhibited deposits of IgE within most Reed-Sternberg cells and their variants. In some, interstitial and extracellular deposits of IgE also were noted, but staining was limited to areas containing histologic evidence of HD. Both patients studied had moderately increased serum IgE levels. Three patients with eosinophilia and IgE exhibited IL-5 messenger RNA as well.

Conclusion.—Some tissue samples of HD contain abundant deposits of IgE. Eosinophilia in HD may reflect both localized deposition of IgE within the tumor and the synthesis of IL-5, possibly by Reed-Sternberg cells infected by the Epstein-Barr virus.

▶ This is an interesting extension of our knowledge about Reed-Sternberg cells with a demonstration of the presence of IgE. As the author comments, this does not establish B-cell origin of Reed-Sternberg cells; the true origin and identity of these cells remain a mystery. It does seem that, by this time, investigators should have been able to get a handle on the central actor in the Hodgkin's drama. This is perhaps a commentary on the difficulties of clinical research and of applying existent methodologies to the characterization of the Reed-Sternberg cell. Perhaps the major difficulty is in getting adequate initial tumor tissue, under the appropriate conditions, for study. Seemingly, a concerted effort to obtain viable sterile Hodgkin's tissue with focused attempts to separate pure populations of Reed-Sternberg cells by immunologic physical and metabolic parameters should result in a population of cells appropriate for definitive classification. This should be achievable by application of molecular genetic and immunologic techniques.—P.J. Quesenberry, M.D.

Hodgkin Disease, Nodular Sclerosis Type: Implications of Histologic Subclassification

Ferry JA, Linggood RM, Convery KM, Efird JT, Eliseo R, Harris NL (Massachusetts Gen Hosp, Boston; Med Practices Evaluation Ctr, Boston)
Cancer 71:457–463, 1993   4–4

Introduction.—It has been suggested in Europe that the subclassification of Hodgkin's disease, nodular sclerosis type (HDNS), may have prognostic significance. Using the same criteria as the British National Lymphoma Investigation (BNLI), Americans have given conflicting results. Patients with HDNS were subclassified for histologic grade, degree

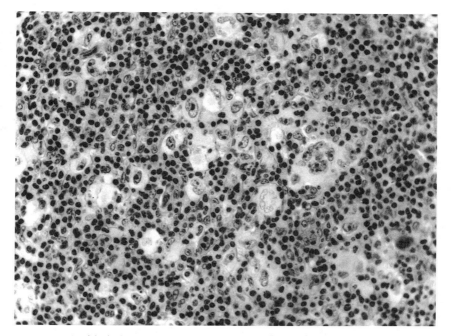

Fig 4–1.—Hodgkin's disease (NSI). Moderate numbers of Reed-Sternberg cells and variants are intermixed with numerous small lymphocytes. (Courtesy of Ferry JA, Linggood RM, Convery KM, et al: *Cancer* 71:457–463, 1993.)

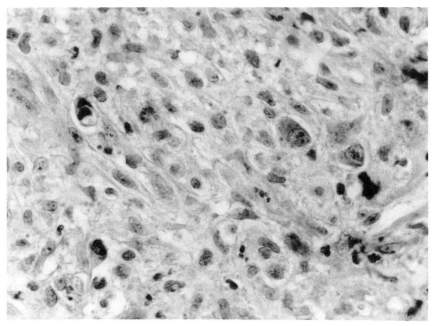

Fig 4–2.—Hodgkin's disease (NSI). There is predominance of bland fibrohistiocytic cells, rare lymphocytes, and a few large atypical cells. Despite the paucity of lymphocytes, this case is classified as NSI because of the small number of atypical cells. (Courtesy of Ferry JA, Linggood RM, Convery KM, et al: *Cancer* 71:457–463, 1993.)

of sclerosis, and presence of necrosis to determine the prognostic significance of these features.

Patients and Methods.—Tumors from 55 female and 24 male patients with a mean age of 27 years were studied. Thirteen patients had stage I disease, 45 had stage II disease, and 21 had stage III disease. Fifty-three patients had not had a relapse; 49 of the 53 were in complete clinical remission. Disease progression or relapse occurred in 26 patients; 17 had successful salvage therapy. The histologic criteria of the BNLI were used in the histologic subclassification of the cellular infiltrate within the nodules.

Findings.—Fifty-eight patients were classified as low grade (NSI) (Figs 4–1 and 4–2) and 21 as high grade (NSII). Twenty of the latter group had prominent areas of lymphocyte depletion (Fig 4–3); only 1 had pleomorphic Reed-Sternberg cells (Fig 4–4). Patients in the NSII subclassification had significantly shorter overall survival, as did those with extensive necrosis, high disease stage, and B symptoms. On multivariate analysis, grade had the strongest effect on survival. All the NSI patients were alive at 5 years, compared with 75% of the NSII group. The only factor significantly associated with risk of relapse was B symptoms; for patients who had relapse, the only predictor of subsequent survival was

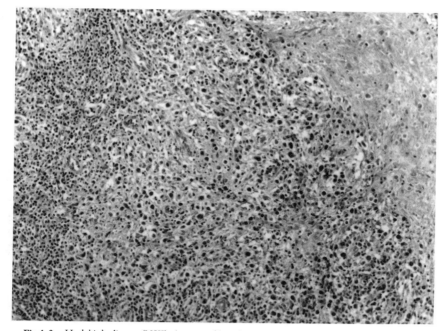

Fig 4–3.—Hodgkin's disease (NSII). An area of lymphocyte depletion is present centrally with a rim of small lymphocytes on the *left* and necrosis in the *upper right.* (Courtesy of Ferry JA, Linggood RM, Convery KM, et al: *Cancer* 71:457–463, 1993.)

the histologic grade. After a first relapse, the 5-year disease-free survival was 94% in the NSI group vs. 11% in the NSII group.

Conclusion.—Among patients with HDNS, the histologic subclassification appears to have clinical relevance. The histologic subtype may be an important consideration in planning therapy. Patients in the NSI subclassification who have a relapse appear to have a more successful salvage and a longer survival than those with the NSII subclassification.

▶ The suggestion that NS histology could be subdivided into 2 groups with quite different prognoses was first made in the late 1960s by Costan Berard. The study by Ferry et al. confirms and extends those observations and mandates that the distinction between the 2 grades of NS be routinely made. Studies of combined modality vs. radiotherapy should be reviewed to investigate whether outcome with the 2 therapeutic approaches is different for each of the NS subtypes.—P.H. Wiernik, M.D.

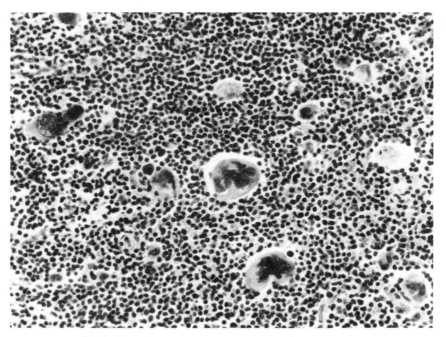

Fig 4–4.—Hodgkin's disease (NSII) with pleomorphic Reed-Sternberg cells. In addition to many Reed-Sternberg cells and variants with the usual morphologic type, this specimen contained the extremely large, bizarre, hyperchromatic cells seen here. (Courtesy of Ferry JA, Linggood RM, Convery KM, et al: *Cancer* 71:457–463, 1993.)

Vanishing Bile Duct Syndrome: A Possible Mechanism for Intrahepatic Cholestasis in Hodgkin's Lymphoma

Hubscher SG, Lumley MA, Elias E (Univ of Birmingham; East Birmingham Hosp; Queen Elizabeth Med Centre, Birmingham, England)
Hepatology 17:70–77, 1993   4–5

Introduction.—Some patients with Hodgkin's lymphoma have an idiopathic intrahepatic cholestasis, the mechanism of which is not well understood. Three patients with Hodgkin's disease had a severe intrahepatic cholestasis of unknown cause.

Patients and Methods.—The patients were 2 men and 1 woman, 26–44 years of age. Two had jaundice, and all had intractable liver damage when they died. The initial impression in all was idiopathic Hodgkin's disease–associated cholestasis. However, on histologic evaluation, advanced vanishing bile duct syndrome was noted in addition to severe cholestasis. Liver specimens obtained within 30 weeks of the onset of jaundice showed the characteristic "burned-out" appearance of the portal tracts, with no periportal changes secondary to chronic cholestasis. Biopsies taken during the course of 1 year from the onset of jaundice revealed progressive periportal damage, with fibrous expansion, marginal ductular proliferation, and copper-associated protein deposition. In each patient's final liver sample, recognizable bile ducts were missing from more than 80% of the small portal tracts.

Conclusion.—Loss of intrahepatic bile ducts may be encountered in patients with Hodgkin's lymphoma. Such a syndrome should be part of the differential diagnosis of Hodgkin's disease–associated intrahepatic cholestasis. Unless bile duct numbers are specifically examined, this diagnosis could easily be missed.

▶ The same studies should be carried out in patients with histiocytic medullary reticulosis, a disease almost always associated with unexplained jaundice and eventual liver failure.—P.H. Wiernik, M.D.

Late Cardiopulmonary Toxicity After Treatment for Hodgkin's Disease

Allavena C, Conroy T, Aletti P, Bey P, Lederlin P (Centre Alexis Vautrin; Clinique Médicale A, Vandoeuvre-Lès-Nancy, France)
Br J Cancer 65:908–912, 1992   4–6

Introduction.—Mantle field irradiation for patients with Hodgkin's disease (HD) may result in cardiac and pulmonary complications, which are often severe. Despite decreases in recent years, these complications are still common. Cardiopulmonary function was studied in patients with HD to determine the effect of mantle field irradiation, alone or in combination with chemotherapy, on cardiac and pulmonary function.

Patients and Methods.—The analysis included 75 patients, aged 50 years or younger, who had received mantle radiotherapy (RT) for HD at least 3 years previously. Nineteen had received RT plus chemotherapy with mechlorethamine, vincristine, procarbazine, and prednisone (MOPP); 42 had received RT plus MOPP and chemotherapy with doxorubicin (Adriamycin), bleomycin, vinblastine, and dacarbazine (ABVD); and 14 received RT only. A control group of healthy subjects was also studied. The patients were evaluated by physical examination, blood cell count, chest radiographs, standard 12-lead ECG, echocardiogram, pulmonary function test, and xenon-133 ventilation-perfusion scintigraphy.

Findings.—None of the patients showed any symptoms of heart disease; 12 had only borderline ECG or echocardiographic abnormalities. Moderate aortic stenosis was present in 1 patient, but this was known before treatment. Four patients had apical or septal hypokinesia and 1 had slight right ventricular dilatation. Moderate to severe abnormalities were noted on the chest radiographs in 16% (12 of 75) of the patients; however, the intensity of these radiographic findings was not significantly correlated with the results of pulmonary function testing, xenon ventilation-perfusion scintigraphy, or clinical examination. Sixty-four percent (29 of 45) of the patients had reduced lung perfusion in the irradiated areas; these patients were asymptomatic. Compared with the control group, the patients had significantly lower resting mean pulmonary function in terms of total and vital capacity. Exercise tolerance, as reflected by blood gas analysis, was below the expected level in only 2 patients, both of whom became dyspneic during low-level exercise. The various test results were not significantly different among the 3 groups of patients.

Conclusion.—In patients with HD, current techniques of mantle field RT seem to result in only minimal cardiopulmonary complications. There were few functional sequelae despite the reduced lung perfusion in the irradiated areas. Studies of treatments for HD should consider not only survival and cure rates but also the reduction of late effects.

▶ The results of this study are contrary to many older reports, especially those concerning patients who were treated with anterior-weighted mantle ports, and those who received a 40-Gy or more midplane dose in 4 weeks. This study demonstrates that improved treatment techniques and lower dosage may have significantly modified cardiopulmonary damage from mantle RT.—P.H. Wiernik, M.D.

Comparison of Psychosocial Adaptation and Sexual Function of Survivors of Advanced Hodgkin Disease Treated by MOPP, ABVD, or MOPP Alternating With ABVD
Kornblith AB, Anderson J, Cella DF, Tross S, Zuckerman E, Cherin E, Henderson ES, Canellos GP, Kosty MP, Cooper MR, Weiss RB, Gottlieb A, Holland JC (Mem Sloan-Kettering Cancer Ctr, New York; Univ of Nebraska, Omaha; Rush-Presbyterian-St Lukes Med Ctr, Chicago; et al)
Cancer 70:2508–2516, 1992   4–7

Purpose.—The major increases in survival with combination chemotherapy in patients with Hodgkin's disease have been achieved at the risk of several long-term side effects. Mechlorethamine, vincristine, procarbazine, and prednisone (MOPP), the most commonly used regimen, causes permanent sterility or menopause, an increased risk of second malignancies, plus other physical and psychological problems observed in cancer survivors. It has been shown that doxorubicin, bleomycin, vinblastine, and dacarbazine (ABVD), alone or alternating with MOPP, can increase survival and decrease gonadal toxicity in patients with advanced Hodgkin's disease. Psychosocial adaptation and psychosexual function in patients treated with MOPP, ABVD, and MOPP alternating with ABVD were compared.

Patients and Methods.—The analysis included 93 disease-free survivors of advanced Hodgkin's disease. There were 56 men and 37 women (median age, 35 years). Patients had been randomly allocated to receive either MOPP, ABVD, or MOPP alternating with ABVD, which had 36-

month failure-free survival rates of 48%, 64%, and 64%, respectively. At least 1 year after completion of the treatment, patients took part in a telephone interview in which their psychological, sexual, family, and vocational functioning were assessed by standardized measures.

Findings.—Surprisingly, there were no significant differences in psychosocial adaptation or psychosexual function according to treatment group. Poorer adjustment was predicted by patient reports of infertility and lower income 1 year before the cancer diagnosis. Most subjects attributed a range of problems to having had cancer, including proven or perceived infertility in 35%, sexual problems in 24%, problems with health and life insurance in 31%, a negative socioeconomic effect in 26%, and conditioned nausea on being reminded of chemotherapy in 51%.

Conclusion.—The use of ABVD or MOPP alternating with ABVD does not appear to offer any significant long-term advantage as opposed to MOPP alone in psychosocial adaptation or psychosexual function among Hodgkin's disease survivors. Regardless of treatment, about one fourth of survivors of Hodgkin's disease have important psychological, physical, sexual, insurance, and socioeconomic problems.

Hodgkin Disease Survivors at Increased Risk for Problems in Psychosocial Adaptation

Kornblith AB, Anderson J, Cella DF, Tross S, Zuckerman E, Cherin E, Henderson E, Weiss RB, Cooper MR, Silver RT, Leone L, Canellos GP, Gottlieb A, Holland JC (Mem Sloan-Kettering Cancer Ctr, New York; Univ of Nebraska, Omaha; Rush-Presbyterian-St Lukes Med Ctr, Chicago; et al)
Cancer 70:2214–2224, 1992   4–8

Introduction.—Although a good deal of work has been done to identify the array of psychosocial problems that may occur in survivors of Hodgkin's disease, there has been little interest in identifying patients at risk for problems in adaptation. Long-term psychosocial adaptation was studied in survivors of advanced Hodgkin's disease to ascertain the nature and extent of these problems and to identify patients at risk of problems.

Patients and Methods.—The sample comprised 273 survivors (60% were men) of advanced Hodgkin's disease who had been treated in clinical trials of the Cancer and Leukemia Group B during a 20-year period. All were currently free of disease and had completed treatment at least 1 year previously. The patients were studied at a median age of 37 years at at average of 6 years after completion of treatment. Questionnaires addressing the patients' psychological, social, vocational, and sexual functioning were mailed to the subjects, followed about 1 week later by a telephone interview.

Findings.—According to the Brief Symptom Inventory, psychological distress was increased by 1 SD over that of healthy subjects. Twenty-two percent had a score 1.5 SD above the norm, which is a suggested criterion for a psychiatric disorder. Other problems reported as a consequence of the disease were denial of life insurance, 31% of patients; denial of health insurance, 22%; sexual problems, 37%; conditioned nausea in response to sights and sounds reminiscent of chemotherapy, 39%; and negative socioeconomic effect, 36%. Problems in psychosocial adaptation were more likely in male patients who earned less than $15,000/yr or were currently unemployed, in unmarried patients, in patients who had had serious illnesses since the completion of treatment, and in less educated patients.

Conclusion.—Problems in psychosocial adaptation appear to be common in survivors of Hodgkin's disease, and many of these patients may require therapy. Risk factors for maladaptation were identified, through which patients could be targeted for additional evaluation at annual medical visits. These patients need services to help them learn their rights and opportunities for insurance and employment.

▶ These 2 articles from the Cancer and Leukemia Group B (Abstracts 4–7 and 4–8) demonstrate the long-term follow-up and supportive care required for patients treated for Hodgkin's disease if they are to be maximally reintegrated into a healthy and happy life-style. Unfortunately, postradiotherapy hypothyroidism was not investigated in these studies. It would be interesting to know whether any of the psychosocial dysfunction observed was related to clinical or subclinical thyroid dysfunction. Certainly, infertility has often resolved after diagnosis and treatment of a hypoactive thyroid after treatment for Hodgkin's disease.—P.H. Wiernik, M.D.

Risk of Second Primary Cancers After Hodgkin's Disease by Type of Treatment: Analysis of 2846 Patients in the British National Lymphoma Investigation
Swerdlow AJ, Douglas AJ, Vaughan Hudson G, Vaughan Hudson B, Bennett MH, MacLennan KA (London School of Hygiene and Tropical Medicine; Univ College and Middlesex School of Medicine, London; Mount Vernon Hosp, Middlesex, England; et al)
BMJ 304:1137–1143, 1992   4–9

Background.—As the survival of patients with Hodgkin's disease improves, the long-term complications of treatment become more important. The risk of second primary cancers during long-term follow-up of patients with Hodgkin's disease was analyzed.

Patients and Methods.—This cohort study included 2,846 patients first treated for Hodgkin's disease between 1970 and 1987. Follow-up was complete in 99.8%.

Findings.—A total of 113 second primary cancers occurred during follow-up. The relative risk of cancer other than Hodgkin's disease was 2.7 when compared with the general population. Significant risks were seen for leukemia; non-Hodgkin's lymphoma; and cancers of the colon, lung, bone, and thyroid. The absolute excess risk related to therapy was higher for solid tumors than leukemia and the lymphomas. The relative risk of leukemia increased shortly after therapy, peaking after 5–9 years. This risk was markedly increased after chemotherapy, combined treatment with radiotherapy and chemotherapy, and relative to the number of courses of chemotherapy. However, it was not significantly increased after radiotherapy. The relative risk of non-Hodgkin's lymphoma increased in the first 5 years after therapy and remained high; however, it showed no clear association with the type or extent of treatment. The relative risk of solid tumors was less elevated initially but increased throughout follow-up. For lung cancer, the relative risk of solid tumors was 8.3 at 10 years or more after the initial diagnosis. The risk of solid tumor increased after radiotherapy and after chemotherapy alone. After chemotherapy, the risk increased significantly with the time since the first treatment.

Conclusion.—The risk of solid tumors, not leukemia, appears to be the major long-term hazard of Hodgkin's disease treatment. This seems to be true after chemotherapy as well as radiotherapy.

▶ The difference between this and other articles on the subject is that, here, chemotherapy as well as radiotherapy seemed to be associated with an increased incidence of solid tumors.—P.H. Wiernik, M.D.

Lung Cancer Following Hodgkin's Disease: A Case-Control Study
Kaldor JM, Day NE, Bell J, Clarke EA, Langmark F, Karjalainen S, Band P, Pedersen D, Choi W, Blair V, Henry-Amar M, Prior P, Assouline D, Pompe-Kirn V, Cartwright RA, Koch M, Arslan A, Fraser P, Sutcliffe SB, Host H, Hakama M, Stovall M (Internatl Agency for Research on Cancer, Lyon, France; Thames Cancer Registry, Sutton, Surrey, England; Ontario Cancer Treatment and Research Found, Toronto; et al)
Int J Cancer 52:677–681, 1992   4–10

Background.—Survivors of Hodgkin's disease have a greatly increased risk of having lung cancer. The roles of chemotherapy, radiotherapy, and other factors in the etiology of lung cancer after Hodgkin's disease were assessed.

Patients and Methods.—Ninety-eight patients with lung cancer were identified among those who had survived for at least 1 year after a diagnosis of Hodgkin's disease. Matched controls numbering 259 were selected from patients with Hodgkin's disease but not lung cancer. Detailed information was abstracted from medical records for each patient and control subject.

Lung Cancer After Hodgkin's Disease by Type of Lung Cancer and Years Since Diagnosis of Hodgkin's Disease

Type of lung cancer	Number of years between diagnosis of Hodgkin's disease and lung cancer						Total
	1	2–3	4–5	6–7	8–9	10+	
Small-cell	2	1	0	0	2	4	9
Squamous-cell	2	7	6	12	7	9	43
Adenocarcinoma	4	2	1	3	3	6	19
Other or unknown	4	0	5	7	6	5	27
Total	12	10	12	22	18	24	98

(Courtesy of Kaldor JM, Day NE, Bell J, et al: *Int J Cancer* 52:677–681, 1992.)

Findings.—Patients treated with chemotherapy alone have about twice the risk of lung cancer development compared with patients treated with both chemotherapy and radiotherapy or radiotherapy alone. No increased risk was associated with a cumulative number of cycles of chemotherapy. Patients treated with radiotherapy alone had an increase in risk related to the estimated radiation dose to the lung. In addition, cigarette smoking was strongly associated with the risk of lung cancer (table).

Conclusion.—All forms of Hodgkin's disease treatment may be carcinogenic to the lung. Chemotherapy in particular is associated with an increased risk that is at least comparable with, and perhaps higher than, the risk associated with radiotherapy.

▶ For more information, see the article by Konits et al. (1).

Reference

1.   Konits PH, et al: *Med Pediatr Oncol* 10:331–338, 1982.

Low-Dose Radiation Therapy and Reduced Chemotherapy in Childhood Hodgkin's Disease: The Experience of the French Society of Pediatric Oncology

Oberlin O, Leverger G, Pacquement H, Raquin MA, Chompret A, Habrand JL, Terrier-Lacombe MJ, Bey P, Bertrand Y, Rubie H, Behar C, Zucker JM, Schaison G, Lemerle J (Institut Gustave Roussy, Villejuif, France; Hôpital Trousseau, Paris; Hôpital Saint Louis, Paris; et al)
J Clin Oncol 10:1602–1608, 1992   4–11

Background.—Chemotherapy and wide-field radiation therapy (RT) produced dramatic therapeutic improvements in childhood Hodgkin's disease when they were first used in the 1960s. Subsequent trials aimed to decrease both treatment modalities without reducing their effectiveness. In 1982, an attempt to reduce both the fields and dose of radiation

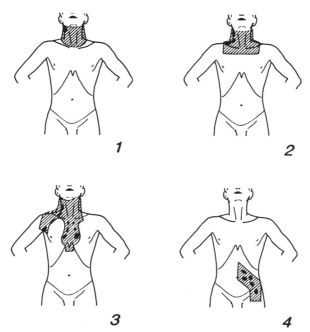

Fig 4–5.—Diagram of the fields according to the initial sites of disease. **1,** upper cervical node. **2,** unilateral cervical nodes. **3,** unilateral cervical and axillar nodes plus mediastinal nodes. **4,** unilateral iliac and inguinal nodes. (Courtesy of Oberlin O, Leverger G, Pacquement H, et al: *J Clin Oncol* 10:1602–1608, 1992.)

and chemotherapy in terms of aggressivity to the gonads and potential carcinogenicity was undertaken in France. Cure rates of cyclic regimens combined with low-dose radiation were assessed after a median 6-year follow-up.

Patients and Methods.—A total of 238 pediatric patients with Hodgkin's disease were included in the study on the basis of initial clinical staging without laparotomy (Fig 4–5). Patients with localized disease were randomized to receive either 4 cycles of doxorubicin (Adriamycin), bleomycin, vinblastine, and dacarbazine (ABVD) or 2 cycles of ABVD alternated with 2 cycles of mechlorethamine, vincristine, procarbazine, and prednisone (MOPP). Patients with more advanced disease received 3 courses of MOPP alternated with 3 courses of ABVD. Patients with good initial results from chemotherapy received 20 Gy of RT limited to the involved sites for localized disease or broader for more advanced disease stages. When a good remission was not obtained, 40 Gy of RT was administered.

Findings.—Ninety-seven percent of the patients were good responders to chemotherapy, and only 11 patients did not achieve a good remission. The response to chemotherapy varied according to the disease stage. The 6-year actuarial survival was 92%, with disease-free survival of 86% (Fig 4–6). The relapse-free survival in patients with localized disease was

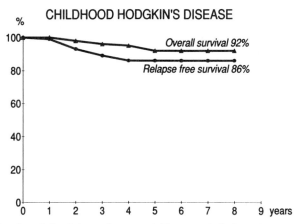

CHILDHOOD HODGKIN'S DISEASE

Overall survival 92%

Relapse free survival 86%

Fig 4–6.—Overall survival and disease-free survival. (Courtesy of Oberlin O, Leverger G, Pacquement H, et al: *J Clin Oncol* 10:1602–1608, 1992.)

90% in the ABVD arm and 87% in the MOPP and ABVD arm. The response to primary chemotherapy was the only prognostic factor for overall survival and disease-free survival.

Conclusion.—In patients with a favorable disease stage, 4 courses of ABVD were equivalent to 4 alternated courses of MOPP plus ABVD. This combined modality therapy permits low-dose RT of 20 Gy, thus reducing post-RT toxicity.

Comparison of High-Dose and Low-Dose Radiation With and Without Chemotherapy for Children With Hodgkin's Disease: An Analysis of the Experience at the Children's Hospital of Philadelphia and the Hospital of the University of Pennsylvania

Maity A, Goldwein JW, Lange B, D'Angio GJ (Children's Hosp of Philadelphia; Univ of Pennsylvania, Philadelphia)
J Clin Oncol 10:929–935, 1992   4–12

Introduction.—The treatment of Hodgkin's disease has markedly improved during the past 3 decades, achieving survival rates as high as 90% in some pediatric populations. However, serious complications, such as soft tissue and skeletal hypoplasia, have been noted in some children as a result of radiation therapy (RT). The data on a previously reported series of children were updated regarding their outcome after low-dose RT and chemotherapy.

Patients and Methods.—A total of 139 patients with Hodgkin's disease who were younger than 18 years of age were followed for 18 years. Included in the present analysis are 109 RT patients, 33 of whom received RT alone as initial treatment, 73 who received RT and chemotherapy, and 12 who received chemotherapy alone initially. The RT included 150–200 centigray (cGy) per day for 5 days a week, with 15 children receiving high-dose (30–40 cGy to each field) RT and 58 receiving low-dose (less than 30 cGy to each field) RT. Several combination chemotherapy regimens were used. Follow-up occurred every 2 or 3 months for the first 2 years and less frequently thereafter.

Results.—The 121 patients demonstrated an actuarial survival rate of 86% during 10 years. Of the 12 patients with progressing disease, 10 experienced an exacerbation during chemotherapy before RT in already affected sites and 2 patients had exacerbations during RT. The 10-year event-free survival (EFS) rate resulted in similar outcomes for all treatment groups. The 10-year EFS did not differ for those with either stage I or stage II disease but was 66% for the patients who received chemotherapy plus RT and 88% for those treated with RT alone. Patients receiving combined treatment had a recurrence rate of 6%, whereas those receiving RT alone had a 5% recurrence rate.

Conclusion.—The results indicate children with Hodgkin's disease who receive low-dose RT and chemotherapy have the same survival and recurrence rates as those who receive the high-dose treatments.

▶ These important studies (Abstracts 4–11 and 4–12) demonstrate that combined modality therapy with reduced radiotherapy dosage is as therapeutic as earlier approaches that used greater RT doses. The long-term complications of therapy in these studies will be of interest. Since the demonstration of a relatively high incidence of cardiac dysfunction in adults who received low-dose anthracycline therapy for childhood leukemia, one must be concerned about the late effects of anthracycline in pediatric Hodgkin's disease.—P.H. Wiernik, M.D.

Extended-Field Radiotherapy Is Superior to MOPP Chemotherapy for the Treatment of Pathologic Stage I-IIA Hodgkin's Disease: Eight-Year Update of an Italian Prospective Randomized Study

Biti GP, Cimino G, Cartoni C, Magrini SM, Anselmo AP, Maurizi Enrici R, Bellesi GP, Bosi A, Papa G, Giannarelli D, Ponticelli P, Papi MG, Rossi Ferrini PL, Biagini C, Mandelli F (Univ "La Sapienza," Rome; Univ Tor Vergata, Rome; Inst for the Study and Treatment of Cancer Regina Elena, Rome; Univ of Florence, Italy)
J Clin Oncol 10:378–382, 1992   4–13

Introduction.—In 1989, extended-field radiation therapy was compared with mechlorethamine, vincristine, procarbazine, and prednisone (MOPP) chemotherapy in the treatment of pathologic stage I–IIA Hodgkin's disease. The preliminary assessment failed to show significant differences in outcome at 5 years, although there was a suggestion that patients relapsing after chemotherapy may have had a worse outcome.

Updated results were available after a median follow-up exceeding 8 years.

Patients and Methods.—Eighty-nine consecutive adult patients with early-stage disease were assigned to receive either radiation therapy or 6 monthly courses of MOPP chemotherapy. The 2 groups were clinically comparable. Irradiation was with a mantle field, followed by periaortic exposure; the dose to involved sites was 40–44 Gy in 5 fractions, whereas uninvolved areas received 36 Gy.

Results.—All 45 irradiated patients and all but 4 of 44 chemotherapy patients achieved a complete response. Twelve patients in each group relapsed. Eight chemotherapy patients died of disease, as did 2 irradiated patients. Three other chemotherapy patients died of a second cancer. The overall survival was significantly longer in the radiation therapy group, but the rates of survival free from progression and without relapse were comparable in the 2 groups.

Conclusion.—Radiation therapy alone remains the best approach to adults with early-stage Hodgkin's disease if prognostic factors are favorable. If chemotherapy continues to be used, better combinations of less toxic agents will be needed.

▶ The results of this study are contrary to those of the National Cancer Institute study. The major point to be derived from both studies is that chemotherapy alone provides another modality for the treatment of early-stage Hodgkin's disease, which may be more important in the Third World than in Europe, parts of Asia, or North America.—P.H. Wiernik, M.D.

Chemotherapy of Advanced Hodgkin's Disease With MOPP, ABVD, or MOPP Alternating With ABVD
Canellos GP, Anderson JR, Propert KJ, Nissen N, Cooper MR, Henderson ES, Green MR, Gottlieb A, Peterson BA (Dana-Farber Cancer Inst, Boston; Univ of Nebraska, Omaha; Harvard School of Public Health, Boston; et al)
N Engl J Med 327:1478–1484, 1992   4–14

Introduction.—For nearly 2 decades, mechlorethamine, vincristine, procarbazine, and prednisone (MOPP) have been the standard therapy for Hodgkin's disease. Three regimens of primary systemic treatment for newly diagnosed advanced Hodgkin's disease in stages IIIA$_2$, IIIB, and IVA or IVB were compared.

Patients and Methods.—The regimens compared were MOPP alone, given for 6 to 8 cycles; MOPP alternated with doxorubicin, bleomycin, vinblastine, and dacarbazine (ABVD), given for 12 cycles; and ABVD alone for 6 to 8 cycles. Of the 361 patients in a first relapse after radiation therapy, 123 were in the first group, 123 were in the second, and 115 were in the third. Patient stratification was based on age, stage, previous radiation, histologic features, and performance status.

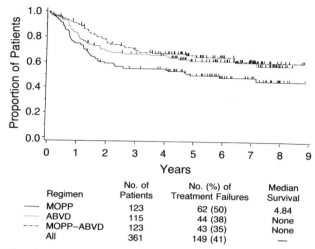

Fig 4–7.—Failure-free survival according to chemotherapeutic regimen. $P = .02$ for the difference between MOPP, ABVD, and MOPP-ABVD. In the column for median years of survival, *none* indicates that the median survival has not yet been reached. (Courtesy of Canellos GP, Anderson JR, Propert KJ, et al: N Engl J Med 327:1478–1484, 1992.)

Regimen	No. of Patients	No. (%) of Treatment Failures	Median Survival
MOPP	123	62 (50)	4.84
ABVD	115	44 (38)	None
MOPP–ABVD	123	43 (35)	None
All	361	149 (41)	—

Results.—The overall response rate was 93%. Complete responses occurred in 77%: 67% in the MOPP group, 82% in the ABVD group, and 83% in the combined treatment group. The rates of failure-free survival at 5 years were 50%, 61%, and 65%, respectively. Failure-free survival was significantly influenced by age, stage, and regimen (Fig 4–7). The 5-year overall survival rate was 66% for the MOPP patients, 73% for the ABVD patients, and 75% for the MOPP-ABVD patients. The MOPP therapy produced more severe bone marrow toxicity than the ABVD therapy and was associated with greater decreases in the prescribed dose.

Conclusion.—In this series, ABVD for 6–8 months was as effective as 12 months of MOPP alternating with ABVD. Both were superior to MOPP alone. The ABVD therapy was the least myelotoxic.

▶ This is one of the most important chemotherapy studies in Hodgkin's disease in many years. It demonstrates the activity of doxorubicin in this disease but does not confirm the Goldie-Coldman hypothesis.—P.H. Wiernik, M.D.

LOPP Alternating With EVAP Is Superior to LOPP Alone in the Initial Treatment of Advanced Hodgkin's Disease: Results of a British National Lymphoma Investigation Trial

Hancock BW, Vaughan Hudson G, Vaughan Hudson B, Bennett MH, MacLennan KA, Haybittle JL, Anderson L, Linch DC (Weston Park Hosp, Sheffield, England; Mount Vernon Hosp, Northwood, England; Univ College and Middlesex School of Medicine, London; et al)

J Clin Oncol 10:1252–1258, 1992

4–15

Introduction.—Cyclical combination chemotherapy with mechlorethamine (Mustine), vincristine or vinblastine, procarbazine, and prednisolone (MOPP or MVPP) has long been established as effective in the treatment of advanced Hodgkin's disease; however, the nausea, vomiting, and phlebitis caused by mechlorethamine may cause considerable morbidity. Similar results, with fewer long-term toxic effects, have been achieved with the substitution of oral chlorambucil (LOPP). A regimen of alternating treatment with doxorubicin (Adriamycin), bleomycin, vinblastine, and dacarbazine and with MOPP has recently been proven superior. Initial treatment with LOPP alone vs. LOPP alternating with etoposide, vinblastine, doxorubicin (Adriamycin), and prednisolone (EVAP) was undertaken.

Patients and Methods.—A total of 594 patients with advanced Hodgkin's disease were randomized to receive either 8 cycles of LOPP or 4 cycles of LOPP alternating with 4 cycles of EVAP. If bulky mediastinal disease was present, initial treatment with radiation therapy was permitted in addition to chemotherapy.

Results.—The overall rate of complete remission (CR) was 57% for patients receiving first-line chemotherapy with LOPP vs. 64% for those receiving LOPP/EVAP; this difference was significant. For patients who received subsequent radiation therapy to residual masses, CR rates were 65% and 75%, respectively; this difference was also significant. Procedure-associated mortality was 1% in patients receiving LOPP and 3% in those receiving LOPP/EVAP. The LOPP/EVAP group had significantly greater actuarial CR relapse-free survival and overall survival. At 5 years, the CR relapse-free rate was 52% in the LOPP arm vs. 72% in the LOPP/EVAP arm; the disease-free survival rate was 32% vs. 42%; and the overall survival rate was 66% vs. 75%.

Conclusion.—This randomized multicenter trial demonstrates the superiority of an alternating regimen of LOPP and EVAP as opposed to LOPP alone as initial treatment for advanced Hodgkin's disease. The LOPP/EVAP regimen is associated with more immediate toxic effects and a modest increase in treatment-related deaths. So far, none of the patients treated in the LOPP/EVAP arm have had second malignancies develop, compared with 7 patients treated in the LOPP arm.

▶ There is increasing evidence that etoposide is an important drug in the treatment of Hodgkin's disease.—P.H. Wiernik, M.D.

Effect of Recombinant Human Granulocyte-Macrophage Colony-Stimulating Factor in Patients With Hodgkin's Disease: A Phase I/II Study

Hovgaard DJ, Nissen NI (Rigshospital, Copenhagen)
J Clin Oncol 10:390–397, 1992

4–16

Background.—Bone marrow toxicity is the main limitation of optimal chemotherapy administration. Whether recombinant human (rh) GM-CSF could prevent myelotoxicity or accelerate hematopoietic recovery after mechlorethamine, vincristine, procarbazine, and prednisone (MOPP) chemotherapy was determined.

Patients and Methods.—Twenty-four patients had Hodgkin's disease. None had been previously treated. In this phase I/II trial, standard MOPP chemotherapy was followed by 5 days of GM-CSF at every other cycle. Patients were sequentially enrolled to receive 1 of 4 dose levels and were randomly assigned to 24-hour continuous intravenous infusion of twice-daily subcutaneous injection of rhGM-CSF.

Findings.—Cycles with rhGM-CSF were associated with significantly higher WBC counts than cycles with MOPP alone. The total number of days of leukopenia and neutropenia was reduced in cycles with rhGM-CSF from 6.3 to .8 and from 5.4 to 1, respectively. All rhGM-CSF dose levels effectively raised the absolute neutrophil count, but only at 8 and 16 µg/kg did this significantly affect chemotherapy scheduling. Adverse reactions were mild and reversible. Such reactions included low-grade fever, chest and bone pain, myalgias, erythema, headache, fatigue, and periorbital edema.

Conclusion.—The administration of rhGM-CSF to patients with Hodgkin's disease improves hematologic recovery after MOPP and appears to be safe. Full-dose chemotherapy can be given on time, resulting in a rise in the overall tolerated dose of myelosuppressive drugs compared with historical controls. Subcutaneous administration was at least as effective as continuous intravenous infusion.

▶ The question is, "What were the response rates compared with the controls?"—P.H. Wiernik, M.D.

High-Dose Salvage Chemotherapy Without Bone Marrow Transplantation for Adult Patients With Refractory Hodgkin's Disease

Tourani JM, Levy R, Colonna P, Desablens B, Leprise P-Y, Guilhot F, Brahimi S, Belhani M, Ifrah N, Sensebe L, Lemevel A, Lotz J-P, Le Maignan C, Andrieu JM (Laennec Hosp, Paris; South Hosp, Amiens, France; Hotel Dieu, Rennes, France; et al)

J Clin Oncol 10:1086–1094, 1992   4–17

Introduction.—Patients with Hodgkin's disease (HD) who do not achieve complete remission (CR), who relapse within the first year, or who have multiple relapses have a poor prognosis. Conventional salvage chemotherapy does not produce a good response in these patients. However, high-dose chemotherapy in combination with bone marrow transplantation (BMT) produces a CR rate of 40% to 80% with a disease-free 3-year survival of about 40%. The results of patients with refractory HD treated with high-dose chemotherapy without BMT were reviewed.

Patients and Methods.—Three courses of high-dose chemotherapy were administered to 39 adult patients with refractory HD. Each cycle of chemotherapy consisted of vindesine, 1 mg/m²/day, administered continuously intravenously from day 1 to 5; adriamycin, 40 mg/m²/day, administered continuously intravenously from day 1 to 3; carmustine, 140 mg/m²/day, from day 3 to 5; and methylprednisolone, 120 mg/m²/day, from day 1 to 5. After the third chemotherapy cycle, irradiation (20 Gy) was performed when possible.

Outcome.—By the end of treatment, 79% of these patients had achieved CR. Among these 31 patients, 10 relapsed with a median time of 3 months. The overall 5-year survival rate was 46%. The main toxicities were hematologic and digestive. Four patients died of treatment-related complications.

Conclusion.—Treatment with high-dose chemotherapy without BMT gave results comparable with treatment with BMT for adult patients with refractory HD. In fact, the timing of intensive chemotherapy appeared to be more important than the presence of BMT. Therefore, it is suggested that intensive chemotherapy regimens be used as the first-line treatment in patients with HD who have poor prognostic factors.

High-Dose Mitoxantrone and Etoposide Conditioning in Autologous Bone Marrow Transplantation for Relapsed Hodgkin's Disease

Lim SH, Baglin TP, Flavell DJ, Flavell SU, Wimperis JZ, Marcus RE (Addenbrooke's Hosp, Cambridge, England; Southampton Gen Hosp, England)

Eur J Haematol 48:110–114, 1992   4–18

Introduction.—Conventional chemotherapy produces complete remission in many patients with advanced-stage Hodgkin's disease (HD), but only about 40% achieve a long, disease-free survival with relapsed patients having a poor outcome. Several alternative agents are under investigation to improve the survival of these patients. High-dose mitoxantrone, a bis-substituted anthraquinone, was used in combination with etoposide before autologous bone marrow transplantation in 6 relapsed patients.

Patients and Methods.—Six relapsed patients with HD, 3 females and 3 males with a medium age of 26.5 years, received high-dose mitoxantrone and etoposide intravenously 9 and 7 days before their bone marrow transplants. The pharmacokinetic studies, cardiotoxicity, and clinical response were assessed.

Results.—Mitoxantrone serum levels peaked soon after the infusion with a median peak of 224.5 ng/mL after the first dose and 330 ng/mL after the second dose. All patients showed mitoxantrone serum levels on the day of the bone marrow transplantation. All patients had febrile neutropenic conditions that complicated the transplantation procedures a median of 5 days after the surgery, with 6 gram-positive organisms isolated from the patients. In addition, all patients developed pancytopenia, which necessitated platelet and blood transfusions. One patient had transient cardiomegaly, but no other signs of cardiotoxicity occurred. Of the 5 patients evaluated for response, 2 patients had a complete remission and 3 had partial remissions. Both complete-response patients relapsed 18 and 23 months afterward, and 2 of 3 partial-response patients have died of HD progression.

Conclusion.—The combined therapy of high-dose mitoxantrone administered with etoposide does not work as a salvage treatment for patients with HD experiencing a relapse. In addition, this combination therapy can lead to prolonged pancytopenia in these patients.

▶ The best treatment for HD with a poor prognosis is still to be determined. These 2 articles (Abstracts 4–17 and 4–18) demonstrate that autologous BMT is not always the answer, although it is generally more successful in HD than in other lymphomas. Randomized trials in which transplant and non-transplant approaches are compared are urgently required in the lymphomas.—P.H. Wiernik, M.D.

The Optimal Timing of Autologous Bone Marrow Transplantation in Hodgkin's Disease Patients After a Chemotherapy Relapse

Desch CE, Lasala MR, Smith TJ, Hillner BE (Virginia Commonwealth Univ, Richmond)
J Clin Oncol 10:200–209, 1992   4–19

Introduction.—A decision analysis model was created to determine the optimal sequence of salvage chemotherapy and autologous marrow transplantation for patients with Hodgkin's disease who have a relapse after primary chemotherapy.

Methods.—The model simulated a patient, aged 25 years, who had a relapse within a year after receiving mechlorethamine, vincristine, pro- carbazine, and prednisone chemotherapy for Hodgkin's disease. Four strategies used marrow transplantation and salvage chemotherapy in vari- ous sequences, whereas a fifth strategy used salvage chemotherapy only. The clinical data were derived from 17 published reports.

Results.—The best strategy appeared to be delaying marrow transplan- tation until the second relapse. The least effective approach was to per- form marrow transplantation in second complete remission. When the terms of the model were altered to simulate advanced disease after the newest combined chemotherapy regimens, immediate marrow transplan- tation was the best approach.

When patients were stratified by the level of risk, marrow transplanta- tion in second relapse proved best for patients relapsing in a good prog- nostic group. When the prognosis was poor, marrow transplantation only in complete remission was best.

Conclusion.—Marrow transplantation should always be considered for patients with Hodgkin's disease who relapse. Most often, marrow transplantation at the time of second relapse will be the best strategy. A comparison of the results of phase II trials on the basis of long-term overall survival on an ongoing basis would be useful.

Non-Hodgkin's Lymphoma

Human Lymphotropic Retroviruses Associated With Mycosis Fungoi- des: Evidence That Human T-Cell Lymphotropic Virus Type II (HTLV- II) as Well as HTLV-I May Play a Role in the Disease
Zucker-Franklin D, Hooper WC, Evatt BL (New York Univ, NY; Centers for Disease Control, Atlanta, Ga)
Blood 80:1537–1545, 1992   4–20

Introduction.—The HTLV-I is known to be causally associated with adult T-cell leukemia. However, its role in mycosis fungoides (MF) still has not been determined. A small percentage of patients with MF have antibodies to the virus. In other patients, cells harbor deleted HTLV-I proviral sequences. Also, particles resembling HTLV-I emerge in cul- tured blood lymphocytes obtained from most patients. Alternatively, dis- parate lymphotropic retroviruses may infect or affect a population of ep- idermotropic lymphocytes, resulting in MF.

Methods and Results.—Heparinized peripheral blood was obtained for study from 9 patients with an unequivocal diagnosis of MF. The cells of 4 patients provided evidence of HTLV-I infection. In the cells of an- other patient, molecular hybridization with HTLV-II–specific pol probes showed HTLV-II. The 103–base pair fragment amplified by the HTLV-

II–specific probe was sequenced and found to have more than 90% homology with the same fragment amplified from cells known to be HTLV-II infected.

Conclusion.—To date, no one has suggested a role for HTLV-II in MF. The findings of HTLV-I, HTLV-II, and their incomplete forms in the cells of patients with MF indicate the possibility of new theories of the pathogenesis of this disease.

Non-Hodgkin's Lymphomas Arising in Patients Successfully Treated for Hodgkin's Disease: A Clinical, Histologic, and Immunophenotypic Study of 14 Cases

Zarate-Osorno A, Medeiros LJ, Longo DL, Jaffe ES (Natl Cancer Inst, Bethesda, Md)
Am J Surg Pathol 16:885–895, 1992   4–21

Introduction.—Patients with complete remission of Hodgkin's disease (HD) are at increased risk of a second malignant neoplasm developing. Although solid tumors and acute leukemias are more common, non-Hodgkin's lymphomas (NHLs) may also develop. Experience with NHL developing after HD was reviewed.

Patients and Methods.—Fourteen patients were selected from a 30-year review of hematopathology files. Ten males and 4 females had NHL after successful treatment of HD. The median age at the diagnosis of NHL was 45 years; median time between the 2 diagnoses was 136 months. Clinically, the patients were comparable with other patients with HD. Twelve patients had nodular sclerosis, 1 had mixed cellularity, and 1 was unclassified. Nine patients underwent immunophenotyping, which showed LeuM1+LCA− Reed-Sternberg and Hodgkin's cells. Treatment for HD was with radiation in 2 patients, chemotherapy in 4 patients, and combination therapy in 8 patients.

Results.—Seventy-nine percent of NHLs were extranodal, often seen as an abdominal mass. There were 6 small noncleaved cell lymphomas, 4 non-Burkitt's and 2 Burkitt's lymphomas; 3 diffuse large-cell lymphomas; and 2 follicular and diffuse large-cell lymphomas. Of the 3 unclassified neoplasms, there was 1 intermediate- and 1 low-grade lymphoma with plasmacytoid differentiation and 1 plasmacytoma. The NHLs all had a typical B-cell lineage immunophenotype and were LeuM1−. Twelve patients were treated with combination chemotherapy, and 7 of them had complete remission; 3 were alive and disease free at 3 years' follow-up.

Discussion.—The clinical, histologic, and immunophenotypic characteristics of 14 patients who had NHL after successful treatment of HD are comparable with those occurring in immunosuppressed patients.

This raises the possibility that immunodeficiency might play a role in the pathogenesis of NHLs occurring after HD.

▶ It would be interesting to know if any of these patients had evidence of the Epstein-Barr virus in their Hodgkin's cells initially and, if so, whether the NHL cells had the same evidence.—P.H. Wiernik, M.D.

Extracorporeal Photopheresis for the Treatment of Cutaneous T-Cell Lymphoma
Zic J, Arzubiaga C, Salhany KE, Parker RA, Wilson D, Stricklin GP, Greer J, King LE Jr (Vanderbilt Univ, Nashville, Tenn)
J Am Acad Dermatol 27:729–736, 1992   4–22

Background.—There are many treatment regimens for cutaneous T-cell lymphoma (CTCL). However, with advanced disease, response rates and patient survival are not sufficient with any current therapy. Extracorporeal photochemotherapy (ECP) has been suggested as an alternative treatment. The results of ECP in 20 patients with CTCL refractory to other treatments were evaluated.

Methods.—The patients received ECP every 3–5 weeks for 6 or more months. All but 1 were in stage T_2 or higher. Extracutaneous disease was present in 8 patients and involved the lymph nodes in 6, bone marrow in 5, and Sézary cells in 6. The time from initial symptoms to diagnosis averaged 5.9 years. The interval between diagnosis and ECP averaged 2.2 years.

Results.—Five patients (25%) obtained a complete response, defined as the disappearance of all lesions. Six patients (30%) had a partial response, defined as disappearance of at least half their lesions. Twenty percent of the patients had disease stabilization, and 25% had disease progression. The only factor predicting who responded and who did not was the number of ECP sessions. By contrast, there was no separate benefit associated with adjunctive chemotherapy or electron beam therapy.

Conclusion.—Long-term ECP may be an effective alternative therapy for CTCL refractory to other treatments. It is likely to be even more useful when combined with other therapeutic modalities.

▶ The authors stated that the study did not provide evidence for the combination of photophoresis with chemotherapy or electron beam therapy, but they indicated that some patients required topical steroids, nitrogen mustard, or methotrexate for optimal control.—P.H. Wiernik, M.D.

Combined Modality Therapy for Primary CNS Lymphoma
DeAngelis LM, Yahalom J, Thaler HT, Kher U (Mem Sloan-Kettering Cancer

Ctr, New York; Cornell Univ, New York)
J Clin Oncol 10:635–643, 1992

4–23

Objective.—Primary CNS lymphoma (PCNSL), an aggressive, non-Hodgkin's lymphoma arising in the brain, spinal cord, or leptomeninges, was once rarely seen. Now, its incidence has increased threefold among apparently immunocompetent patients. Treatment with whole-brain radiotherapy (RT) and corticosteroids has yielded a median survival of 15–18 months. For patients with recurrent PCNSL, chemotherapy has been of value.

Patients and Methods.—Thirty-one patients with non-AIDS PCNSL were treated with a combined regimen of chemotherapy and cranial irradiation as their initial therapy. After placement of an Ommaya reservoir, patients received pre-RT systemic methotrexate, 1 g/m², along with six 12-mg doses of methotrexate via the Ommaya reservoir. They then received intracranial RT, consisting of 4,000 centigray (cGy) of whole-brain RT plus a 1,440-cGy boost. This was followed by 2 cycles of cytarabine, each course consisting of 2 doses of 3 g/m² separated by 24 hours and infused during 3 hours. At the same time, another 16 patients were treated with RT alone. These patients either declined chemotherapy or began RT treatment before consultation. All of these patients would have been eligible for the combination regimen.

Results.—Of 22 patients who were assessable after methotrexate but before the start of RT, 14 had a partial remission, 3 had a minor response, and 5 had stable disease. The median time to recurrence was 41 months in the combination therapy group compared with 10 months in the RT-only group. The median survival was 42.5 months in the combination therapy group vs. 21.7 months in the RT-only group, although this difference was nonsignificant because of the small sample size. Survival was improved by the administration of systemic chemotherapy for patients in the RT-only group.

Conclusion.—The combination of chemotherapy with cranial RT appears to significantly improve disease-free survival and contributes to overall survival as initial treatment for PCNSL. This combination should be considered for all patients with non-AIDS PCNSL. If further research can enhance the efficacy of chemotherapy, PCNSL may become the first primary brain tumor that is treatable with chemotherapy alone.

▶ This is an important therapeutic contribution to this rare disease that seems to be increasing in frequency.—P.H. Wiernik, M.D.

Phase II Trial of Fludarabine Phosphate in Lymphoma: An Effective New Agent in Low-Grade Lymphoma

Redman JR, Cabanillas F, Velasquez WS, McLaughlin P, Hagemeister FB, Swan F Jr, Rodriguez MA, Plunkett WK, Keating MJ (Univ of Texas, MD Anderson Cancer Ctr, Houston)

J Clin Oncol 10:790–794, 1992

4–24

Introduction.—The purine nucleoside fludarabine phosphate (FAMP) is being tested for use as an antineoplastic agent. The use of high-dose FAMP in patients with acute leukemia resulted in severe CNS toxicity. This was used at a lower dose to determine its effectiveness against relapsed lymphoma.

Patients and Methods.—Eighty-four patients with lymphoma entered the study during a 3.5-year period. Of these, 67 were evaluable. Their median age was 56 years, and they had received a median of 3 regimens of chemotherapy before treatment with FAMP. Treatment with FAMP began at a dosage of 25 mg/m² given intravenously for 30 minutes daily for 5 days every 3–4 weeks.

Results.—The response rates were 62% for follicular small cleaved-cell lymphoma, 80% for follicular mixed small- and large-cell lymphoma, and 100% for follicular large-cell lymphoma. Lower response rates were noted for small lymphocytic lymphoma and transformed lymphoma, 33%; mycosis fungoides, 40%; and Hodgkin's disease, 25%. None of the 20 patients with other intermediate- or high-grade lymphomas responded. The overall response rate was 37%, including 5 complete and 23 partial responses. Most toxic complications were hematologic and infectious in nature, with no serious gastrointestinal, hepatic, renal, or neurologic toxicities.

Conclusion.—This phase II trial shows that FAMP has major activity in follicular lymphoma. Its differential effect on low- vs. intermediate- and high-grade lymphoma calls for fundamental research. Future clinical studies should use FAMP in varying dosage schedules and in combination chemotherapeutic regimens.

▶ I have observed complete and durable responses in patients with low-grade lymphoma who have failed treatment with vincristine, doxorubicin, dexamethasone, and CVP. Fludarabine is a major new drug for this disease.—P.H. Wiernik, M.D.

Interferon Alfa Combined With Cytotoxic Chemotherapy for Patients With Non-Hodgkin's Lymphoma

Smalley RV, Andersen JW, Hawkins MJ, Bhide V, O'Connell MJ, Oken MM, Borden EC (Univ of Wisconsin, Madison; Dana-Farber Cancer Inst, Boston;

Georgetown Univ, Washington, DC; et al)
N Engl J Med 327:1336–1341, 1992

4–25

Introduction.—Interferon-alfa has been found to be as effective as an antitumor agent in patients with low-grade non-Hodgkin's lymphoma. However, its efficacy in patients with intermediate-grade non-Hodgkin's lymphoma has not been as well studied. The efficacy of adding interferon-alfa to cytotoxic chemotherapy in patients with clinically aggressive, low-grade non-Hodgkin's lymphoma and histologic variants of intermediate-grade non-Hodgkin's lymphoma, excluding diffuse histiocytic lymphoma, was assessed.

Patients and Methods.—A total of 291 patients were assigned randomly to receive cyclophosphamide, vincristine, prednisone, and doxorubicin or to receive this regimen plus recombinant interferon-alfa. Treatment was delivered in 8–10 cycles every 4 weeks.

Results.—Although the regimens yielded comparable objective results, the interferon regimen more effectively prolonged the time to treatment failure and duration of complete response. When outcomes were adjusted for important covariates, interferon-alfa also had a greater effect on overall survival (Fig 4–8).

Conclusion.—Interferon added to the 4-drug doxorubicin-based chemotherapy regimen proved to be an effective antitumor agent in patients with clinically aggressive low- or intermediate-grade non-Hodgkin's lymphoma. The addition of interferon was associated with prolonged, relapse-free survival and overall survival rates.

▶ It seems clear now that interferon-alpha can prolong remission duration and survival in low- and intermediate-grade lymphoma.—P.H. Wiernik, M.D.

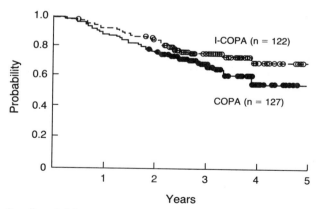

Fig 4–8.—Overall survival in treatment groups. Twenty-seven patients died in the cyclophosphamide, vincristine, prednisone, doxorubicin plus interferon-alpha-2a (*I-COPA*) group, and 41 died in the cyclophosphamide, vincristine, prednisone, doxorubicin (*COPA*) group. (Courtesy of Smalley RV, Andersen JW, Hawkins MJ, et al: *N Engl J Med* 327:1336–1341, 1992.)

Granulocyte Colony-Stimulating Factor to Prevent Dose-Limiting Neutropenia in Non-Hodgkin's Lymphoma: A Randomized Controlled Trial

Pettengell R, Gurney H, Radford JA, Deakin DP, James R, Wilkinson PM, Kane K, Bentley J, Crowther D (Christie Hosp NHS Trust, Manchester, England; Amgen-Roche, Cambridge, England)
Blood 80:1430–1436, 1992   4–26

Introduction.—The potential benefits of accelerated neutrophilic recovery were examined in patients with high-grade non-Hodgkin's lymphoma who received G-CSF in addition to weekly vincristine, adriamycin, prednisolone, etoposide, cyclophosphamide, and bleomycine (VAPEC-B) chemotherapy.

Patients and Methods.—Of 80 patients, 39 received chemotherapy alone, whereas 41 received G-CSF in addition in a daily subcutaneous dose of 230 $\mu g/m^2$. All patients received ketoconazole and cotrimoxazole prophylactically. Chemotherapy was given for 11 weeks.

Results.—Neutropenia occurred significantly less often in patients given G-CSF in addition to chemotherapy. Treatment delay was less evident in the G-CSF group, and these patients received more intensive treatment. Ninety percent of patients given G-CSF and 92% of controls had a complete or partial tumor response. There were no significant differences in overall or disease-free survival rates. Musculoskeletal pain was the only possible side effect of G-CSF administration.

Discussion.—Large randomized studies are needed, but this trial demonstrated a significant reduction in neutropenia with fewer and shorter treatment delays in patients with non-Hodgkin's lymphoma who received G-CSF in conjunction with chemotherapy.

▶ The growth factor had limited impact on outcome in this study.—P.H. Wiernik, M.D.

Survival After Relapse of Low-Grade Non-Hodgkin's Lymphoma: Implications for Marrow Transplantation

Weisdorf DJ, Andersen JW, Glick JH, Oken MM (Univ of Minnesota, Minneapolis; Dana-Farber Cancer Inst, Boston; Univ of Pennsylvania, Philadelphia)
J Clin Oncol 10:942–947, 1992   4–27

Objective.—Advances in treatment of non-Hodgkin's lymphomas (NHLs) have been unable to prevent continuing and late disease recurrence; median survival in patients with low-grade NHLs is only 7 to 10 years. Initial chemotherapy for lymphoma was analyzed to determine factors predicting short survival after relapse, with the goal of identifying candidates for intensive investigation and bone marrow transplantation.

Methods.—From 3 sequential phase III studies of induction chemotherapy, patients were drawn who had previously untreated NHLs of favorable histology. Of the 1,063 patients entered into the studies, the current analysis included 466 patients who achieved an initial complete response (CR) or partial response (PR) and had a subsequent relapse. Median follow-up was 13 years. A training set consisting of two thirds of the patients was used in a multivariate regression analysis, which was verified in the remaining one third of the patients as a validation set.

Results.—Factors associated with longer survival after relapse were age younger than 60 years, CR, and duration of response. Multivariate analysis suggested that survival was shorter in patients aged 60 or older, regardless of whether they had a CR or the duration of their response. The median survival in patients younger than 60 years with an initial CR lasting more than 1 year was 6 years; corresponding figures were 4 years for patients with a PR of more than 1 year and only 2 years for patients with a response of 1 year or less. Compared with the age-adjusted population mortality rates, mortality of even the most favorable NHL group was increased 10-fold.

Conclusion.—Patients with low-grade NHLs who have a response period of 1 year or less appear to have poor survival after relapse. Therefore, these patients may be suitable candidates for salvage therapy including bone marrow transplantation. The survival after relapse is better for patients with greater initial responses. Future studies attempting to demonstrate a survival advantage must include long follow-up and control group comparisons.

Autologous Versus Allogeneic Bone Marrow Transplantation for Non-Hodgkin's Lymphoma: A Case-Controlled Analysis of the European Bone Marrow Transplant Group Registry Data

Chopra R, Goldstone AH, Pearce R, Philip T, Petersen F, Appelbaum F, De Vol E, Ernst P (Univ College and Middlesex School of Medicine, London; Centre Leon Berard, Lyons, France; Fred Hutchinson Cancer Ctr, Seattle; et al)
J Clin Oncol 10:1690–1695, 1992   4–28

Objective.—One of the difficulties in comparing allogeneic bone marrow transplantation (alloBMT) and autologous bone marrow transplantation (ABMT) regimens in lymphoma is the disparity between the 2 groups in patient characteristics. The effectiveness of alloBMT was compared with that of ABMT in patients with non-Hodgkin's lymphoma.

Patients.—Of 938 patients with ABMT who were enrolled in the European Bone Marrow Transplant Group, 101 were matched with the same number of patients with alloBMT (among 122 having this procedure). The groups were matched for age, gender, interval between diagnosis and transplantation, and several prognostic factors (clinical status at the time of transplantation, stage of disease, type of histology, conditioning therapy).

Findings.—Progression-free survival rates were 49% at a median follow-up of 31 months for patients who had alloBMT and 46% at a median follow-up of 48 months for those who had ABMT. The overall rates of relapse and progression were 23% and 38%, respectively, not a significant difference. Relapse was less frequent after alloBMT in patients with lymphoblastic lymphoma, but progression-free survival was not significantly more frequent, and there was a higher procedure-related mortality with alloBMT (24% vs. 10%). Patients with chronic graft-vs.-host disease relapsed and progressed significantly less often than the others.

Conclusion.—In patients with non-Hodgkin's lymphoma, ABMT may provide results comparable with those of alloBMT with less morbidity. However, alloBMT may be preferable for younger patients with lymphoblastic lymphoma.

▶ These studies (Abstracts 4–27 and 4–28) help to define which patients with lymphoma should be considered for transplantation and what type of transplant should be offered.—P.H. Wiernik, M.D.

Multiple Myeloma

P-Glycoprotein Expression in Human Plasma Cell Myeloma: Correlation With Prior Chemotherapy

Grogan TM, Spier CM, Salmon SE, Matzner M, Rybski J, Weinstein RS, Scheper RJ, Dalton WS (Univ of Arizona, Tucson; Free Univ, Amsterdam)
Blood 81:490–495, 1993   4–29

Background.—P-glycoprotein (PGP) expression may occur in patients with multidrug resistant (MDR) myeloma. P-glycoprotein is known to serve as an efflux pump, protecting the neoplastic cells, but it is unknown whether PGP expression might be related to previous exposure to cytotoxic drugs. The expression of PGP was assessed in treated and nontreated patients to determine whether it might be related to the specific type and amount of drug exposure.

Methods.—The analysis included 106 consecutive bone marrow samples from 104 patients with myeloma. The specimens were taken either before or after therapy and at the time of clinical relapse. All samples were assessed by an immunocytochemical assay using an MDR-1–specific monoclonal antibody.

Findings.—Only 6% of previously untreated patients expressed PGP, compared with 43% of previously treated patients. Fifty percent of patients receiving more than 20 mg of vincristine and 83% of those receiving more than 340 mg of doxorubicin expressed PGP. Of 11 patients who received both drugs in those amounts, all expressed PGP. Eighty-eight percent of plasma cells in patients treated with doxorubicin were PGP-positive, compared with 65% of those in patients not receiving doxorubicin. On the basis of those results, a predictive mathematical model from which to generate dose-related normograms for PGP expression was developed. Disease duration did not appear to be a significant variable, as the mean of 33 months in PGP-negative patients had overlapping confidence limits with the mean of 42 months in PGP-positive patients. The expression of PGP was not correlated with other clinical or immunophenotypic factors.

Conclusion.—This study demonstrates a strong relationship between PGP expression in myeloma and previous drug treatment. The expression of PGP is highly related to previous treatment with vincristine and doxorubicin, especially treatment with both drugs at high doses. Patients who relapse after receiving relatively high doses appear very likely to have MDR expression.

▶ This study may be used as an argument for not using the vincristine, doxorubicin, dexamethasone regimen as initial therapy.—P.H. Wiernik, M.D.

C-Reactive Protein and β-2 Microglobulin Produce a Simple and Powerful Myeloma Staging System

Bataille R, Boccadoro M, Klein B, Durie B, Pileri A (Hopitaux de Nantes, France; Univ of Torino, Italy; Charing Cross Hosp, London)
Blood 80:733–737, 1992   4–30

Introduction.—There is still no wholly sufficient procedure for staging multiple myeloma (MM). The 2 most widely used methods are the Durie and Salmon and the serum β_2-microglobulin (β_2M) systems, which mainly reflect tumor burden. Other useful parameters (e.g., myeloma cell

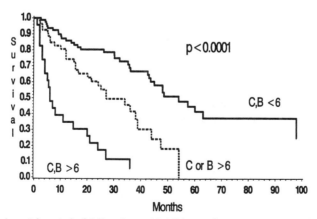

Fig 4–9.—Actuarial survival of 162 patients with MM according to serum CRP and β_2M levels at diagnosis. C, B < 6 = CRP and β_2M < 6 mg/L; C or B ≥ 6 = CRP or β_2M ≥ 6 mg/L; C, B ≥ 6 mg/L = CRP and β_2M ≥ 6 mg/L. (Courtesy of Bataille R, Boccadoro M, Klein B, et al: *Blood* 80:733–737, 1992.)

proliferative activity) are more complex and time-consuming. It has been found that IL-6 is a major growth factor for MM. The activity of IL-6 is reflected by serum C-reactive protein (CRP) concentration.

Methods.—An enzyme-linked immunosorbent assay was used to measure the serum CRP level in 52 patients with monoclonal gammopathy of undetermined significance and 162 patients with MM. Forty-nine CRP measurements were made during remission and 33 were made at relapse. The prognostic value of serum CRP level in MM was analyzed by survival analysis, and it was correlated with other prognostic factors (e.g., bone marrow myeloma cells and serum β_2M levels).

Findings.—At diagnosis, patients with monoclonal gammopathy of undetermined significance had a median serum CRP level of .7 mg/L compared with 3.75 mg/L for patients with MM. Serum CRP proved to be a highly significant prognostic factor and was independent of serum β_2M. Together, the 2 measurements could be used to stratify patients with MM into 3 groups. The low-risk group, who had CRP and B$_2$M less than 6 mg/L, composed 50% of the patients. Thirty-five percent had CRP or β_2M of 6 mg/L or more and were classified as intermediate risk. Fifteen percent of the patients had both measurements at 6 mg/L or more and were classified as high risk. The median survival was 36 months for all patients with MM, 54 months for the low-risk group, 27 months for the intermediate-risk group, and 6 months for the high-risk group (Fig 4–9).

Conclusion.—As an indicator of IL-6 activity, the serum CRP level appears to be a powerful new prognostic factor for patients with MM. The authors propose combining it with β_2M to provide a strong prognostic staging system. Both measures are rapid, simple, reliable, and economical.

▶ It should be remembered that renal disease and interferon therapy can result in an elevated β_2M level that is inaccurate with respect to myeloma staging.—P.H. Wiernik, M.D.

Curability of Solitary Bone Plasmacytoma
Dimopoulos MA, Goldstein J, Fuller L, Delasalle K, Alexanian R (Univ of Texas, Houston)
J Clin Oncol 10:587–590, 1992   4–31

Background.—Approximately 5% of patients with myeloma have a solitary bone plasmacytoma (SBP) as their sole disease feature. Local radiotherapy is generally effective for the primary lesion, although a majority of patients have multiple myeloma. Therefore, the SBPs are considered to be a manifestation of systemic disease, and, hence, incurable. The criteria for identifying solitary disease have varied. Long-term results post–treatment have varied significantly, and the potential for cure remains uncertain.

Patients and Methods.—After pathologic confirmation, 45 patients with plasma-cell myeloma were found to have an SBP. Each of these patients received megavoltage irradiation of at least 3000 centigray. The radiotherapy fields encompassed all gross disease with generous margins of normal tissue.

Results.—Permanent control of disease at the involved sites was achieved in all but 2 patients. However, 46% of the patients had multiple myeloma, and two thirds of these patients did so within 3 years, which indicated an understaging of the extent of the disease at diagnosis. In 30% of the patients, myeloma protein disappeared and there has been no disease recurrence. All patients have experienced a mean survival rate of 13 years, and at 10 years, the myeloma-specific survival fraction was 53%.

Conclusion.—Patients with myeloma protein that disappears with radiotherapy have a good chance for long-term stability and, therefore, have no need for adjuvant therapy. However, adjuvant therapy could be useful for patients who have either persistent myeloma protein or nonsecretory disease and who may be at high risk of having multiple myeloma. Interferon-alfa has been clinically promising and should be considered for use in patients who are newly diagnosed and likely to progress after radiotherapy for SBP.

▶ Why not treat those patients with persistent myeloma protein after radiotherapy with induction chemotherapy rather than interferon?—P.H. Wiernik, M.D.

Low-Risk Intensive Therapy for Multiple Myeloma With Combined Autologous Bone Marrow and Blood Stem Cell Support

Jagannath S, Vesole DH, Glenn L, Crowley J, Barlogie B (Univ of Arkansas, Little Rock; Fred Hutchinson Cancer Research Ctr, Seattle)
Blood 80:1666–1672, 1992   4–32

Introduction.—For most patients with multiple myeloma (MM) who are receiving intensive chemotherapy, autologous stem cell support is favored rather than allogeneic transplantation; however, the duration of bone marrow aplasia is directly related to the occurrence of life-threatening complications. It has been suggested that the combined use of bone marrow and blood stem cells can accelerate hematopoietic engraftment. Peripheral blood stem cell (PBSC) collection was done in patients with MM while investigating double transplantation.

Patients and Methods.—The collection of PBSCs was attempted in 75 previously treated patients with symptomatic MM. All were aged 70 years or younger, had a performance status not less than 2, and had no organ compromise. The PBSCs were collected after the administration of high-dose cyclophosphamide (HD-CTX; 6 g/m²), with or without GM-CSF. Melphalan in a dose of 200 mg/m² was subsequently given to 57 patients, and melphalan (140 mg/m²) and total body irradiation (850 centigray) were given to 3 patients; all 60 were supported by both autologous bone marrow and PBSCs. The GM-CSF was given after transplantation in 38 patients.

Results.—Good mobilization, i.e., more than 50 GM-CFUs per 10⁵ mononuclear cells, was obtained for patients whose previous chemotherapy did not exceed 1 year and in whom GM-CSF was used after HD-CTX. Good mobilization was also associated with rapid platelet recovery to 50,000/μL within 2 weeks. The 37 patients who had good PBSC collection proceeded to hematologic recovery within 2-weeks. Neutrophils recovered within 2 weeks, making post–HD-CTX and post-transplant infectious complications manageable; there was only 1 treatment-related death after HD-CTX. The overall cumulative response rate was 68% (51/75), and the 12-month event-free and overall survival was projected at 85%.

Conclusion.—This experience suggests that double transplantation with both bone marrow and PBSCs, along with GM-CSF, is safe and effective for patients with MM, particularly those with less than 1 year of previous therapy. Complete hematologic recovery is obtained in more than 80% of the patients within 1 month. This means that patients who have post-transplant relapse will have adequate hematopoietic reserve for additional chemotherapy.

▶ These are provocative data suggesting that patients younger than age 70 can safely undergo high-dose chemotherapy and significantly benefit from it. The time is ripe for a prospective comparison of this approach with a standard one.—P.H. Wiernik, M.D.

Treatment of Waldenstrom Macroglobulinemia With 2-Chlorodeoxyadenosine

Dimopoulos MA, Kantarjian H, Estey E, O'Brien S, Delasalle K, Keating MJ, Freireich EJ, Alexanian R (Univ of Texas, Houston)
Ann Intern Med 118:195–198, 1993   4-33

Purpose.—Waldenström's macroglobulinemia, a low-grade lymphoid malignancy composed of mature plasmacytoid lymphocytes that produce a monoclonal IgM, is generally treated by combination chemotherapy with alkylating agents and steroids. A response is obtained in about half of previously untreated patients. The deoxyadenosine analogue 2-chlorodeoxyadenosine (2-CdA) has proven to be an effective treatment for several lymphoid malignancies, most notably hairy-cell leukemia.

Patients and Methods.—An uncontrolled phase II trial of 2-CdA was conducted in the treatment of Waldenström's macroglobulinemia. The subjects were 29 consecutive, symptomatic patients, 9 of whom had received no previous treatment. All received 2 courses of 2-CdA in a continuous intravenous infusion of .1 mg/kg/day for 7 days.

Results.—A response was obtained in 59% of the patients, with 1 patient achieving a complete response. All patients with a new diagnosis responded, as did 40% of the rest. All responding patients had rapid symptomatic relief, including 1 patient each with cryoglobulinemia and peripheral neuropathy. The median time to 50% reduction of IgM synthesis in previously untreated patients was 1 month. Only 1 relapse has occurred after a median follow-up of 7 months. Treatment was well tolerated. The only case of serious toxicity was in a patient who was severely pancytopenic before and after treatment and died on day 70 with aspergillus pneumonia.

Conclusion.—2-Chlorodeoxyadenosine appears to be an effective treatment for most patients with Waldenström's macroglobulinemia. Toxicity is minimal. The several agents with demonstrated effectiveness against this disease are not cross-resistant, so sequential treatment should be studied to achieve more pronounced and durable remissions.

▶ Here is yet another disease in which this drug may become the treatment of choice.—P.H. Wiernik, M.D.

Chronic Leukemias

HAIRY-CELL LEUKEMIA

A Single Cycle of 2-Chlorodeoxyadenosine Results in Complete Remission in the Majority of Patients With Hairy Cell Leukemia
Tallman MS, Hakimian D, Variakojis D, Koslow D, Sisney GA, Rademaker AW, Rose E, Kaul K (Northwestern Univ, Chicago; RW Johnson Pharmaceutical Research Inst, Raritan, NJ)
Blood 80:2203–2209, 1992   4–34

Introduction.—Hairy-cell leukemia (HCL) may be treated by splenectomy, which does not produce pathologic remission; interferon-alpha, which produces mainly partial remissions; or 2-deoxycoformycin (2-DCF), which produces complete remission (CR) but is cytotoxic. The purine analogue 2-chlorodeoxyadenosine (2-CdA), which is resistant to adenosine deaminase, produces CR with minimal toxicity.

Patients and Methods.—Twenty-six patients with HCL, median age 48 years, were treated during a 1-year period. Fifteen patients had not received any previous treatment; 4 had been treated with interferon-alpha alone; 3 with splenectomy alone; 2 with splenectomy followed by interferon-alpha; and 2 with splenectomy, then interferon-alpha, then 2-

DCF. Patients received 2-CdA at a dosage of .1 mg/kg/day for 7 days by continuous infusion.

Results.—Twenty patients were assessable at 3 months. With a single course of therapy, the CR rate was 80%; the rest of the patients achieved partial remission (PR). The peripheral blood count recovered in all 4 patients with PR, but 3 had residual HCL bone marrow and 1 had residual splenomegaly. Responses were just as good in patients with bulky adenopathy, massive splenomegaly, and severe pancytopenia as in those with only modest marrow involvement. A CR was obtained in 2 of 3 patients with residual marrow disease after a second course of treatment with 2-CdA, for a 90% CR rate. At a median follow-up of 1 year, none of the complete responders had relapse. Among the toxic effects were myelosuppression and culture-negative fever; the only infectious complication was community-acquired pneumonia.

Conclusion.—A single-cycle of 2-CdA induces CR in the vast majority of patients with HCL, regardless of whether they have been previously treated. The treatment, which is easy to administer and has minimal toxicity, is quickly becoming the choice for the uncommon chronic lymphoproliferative disorder of HCL.

▶ This important study demonstrates that the discovery of a new drug can be more important in treating cancer than kinetic hypotheses or molecular biology. New drug development is still the most productive activity in cancer treatment research.—P.H. Wiernik, M.D.

CHRONIC LYMPHOCYTIC LEUKEMIA

Listeriosis in Patients With Chronic Lymphocytic Leukemia Who Were Treated With Fludarabine and Prednisone

Anaissie E, Kontoyiannis DP, Kantarjian H, Elting L, Robertson LE, Keating M (Univ of Texas, Houston)
Ann Intern Med 117:466–469, 1992   4–35

Background.—*Listeria monocytogenes* will cause infection in individuals with defective cell-mediated immunity. Vulnerable populations include the elderly, cancer and AIDS patients, and transplant recipients. Even though chronic lymphocytic leukemia is the most common leukemia in the West, few of these patients have listeriosis. However, an increased incidence of listeriosis has been noted in these patients who have been treated with combination therapy (prednisone and fludarabine).

Patients and Methods.—This retrospective cohort study comprised 795 patients diagnosed with chronic lymphocytic leukemia. Data were gathered from routine hospital-wide infection surveillance to determine the incidence of listeria sepsis among these patients. Combination chemotherapy was given to 208 of these patients.

Results.—Seven of 208 patients who received the combination chemotherapy subsequently developed listeriosis compared with none of the 387 patients who received conventional chemotherapy. The increased incidence of listeriosis coincided with the introduction of the drug fludarabine. However, none of the 160 patients who received only fludarabine had listeriosis. Also, in patients who received the combination treatment, a dramatic reduction in CD4 cells accompanied by listeriosis development was noted.

Conclusion.—An increased risk of listeriosis development was noted in patients with chronic lymphocytic leukemia who received the combination chemotherapy of prednisone and fludarabine. The risk may be even higher among those patients who had received previous treatment with other immunosuppressive medications. Indications are that CD4 cell depletion might have a role in listeriosis development. Therefore, dosage-schedule modification of the fludarabine-prednisone combination is recommended. In addition, antibacterial prophylaxis and food restrictions (those items know to contain *L. monocytogenes*) are advised.

▶ Fludarabine is an extremely valuable but very immunosuppressive drug. Treatment with fludarabine-cytarabine combinations in patients with acute myeloid leukemia at the same institution has resulted in a high rate of infections not commonly seen in these patients treated with other-than-marrow transplantation.—P.H. Wiernik, M.D.

Response Assessment in Chronic Lymphocytic Leukemia After Fludarabine Plus Prednisone: Clinical, Pathologic, Immunophenotypic, and Molecular Analysis
Robertson LE, Huh YO, Butler JJ, Pugh WC, Hirsch-Ginsberg C, Stass S, Kantarjian H, Keating MJ (Univ of Texas, Houston)
Blood 80:29–36, 1992   4-36

Background.—The recent identification of several active agents and treatment regimens for chronic lymphocytic leukemia (CLL) has generated a renewed interest in CLL clinical research. The CLL treatment response according to clinical, pathologic, immunophenotypic, and molecular features was evaluated, and the clinical relevance of these findings was considered.

Patients and Methods.—Of a total of 159 patients, 81 had advanced Rai stage III or IV, and 78 had progressive Rai stage 0 to II. Each patient was treated with intravenous fludarabine (30 mg/m^2) and oral prednisone (30 mg/m^2) for 5 days. Thirty-six participants were previously untreated.

Results.—After the medication regimens, complete response (CR) rates were 12%, nodular complete response (nCR), 30%, and partial response (PR), 18%. Of those patients who achieved CR or nCR rates, less than 30% of nucleated cells were lymphocytes in bone marrow aspirates. However, residual nodular and/or interstitial lymphocyte involvement was noted in patients who had nCR during marrow biopsy examination. In patients who had CR, no leukemic infiltration was noted on bone marrow examination. In the CR and nCR groups, the comparison of time to progression revealed a projected 87% vs. 55% progression-free survival at 2 years. Flow cytometry (measuring CD5 and surface immunoglobulins on B cells) detected no residual disease after 6 courses of treatment in 89% of the CR, 51% of the nCR, and 19% of the PR patients. In those patients who partially responded and had no flow cytometry-detectable disease, residual disease was restricted to lymphadenopathy. At 2 years, the time to progression was longer in CR and nCR patients with no flow cytometry–detectable disease (84% vs. 39% progression-free survival). Post-treatment immunoglobulin gene rearrangement investigation (using JH, kappa–light chain JK region, and lambda–light chain CΛ region probes) showed a return to the germline configuration in 5 of 7 CR, and 2 of 8 nCR patients. These molecular studies agreed with the dual-parameter immunophenotype results. No relapses have occurred in patients who reverted to a germline DNA pattern after treatment.

Conclusion.—The lack of detectable residual disease is achievable in CLL with fludarabine. Bone marrow biopsies, in conjunction with B-cell surface antibody and CD5 characterization, may be used to predict the quality of the treatment response.

▶ This study suggests that the quality of the response after fludarabine and prednisone is better than what was achievable before the introduction of this regimen. In an effort to build on this observation, an intergroup study coordinated by the Cancer and Leukemia Group B has been mounted to prospectively test the relative merits of fludarabine, chlorambucil, and a combination of the 2 agents.—P.H. Wiernik, M.D.

Induction of Apoptotic Cell Death in Chronic Lymphocytic Leukemia by 2-Chloro-2'-Deoxyadenosine and 9-β-D-Arabinosyl-2-Fluoroadenine
Robertson LE, Chubb S, Meyn RE, Story M, Ford R, Hittelman WN, Plunkett W (Univ of Texas, Houston)
Blood 81:143–150, 1993   4–37

Background.—The purine nucleoside analogues 2-chloro-2'-deoxyadenosine (CldAdo) and 9-β-D-arabinosyl-2-fluoroadenine (F-ara-A) have exhibited potent activity against low-grade lymphocytic malignancies. Both analogues were cell cycle specific and require DNA synthesis for their cytotoxic effects. The low proliferative rate of chronic lymphocytic leukemia (CLL) cells has suggested that programmed cell death (apoptosis) may be involved in the cytotoxic actions of CldAdo and F-ara-A. Lymphocytes from patients with CLL were exposed to CldAdo and F-ara-A for 24 to 72 hours.

Findings.—Features of apoptosis were evident after exposing cells to either purine nucleotide, and there was evidence that DNA was cleaved into nucleosome-sized multimers. Drug-related DNA fragmentation was both time and dose dependent. Induced and spontaneous DNA fragmentation were prevented by chelating intracellular calcium, but not by inhibiting macromolecular synthesis with actinomycin D, cycloheximide, and puromycin. Less DNA fragmentation was found in B leukemic cells from patients with treatment-resistant disease.

Conclusion.—The purine nucleoside analogues CldAdo and F-ara-A induce apoptotic death of CLL cells.

▶ Here are 2 additional drugs that deserve further study in CLL.—P.H. Wiernik, M.D.

Response to 2-Chlorodeoxyadenosine in Patients With B-Cell Chronic Lymphocytic Leukemia Resistant to Fludarabine
Juliusson G, Elmhorn-Rosenborg A, Liliemark J (Huddinge Hosp, Sweden; Karolinska Inst, Stockholm)
N Engl J Med 327:1056–1061, 1992   4–38

Introduction.—Fludarabine, a halogenated nucleoside analogue, yields a high rate of complete remission in patients with untreated B-cell chronic lymphocytic leukemia (CLL). However, life expectancy is decreased and outcome is very poor in patients whose disease has proved refractory to primary treatment. Four consecutive patients with CLL who failed to respond to fludarabine but who responded well to 2-chlorodeoxyadenosine, another halogenated nucleoside analog, were reported.

Patients and Results.—The patients all had inadequate responses to second-line or subsequent fludarabine treatment. One patient, who had progressing lymphocytosis, anemia, and thrombocytopenia despite receiving 10 courses of fludarabine, went into complete remission after 2-chlorodeoxyadenosine treatment. Good partial remissions were achieved in 2 patients with less-than-partial remissions after 6 courses of fludarabine. The fourth patient had Coombs'-positive hemolytic anemia with no response to 3 courses of fludarabine. In this case, 2-chlorodeoxyadenosine resulted in partial remission with resolution of hypogammaglobulinemia.

Discussion.—For some patients with advanced CLL, 2-chlorodeoxyadenosine appears to be an effective therapy. Despite their similar structures, this drug does not appear to show cross-resistance with fludarabine. Further evaluations of 2-chlorodeoxyadenosine in patients with CLL that is highly resistant to chemotherapy are needed.

▶ This important article indicates that drugs with the same presumed mechanism of action may not be cross-resistant. Both of these drugs are important new discoveries in CLL treatment. However, both should be used with caution because they can lead to permanent and major myelosuppression.—P.H. Wiernik, M.D.

Chronic Myelocytic Leukemia

The ABL-BCR Fusion Gene Is Expressed in Chronic Myeloid Leukemia
Melo JV, Gordon DE, Cross NCP, Goldman JM (Royal Postgraduate Med School, London)
Blood 81:158–165, 1993   4–39

Introduction.—Chronic myeloid leukemia (CML) appears to result from the presence of the Philadelphia (Ph) chromosome and the t(9;22) (q34;q11) reciprocal translocation. The BCR-ABL hybrid gene participates in the pathogenesis of the disease, but questions remain about the reciprocal chimeric gene ABL-BCR on chromosome 9q+. Reverse transcription and PCR amplification were done in cells from BCR-ABL–positive patients and 5 CML cell lines to determine the gene's role in the disease process.

Patients and Methods.—The PCR amplification and reverse transcription methods were applied to cell samples from 44 patients with CML, 20 of whom had the chronic phase of CML, and 24 of whom had the blast crisis episode. The usual Ph and 9q+ chromosomes were demonstrated in 38 patients. Five BCR-ABL–positive cell lines were also studied from patients with CML in blast crisis.

Results.—The BCR-ABL amplification studies found the b2a2- and b3a2-type transcripts. Patients in the chronic phase included 45% expressing only b2a2 and 50% expressing only b3a2 BCR-ABL transcripts. Those in blast crisis had 59% b2a2 only- and 38% had b3a3-only gene transcripts. All patients also had the normal BCR allele. Some 34 of the 49 patients (69%), including 2 Ph-negative patients and 1 patient without the 9q+ chromosome, demonstrated ABL-BCR amplification of the Ib-BCR type; 6 of the patients also expressed the Ia-BCR type. These results showed 3 types of ABL-BCR expressions: 12 at the Ib-b4 junction, 19 at the Ib-b3 junction, and 3 with double transcripts at Ib-b4 and Ib-b3. In 27 patients (79%), the junction type of the ABL-BCR gene mirrored the reciprocal of the BCR-ABL gene. In 4 products of the ABR-BCL gene in coding studies, the sequences exactly matched the ABL exon Ib[24] or Ia[25].

Conclusion.—In the Ph-positive CML cells, the coding sequences for the ABL and the BCR genes become disrupted because of a reciprocal exchange of material between chromosomes 9 and 22. The gene product of this DNA exchange may cause a deregulation of the guanosine triphosphatase–activating protein function of the BCR gene.

▶ Is the expression of this fusion gene modified by interferon?—P.H. Wiernik, M.D.

Treatment of Advanced Stages of Philadelphia Chromosome-Positive Chronic Myelogenous Leukemia With Interferon-α and Low-Dose Cytarabine
Kantarjian HM, Keating MJ, Estey EH, O'Brien S, Pierce S, Beran M, Koller C, Feldman E, Talpaz M (MD Anderson Cancer Ctr, Houston)
J Clin Oncol 10:772–778, 1992   4–40

Introduction.—The course of chronic myeloid leukemia (CML) progresses relentlessly from the indolent or chronic phase to the resistant accelerated and blastic phases. Conventional treatment with hydroxyurea or busulfan effectively controls disease evolution in the chronic phase but has little impact on disease evolution in the terminal phases. The efficacy of interferon-alpha (INF-α) and low-dose cytarabine (ara-C) in combination chemotherapy was assessed in patients with CML.

Patients and Methods.—Sixty patients in the advanced phases of Philadelphia chromosome–positive CML were treated with INF-α, 5×10^6 units/m² surface area every day, and low-dose ara-C, 15 mg/m² every day, for 2 weeks every 4 weeks until remission, then for 1 week every month for maintenance. Forty patients were in the late chronic phase of disease, and 20 were in the accelerated phase. The outcomes of these

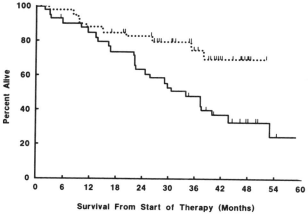

Survival From Start of Therapy (Months)

Fig 4–10.—Survival of patients in the late chronic phase of CML treated with INF-α and ara-C (*dotted line*) or with INF-α alone (*solid line*). (Courtesy of Kantarjian HM, Keating MJ, Estey EH, et al: *J Clin Oncol* 10:772–778, 1992.)

patients were compared with those of 58 patients who had been treated previously with INF-α alone in the same doses.

Results.—Patients receiving INF-α plus ara-C in the late chronic phase had better complete hematologic response rates (55% and 28%, respectively) than those given INF-α alone. In this group, there was also a trend toward better Philadelphia chromosome suppression and a longer survival for those given combined therapy. These differences did not seem to be attributable to imbalances in prognostic factors between groups. In patients in the accelerated phase, adding ara-C to INF-α treatment did not improve the response rate. Differences in survival were explained by different patient characteristics. Twenty-five percent of patients had suppression of clonal evolution. Those with clonal evolution as the only criterion for disease acceleration had a longer survival than patients with other or additional accelerated-phase criteria (Fig 4–10).

Conclusion.—The results of combined INF-α and ara-C treatment in patients in late chronic-phase CML are promising. The efficacy of this treatment in early chronic-phase CML should be evaluated.

▶ We have had success with interferon plus plicamycin in advanced stages of CML.—P.H. Wiernik, M.D.

Polyclonal Hematopoiesis in Interferon-Induced Cytogenetic Remissions of Chronic Myelogenous Leukemia

Claxton D, Deisseroth A, Talpaz M, Reading C, Kantarjian H, Trujillo J, Stass S, Gooch G, Spitzer G (Univ of Texas, Houston)
Blood 79:997–1002, 1992   4–41

Objective.—For patients with early chronic myeloid leukemia (CML), interferon (INF) therapy can produce a partial or complete cytogenetic remission. After complete remission, patients may continue therapy for years with only diploid metaphases on bone marrow examination.

Observations.—Using X-linked polymorphic markers, the investigators analyzed cells from 5 female patients in major cytogenetic remission from CML during INF therapy. According to clonality analysis using the *Bst* XI phosphoglycerate kinase gene polymorphism, granulocytes were nonclonal during remission in all patients. For each patient, 2 separate specimens obtained during treatment and at least 1 T-cell line were assessed. Densitometry results confirmed that relative intensity of band A1 values of remission samples and T cells were within a close range of one another. One patient with incomplete remission at the time of sampling had rearrangement on *bcr*-region studies.

Conclusion.—In patients with INF-induced remissions of CML, granulopoiesis appears to be nonclonal. The findings confirm the presence of residual and apparently normal hematopoietic progenitors with the ability to stably reconstitute the bone marrow in this disorder.

▶ Here is further evidence that INF therapy changes the biology of the disease.—P.H. Wiernik, M.D.

Chronic Myelogenous Leukemia in the Lymphoid Blastic Phase: Characteristics, Treatment Response, and Prognosis
Derderian PM, Kantarjian HM, Talpaz M, O'Brien S, Cork A, Estey E, Pierce S, Keating M (MD Anderson Cancer Ctr, Houston)
Am J Med 94:69–74, 1993   4–42

Background.—The prognosis appears to be poor in patients with chronic myeloid leukemia (CML) in the blastoid phase. Twenty-five percent of these patients have lymphoid blastic morphology. The clinical and laboratory features and the outcomes of patients with CML in the lymphoid blastic phase were evaluated.

Patients and Methods.—Of 296 patients with CML blastic-phase disease seen during a 24-year period, 68 had CML lymphoid blastic-phase disease. The pretreatment characteristics, treatment responses, and survival rates of this patient group were compared with those of patients with myeloid or undifferentiated blastic-phase CML.

Findings.—The median age was 40 years in the lymphoid disease group and 52 years in the other 2 groups. The lymphoid group also had significantly less anemia, lower white blood cell and peripheral blast counts, higher marrow blast percentages, lower lactic dehydrogenase levels, and higher albumin levels. Forty percent of the lymphoid group had accelerated-phase CML before the blastic phase, compared with 54% of those in other morphologic groups. In the lymphoid group, 97% of patients had the common acute lymphocytic leukemia antigen; they also had a lower incidence of trisomy 8 and isochromosome 17 abnormalities. The incidence of lymphoid blastic-phase disease was not increased in the last decade of the experience. Lymphoid disease was no more common in patients with chronic-phase CML treated with alpha-interferon. The chemotherapeutic response rate in the lymphoid group during the first salvage was 49% vs. less than 20% for the other groups. The complete response rate to the combination of vincristine, Adriamycin, and dexamethasone was 61%. The median survival was 9 months in the lymphoid group vs. 3 months in the others.

Conclusion.—Among patients with blastic-phase CML, those with lymphoid disease have different clinical and laboratory features. It is extremely important to differentiate patients with lymphoid transformation because their treatment and prognosis are different. Therapy is similar to that of acute lymphocytic leukemia. The survival benefit of lymphoid morphology does not last long, so plans for bone marrow transplantation or experimental treatments should be implemented rapidly.

▶ The lymphoid type of blast crisis in CML is responsive to acute lymphoid leukemia–type therapy. However, the responses with that therapy in this type of blast crisis are usually brief. On the other hand, patients with lymphoid blast crisis survive longer than patients with myeloid blast crisis irrespective of therapy. The bottom line is that patients with lymphoid blast crisis should not be excluded from trials of new treatments for blast crisis simply because they may briefly respond to acute lymphoid leukemia–type therapy, but they must be evaluated separately from other patients with blast crisis with respect to survival, because their prognosis for survival is better.—P.H. Wiernik, M.D.

Phase II Study of Mitoxantrone and 5-Azacytidine for Accelerated and Blast Crisis of Chronic Myelogenous Leukemia: A Study of the Eastern Cooperative Oncology Group

Dutcher JP, Eudey L, Wiernik PH, Paietta E, Bennett JM, Arlin Z, Kellermeyer R, Rowe J, O'Connell M, Oken M, Cassileth PA (Albert Einstein Cancer Ctr, Bronx, NY; Dana-Farber Cancer Inst, Boston; Univ of Rochester, NY; et al)
Leukemia 6:770–775, 1992   4–43

Background.—Once chronic myeloid leukemia (CML) enters the acute blastic phase, it is highly resistant to available cytotoxic therapies. It has been suggested that the anthraquinone mitoxantrone and the primidine analogue 5-azacytidine might be active in the blast crisis of CML. Whether a combination of these 2 agents is better therapy than either 1 alone was examined.

Methods.—Forty evaluable adult patients in blast crisis or the accelerated phase of CML were treated with mitoxantrone, 12 mg/m²/day for 3 days, and 5-azacytidine, 150 mg/m²/day for 5 days. The bone marrow response was assessed on day 14 to determine the need for a second course; subsequent specimens were obtained to determine the response to therapy.

Results.—The main toxic effects were hematologic in nature, with prolonged pancytopenia in some cases. There were 22 deaths during induction, 13 from disease and 9 from aplasia. There was a 23% overall response rate, with 5 complete responders, 2 partial responders, and 2 patients showing hematologic improvement. When assessed, the cytogenetic and immunophenotypic characteristics of the leukemia were correlated with the patient's response and survival; however, they had no predictive value once the patient was in blast crisis. The response was predicted to some extent by the initial platelet count, hemoglobin, and lower WBC count. Prolonged survival was predicted by lack of liver involvement, lower WBC count, and higher platelet count. One third of the responders remained alive at 1 year, although response and survival were not strongly correlated.

Conclusion.—The described regimen of mitoxantrone and 5-azacytidine appears to have antileukemic activity for patients in the blast crisis of CML. Mitoxantrone, alone or in combination with cytosine arabinoside or 5-azacytidine, remains an appropriate treatment for these patients until more effective regimens become available.

▶ This regimen was based on earlier encouraging results with a combination of etoposide and 5-azacytidine in our group. The results with the present regimen are not as good. We have had much better early results with a combination of mitoxantrone and carboplatin, which deserves further study.—P.H. Wiernik, M.D.

Treatment of Chronic Myeloid Leukemia With Allogeneic Bone Marrow Transplantation After Preparation With BuCy2

Biggs JC, Szer J, Crilley P, Atkinson K, Downs K, Dodds A, Concannon AJ, Avalos B, Tutschka P, Kapoor N, Brodsky I, Topolsky D, Bulova SI, Copelan EA (St Vincent's Hosp, Sydney, Australia; Alfred Hosp, Melbourne, Australia; Ohio State Univ, Columbus; et al)
Blood 80:1352–1357, 1992   4–44

Introduction.—In patients with chronic myeloid leukemia (CML), allogeneic bone marrow transplantation (BMT) after high-dose chemotherapy and total body irradiation has resulted in a cure for at least half of the patients who undergo transplantation while in the chronic phase. More recently, an irradiation-free regimen consisting of oral busulfan and intravenous cyclophosphamide (BuCy) for 4 days was associated with a low relapse rate but a high incidence of transplant-related mortality. Reducing the dose of cyclophosphamide and giving it during 2 days (BuCy2) might reduce the incidence of treatment-related complications. The results of using this conditioning regimen in 115 patients with CML were reported.

Patients and Methods.—There were 68 men and 47 women, median age 35 years, all with Philadelphia chromosome–positive CML. Sixty-two patients underwent transplantation in the chronic phase, 26 in the accelerated phase, and 27 in blast transformation. The BuCy2 regimen consisted of busulfan, 4 mg/kg for 4 days, and cyclophosphamide, 60 mg/kg on each of 2 days. This was followed by histocompatible sibling allogeneic BMT 24 to 48 hours later.

Results.—The 3-year actuarial survival rate was 58% for those in the chronic phase, 41% for those in the accelerated phase, and 25% for those in blast transformation. Corresponding probabilities of relapse were 3%, 12%, and 27%. Transient cytogenic relapse occurred in just 2 patients who underwent transplantation while in the chronic phase; 1 of them died of transplant-related complications and the other remains cytogenically normal after nearly 2 years. The survival rate was 70% for patients who received their transplant within 1 year of diagnosis in the chronic phase, compared with 40% when the transplant was done more than 1 year after the diagnosis. This difference, resulting from transplant-related complications, was correlated with prior exposure to high doses of busulfan.

Conclusion.—In patients with CML undergoing allogeneic EMT, the BuCy2 conditioning regimen yields survival and mortality figures similar to those expected with regimens including total body irradiation. The relapse rate may be lower than that with radiation, but a larger analysis would be required to establish this.

▶ The suggestion that this regimen may be associated with fewer relapses than regimens that include radiotherapy is certainly worthy of further study.—P.H. Wiernik, M.D.

Molecular Remission Occurring After Donor Leukocyte Infusions for the Treatment of Relapsed Chronic Myelogenous Leukemia After Allogeneic Bone Marrow Transplantation

Drobyski WR, Roth MS, Thibodeau SN, Gottschall JL (Med College of Wisconsin, Milwaukee; Univ of Michigan, Ann Arbor; Mayo Clinic and Mayo Found, Rochester, Minn)

Bone Marrow Transplant 10:301–304, 1992   4–45

Introduction.—Several patients with chronic myeloid leukemia (CML) in relapse have remitted after receiving infusions of donor leukocytes. However, it is not clear whether this treatment leads to complete molecular remission.

Case Report.—Woman, 34, had Philadelphia chromosome (Ph[1])-positive CML in the accelerated phase and received a T-cell–depleted bone marrow transplant from an HLA-identical sister. Mild graft-vs.-host disease developed despite the use of anti-CD3 monoclonal antibody. Relapse was evident cytogenetically a year after transplantation, and hematologic relapse soon followed. A second marrow transplant containing T cells was given, but the patient relapsed again and exhibited multiple cytogenetic abnormalities in addition to Ph[1]. Treatment with interferon-alpha was poorly tolerated. About 1-month after relapse, 3 leukocyte infusions were given, using cells taken from the second marrow donor. Pancytopenia developed 7 weeks later, when there was evidence of mixed chimerism. Complete donor chimerism and persistent leukemia were documented 2 weeks later. Granulocyte-CSF was then given. After an eruption of graft-vs.-host-disease, marrow studies showed complete elimination of the leukemia clone. The patient remained in complete remission 48 weeks after white cell infusion.

Conclusion.—Leukocyte infusions may be an effective type of adoptive immunotherapy, leading to sustained molecular remission of CML. Some relapses after marrow transplantation may represent a suboptimal graft-vs.-leukemia reaction.

Hematologic Relapse of Chronic Myelogenous Leukemia Following Allogeneic Bone Marrow Transplantation: Apparent Graft-Versus-Leukemia Effect Following Abrupt Discontinuation of Immunosuppression

Collins RH Jr, Rogers ZR, Bennett M, Kumar V, Nikein A, Fay JW (Baylor Univ, Dallas; Univ of Texas, Dallas)
Bone Marrow Transplant 10:391–395, 1992   4–46

Background.—The anti-leukemia efficacy of allogeneic bone marrow transplantation may reflect actions of the immune cells that are transferred. Relapse is more frequent in recipients of syngeneic or T-cell–depleted grafts and less frequent in those in whom graft-vs.-host disease (GVHD) occurs. Immunosuppressive measures intended to prevent GVHD may conceivably inhibit the development of a graft-vs.-leukemia (GVL) effect.

A Pilot Trial.—Cyclosporine immunosuppression was stopped in 2 patients with a hematologic relapse of chronic myelogenous leukemia (CML) after allogeneic bone marrow transplantation. Both patients rapidly entered complete hematologic and cytogenetic remission and have remained in remission, 1 for 30 months and 1 for 22 months after marrow transplantation. In 1 patient, resolution of leukemia was associated with the development of GVHD. The second patient exhibited lytic activity against autologous CML cells that increased with IL-2.

Conclusion.—Withdrawal of immunosuppression could prove helpful when CML recurs after bone marrow transplantation. Serial studies of T-cell and natural killer cell–mediated activity against potential GVL target antigens may elucidate the mechanisms of GVL.

▶ Can "donor" leukocytes given *instead* of allogeneic bone marrow transplant produce GVHD equivalent to that of allogeneic bone marrow transplant and yield similar therapeutic results?—P.H. Wiernik, M.D.

Unrelated Donor Marrow Transplantation Therapy for Chronic Myelogenous Leukemia: Initial Experience of the National Marrow Donor Program

McGlave P, Bartsch G, Anasetti C, Ash R, Beatty P, Gajewski J, Kernan NA (Univ of Minnesota, Minneapolis; Fred Hutchinson Cancer Research Ctr, Seattle; Med College of Wisconsin, Milwaukee; et al)

Blood 81:543–550, 1993   4–47

Purpose.—Marrow transplantation is the only proven cure for chronic myeloid leukemia (CML), but most eligible patients lack a suitable related donor. The identification of suitable unrelated donors has been facilitated by the National Marrow Donor Program (NMDP). The results of the first 196 transplants performed in patients with CML using donor marrow obtained by the NMDP were analyzed.

Patients and Methods.—The procedures were done during a 3-year period at 21 marrow transplant centers affiliated with the NMDP. The median time from initiation of the search to transplantation was 8 months. The patients were 121 males and 75 females (median age, 33 years). One hundred fifteen patients underwent transplantation when in the chronic phase, 51 in the accelerated phase, 14 in blast crisis, and 16 in a subsequent chronic phase. The marrow was identical at the HLA A, B, and DR loci in 133 patients and 1 locus apart in 63. Preparative therapy consisted of high-dose chemotherapy and total body irradiation in 169 patients and chemotherapy only in 27. Non–T cell–depleted marrow was used in 161 patients.

Outcome.—Engraftment was successful in 174 patients in a median of 22 days. Graft failure occurred in 22 patients and an additional 10 patients had late graft failure. There was a .54 incidence of grade III or IV acute graft-vs.-host disease (GVHD) and a .52 incidence of extensive chronic GVHD. Both types of GVHD were less common with T-cell–depleted marrow. The 2-year actuarial incidence of hematologic relapse was .11. The 2-year disease-free survival was .45 in patients with transplantation in the first chronic phase within 1 year of diagnosis, .36 for those in the first chronic phase after 1 year of diagnosis, .27 for those in the accelerated phase, .22 for those in the subsequent chronic phase, and 0 for those in blast crisis. Factors independently associated with disease-free survival included transplantation with HLA-matched marrow, younger age, and transplantation in the first chronic phase. At 1 year, 50% of survivors had normal activity levels, 41% had mild impairment, and 9% had severe impairment.

Conclusion.—For patients with CML, marrow transplantation with HLA-matched unrelated donor marrow is facilitated by the NMDP. Prolonged, disease-free survival can be attained in some patients, particularly younger patients with transplantation early in the course of disease with HLA A- , B- , and DR-matched marrow. The treatment is associated with a high incidence of graft failure, acute and chronic GVHD, and long convalescence.

MYELODYSPLASIA

Circulating CD34+ Cells: An Adverse Prognostic Factor in the Myelodysplastic Syndromes

Sullivan SA, Marsden KA, Lowenthal RM, Jupe DM, Jones ME (Univ of Tasmania; Royal Hobart Hosp; Menzies Ctr for Population Health Research, Hobart, Tasmania, Australia)
Am J Hematol 39:96–101, 1992   4–48

Introduction.—The myelodysplastic syndromes (MDSs) are a group of 5 hematologic disorders, characterized by bone marrow dysplasia and varying degrees of anemia, leukopenia, and thrombocytopenia, that in many cases transform to acute myeloid leukemia (AML). Some laboratory parameters have been shown to have prognostic significance. The significance of the presence of CD34+ cells, the human progenitor cell antigen, in bone marrow is debatable.

Methods.—Sixty-two patients with MDS identified in the course of a 2-year epidemiologic survey of MDS in southern Tasmania were tested for the presence of CD34 in the peripheral blood. The Bournemouth score and bone marrow CFU-GM colony growth were also assessed. The CD34+status was compared with these other variables as prognostic indicators of transformation to AML and patient survival.

Results.—Twenty-three patients had circulating CD34+ cells. Nine of these patients went on to have AML, compared with none of the 39 CD34-negative patients. At the end of 2 years, 11 of the CD34+ group vs. 6 of the CD34-negative groups were dead. The Bournemouth score was also associated with development of AML and death—these were the only 2 significant prognostic indicators of either poor outcome.

Conclusion.—In patients with MDS, circulating CD34+ cells appear to be associated with progression to AML and poor survival. The CD34+ status is a better prognostic indicator than either cytogenetic data or CFU-GM colony growth. The CD34 test does not require bone marrow biopsy and, thus, may be especially useful for elderly patients.

▶ The association of CD34+ with transformation to AML is a new important finding. The CD34+ MDS should be considered a new MDS classification that may be more meaningful than the French-American-British subtypes.—P.H. Wiernik, M.D.

Primary Myelodysplastic Syndromes: Analysis of Prognostic Factors in 235 Patients and Proposals for an Improved Scoring System
Aul C, Gattermann N, Heyll A, Germing U, Derigs G, Schneider W (Heinrich Heine Univ, Düsseldorf, Germany)
Leukemia 6:52–59, 1992   4–49

Introduction.—The myelodysplastic syndromes (MDSs) a heterogenous group of bone marrow disorders, apparently result from the malignant transformation of a multipotent stem cell. The MDSs are heterogenous in their hematologic manifestations and in the survival of individual patients: some succumb to complications of bone marrow failure or transformation to acute myeloid leukemia within months of diagnosis, whereas others may survive for many years. The prognostic importance of an increased medullary blast cell count is generally agreed on, but the independent value of other variables as predictors of outcome is controversial. A survival analysis of 235 consecutive patients with primary MDSs and a proposal for an improved scoring system that is useful for all subgroups of MDSs and contains valid prognostic information were reviewed.

Patients and Methods.—This retrospective study analyzed 235 untreated patients with primary MDSs diagnosed between 1970 and 1986. Besides the well-known French-American-British (FAB) classification of MDS, a supplementary group with pure sideroblastic anemia (PSA), characterized by nonerythroid cells lacking dysplastic feaures, was added. The study population had a median age of 72 years and included 55 patients with refractory anemia (RA), 53 with RA with excess of blasts (RAEB), 40 with PSA, 33 with RA with ring sideroblasts (RARS), 29 with RAEB in transformation, and 25 with chronic myelomonocytic leukemia (CMML). Twenty-eight parameters, including clinical, laboratory, and morphologic characteristics, were investigated with univariate and multivariate analysis for their relationship to survival and transformation to acute myeloid leukemia.

Results.—For the entire series, the probability of survival was 59% at 1 year after diagnosis and 24% at 5 years; the actuarial risk of leukemic transformation was 21% at 1 year and 36% at 5 years. Unfavorable prognostic indicators as shown by univariate analysis included age > 70 years, poor performance status, lymphadenopathy, hemoglobin $\leq$ 9 g/dL, platelet count $\leq 100 \times 10^9$/L, lactate dehydrogenase (LDH) ≥ 200 units/L, advanced FAB subtype, severe dysgranulopoiesis, and dysmegakaryopoiesis. Among patients with a low medullary blast count, those with PSA had the best survival, 59% at 5 years, whereas patients with RARS had an 18% survival and those with RA had a 22% survival at 5 years. Serum LDH levels were an important risk determinant. Few factors, including the presence of Auer rods and micromegakaryocytes and the degree of dysgranulopoiesis, predicted leukemic transformation. Multivariate analysis showed that the medullary blast cell count was the most significant prognostic factor for survival, with LDH as the second most important covariate and PSA as an independent prognostic variable. This analysis showed that the prognostic weight of the original FAB classification can largely be replaced by another simple scoring system. In this system, a score of unity was allocated for each of the following: bone marrow blasts $\geq$ 5%, LDH > 200 units/L, hemoglobin $\leq$ 9 g/dL, and platelets $\leq$ 100 $\times$ 10⁹/L. Patients with a score of 0 had a cumulative 2-year survival of 91%, whereas those with a score of 3 or 4 had a 2-year survival as low as 9%. The actuarial risk of acute myeloid leukemia also correlated well with the score.

Conclusion.—The proposed scoring system appears reasonably simple but reliable enough for clinical decision-making. Unlike the Bournemouth score, this system can identify patients with RA and RARS who have an unfavorable prognosis despite no excess of blasts and, if LDH levels are included, can accurately assess patients with CMML who are otherwise given overly optimistic prognoses.

▶ It will be interesting to see whether the scoring system developed in this retrospective study survives a prospective test.—P.H. Wiernik, M.D.

Acute Leukemias

ACUTE MYELOID LEUKEMIA

Occupational Risk Factors for Acute Leukaemia: A Case-Control Study

Richardson S, Zittoun R, Bastuji-Garin S, Lasserre V, Guihenneuc C, Cadiou M, Viguie F, Laffont-Faust I (INSERM U 170, Villejuif, France; Hôtel-Dieu, Paris; Laboratoire de statistiques Médicales, Paris; et al)
Int J Epidemiol 21:1063–1073, 1992   4-50

Objective.—Because the role of various exposures in acute leukemia is ambiguous, 185 patients older than age 30 years with acute leukemia were examined. They were matched for age, sex, ethnicity, and site of residence with 561 controls seen in the same 4-year period.

Findings.—Professional exposure to ionizing radiation was not found in excess among cases, but there was a significant relationship between acute leukemia and high or medium levels of exposure to benzene. Exposure to high or medium levels of exhaust gas for more than 10 years also was a risk factor. Significant odds ratio values also were found for exposure to insecticides or weed killers, or both, and for exposure to electric and magnetic fields (EMFs). Exposure to benzene and to EMFs was associated with myelogenous subtypes of leukemia. Pesticide-related cases included both lymphoblastic and myeloblastic leukemias.

Conclusion.—These findings support a role for benzene, pesticides, and EMFs as leukemogenic agents.

▶ The literature on pesticides and EMFs is controversial, but this well-conducted study adds to the data that implicate both as causes of acute leukemia. This study also suggests that relatively high-level exposure to benzene is related to the cause of acute myeloid leukemia, and, contrary to some other studies, a relationship between benzene exposure and acute lymphoblastic leukemia was noted.—P.H. Wiernik, M.D.

Distinct Cytogenetic and Clinicopathologic Features in Acute Myeloid Leukemia After Occupational Exposure to Pesticides and Organic Solvents
Fagioli F, Cuneo A, Piva N, Carli MG, Previati R, Balboni M, Tomasi P, Cariani D, Scapoli G, Castoldi G (Univ of Ferrara, Italy)
Cancer 70:77–85, 1992   4–51

Introduction.—Cytotoxic drugs and radiation exposure are acknowledged leukemogenic agents, but the role of other myelotoxic agents present in the environment is ill-defined. Two groups of patients—exposed or unexposed to pesticides or organic solvents—were assessed to better define the role of environmental exposure in the genesis of acute myeloid leukemia (AML).

French-American-British Classes, Clinical Features at Presentation, Response to Chemotherapy, and Survival in Patients With AML Exposed to Pesticides or Organic Solvents and Patients Not Exposed

	Exposed		Not exposed
	Pesticides	*Solvents*	
FAB subtypes *	M1(1); M2(6); M4(6); M5(2); M6(1); M7(2)	M1(1); M2(1); M3(1); M4(1); M5(2); M6(1)	M1(3); M2(8); M3(2); M4(12); M5(8); M6(1)
Age (yr)	50–82 (68)	32–74 (55)	14–79 (66)
Hemoglobin value (g/dl)	5.0–10.5 (9)	5.4–9.5 (7.6)	5.6–13.7 (8.9)
Leukocyte count (×10⁹/l)	2.1–83.9 (6.6)	1.3–11.0 (4.8)	1.0–249.0 (15.6)
Platelet count (×10⁹/l)	20.0–488.0 (85)	18–243.0 (85)	26.0–240.0 (71)
% bls (PB)	4–80 (32)	3–70 (30)	2–95 (64)
% bls (BM)	30–90 (45)	34–85 (58)	35–90 (70)
CR†	1/13	0/6	14/29
Survival (mo)	1–78+ (1,5)	1–8 (2)	1–36+ (8)

Abbreviations: FAB, French-American-British; CR, complete response; bls, blasts; PB, peripheral blood; BM, bone marrow.
Note: Results are reported as variation ranges; median values are given in parentheses.
* Number of cases in each FAB category.
† Number of complete remissions/number of patients treated with myeloablative chemotherapy.
(Courtesy of Fagioli F, Cuneo A, Piva N, et al: Cancer 70:77–85, 1992.)

Patients and Methods.—Fifty-nine patients with de novo AML had bone marrow smears available for cytologic review and assessable immunologic and cytogenetic data. On the basis of an interview about occupational history and hobbies, 25 patients were categorized as exposed and 34 as unexposed. Seven of the exposed patients had prolonged contact with organic solvents and 18 with pesticides. The median age was similar for the 2 groups, but the male-female ratio was greater in the exposed group (3.2 vs. .9).

Results.—Exposed patients had lower leukocyte counts and lower blast-cell percentages in their bone marrow. The French-American-British system subtypes of erythroleukemia and megakaryoblastic leukemia were seen more frequently among exposed patients. Complete remission with conventional chemotherapy was achieved in only 1 of 19 exposed patients, compared with 14 of 29 unexposed patients. The overall median survival was 2 months in the exposed group and 8 months in the unexposed group (table). Clonal chromosome aberrations were detected in 22 of 25 exposed patients and in 10 of 34 unexposed patients. Myelodysplasia involved multiple cell lineages in all assessable exposed patients; among unexposed patients, morphologic aberrations of the non-blast cell populations were confined to a minority of cells.

Conclusion.—Acute myeloid leukemia in patients professionally exposed to pesticides and organic solvents may represent a distinct cytogenetic and clinicopathologic entity. Patients with AML after chemotherapy for another tumor have similar features, suggesting that common transformation pathways may underlie leukemogenesis induced by cytotoxic drugs and certain environmental exposures.

▶ Contrary to the article by Richardson et al. (Abstract 4–50), this study found a clear relationship between cytogenetics and leukemia related to chemical exposure. This study is supported by many others in the literature that yielded similar results.—P.H. Wiernik, M.D.

Involvement of a Homolog of Drosophila Trithorax by 11q23 Chromosomal Translocations in Acute Leukemias

Tkachuk DC, Kohler S, Cleary ML (Stanford Univ, Calif)
Cell 71:691–700, 1992   4–52

Introduction.—The molecular rearrangements associated with chromosomal translocations found in patients with various leukemias suggest that several newly discovered proteins may play a role in leukemogenesis, particularly 1 located in chromosome band 11q23. A gene was identified that participated in recurring 11q23 leukemic translocations and coded for a very large protein that is a homolog of the *Drosophila* trithorax protein.

Methods.—With fusion transcript methods for the t(11;19) locus, the recurring 11q23 translocation code was defined. Other current standard molecular methods, including nucleotide sequence analysis, Southern and Northern blot analyses, gene cloning in several cell cultures, and computer analyses to align the human trithorax protein (HRX) and trithorax proteins, were used.

Results.—In identifying the transcription unit at the 11q23 translocation site, a genomic DNA fragment at the 3' end of the 92-kb Notl fragment hybridized with the transcripts in several cell lines. The 11q23 gene mapped to both sides of the 11q23 break point cluster region. When compared with *Drosophila* trithorax, the nucleotide sequence assessment of this complementary DNA (cDNA) showed an open reading frame of 11,904 nucleotide which coded for a predicted protein of 3,968 amino acids. The homology search of the Swiss protein data base demonstrated this predicted protein to be significantly similar to the *Drosophila* trithorax protein. In addition, 2 other regions were divergent homologs of the amino-terminal hook area and included amino acids 217-227 and 301-309. Only 4.6 kb of the eleven-nineteen leukemia cDNA was cloned, but sequence comparisons of the protein found no significant similarities to previously identified proteins.

Conclusion.—Human multilineage leukemias appear to disrupt a homolog of the *Drosophila* developmental protein trithorax via chromosomal translocations. This may occur through DNA binding within the minor groove of the protein at the amino-terminal hook sites.

▶ This is a fascinating finding.—P.H. Wiernik, M.D.

Cytogenetics for Detection of Minimal Residual Disease in Acute Myeloblastic Leukemia

Freireich E, Cork A, Stass SA, McCredie KB, Keating MJ, Estey EH, Kantarjian HM, Trujillo JM (Univ of Texas, Houston)
Leukemia 6:500–506, 1992   4–53

Background.—Most patients with acute myeloid leukemia (AML) have cytogenetic abnormalities. The continued presence rate of these anomalies in patients with AML who were experiencing complete morphologic and hematologic remission was examined. A correlation between the persistence of cytogenetic abnormality and patient prognosis was made.

Patients.—Study participants included patients with AML from the favorable (inv 16, t[8;21], and t[15;17]) and unfavorable (+8, −5, −7, and Philadelphia-positive) cytogenetic categories. Seventy-one patients had metaphase spreads in remission marrows that were assessable, and 20 of these (28%) had 1 or more abnormal metaphases, matching that found in the pretreatment marrow.

Results.—Within 78 weeks, all 20 of the patients with abnormal metaphase relapsed. Therefore, no false-positives occurred in this study. In 51 patients, diploid metaphases only were noted in the complete remission marrow: 25 relapsed and 21 remained in continuous complete remission, indicating a 49% false-negative rate. Thus, continuous complete remission is not guaranteed by the lack of chromosomally abnormal bone marrow cells. The favorable cytogenetic groups had the most useful cytogenetic studies; the least useful studies were in the unfavorable groups. Outcome or recurrence risks were not affected by the persistence of pretreatment marrow normal metaphases. Analogous cytogenetic anomalies (found in the pretreatment marrow) or the same abnormality with additional chromosomal changes were found in 25 of 34 assessable patients who experienced relapse after remission.

Conclusion.—An objective mode for residual leukemia detection is provided via cytogenetic examinations of complete remission bone marrow samples in patients with AML. Moreover, this method aids in identifying patients with prolonged disease-free survival potential.

▶ Several studies have demonstrated the feasibility of detecting minimal residual disease in AML, but this is the first one to my knowledge that shows a relationship between the presence or absence of minimal residual disease and disease-free survival.—P.H. Wiernik, M.D.

Phenotypical Characteristics of Acute Myelocytic Leukemia Associated With the t(8;21) (q22;q22) Chromosomal Abnormality: Frequent Expression of Immature B-Cell Antigen CD19 Together With Stem Cell Antigen CD34
Kita K, Nakase K, Miwa H, Masuya M, Nishii K, Morita N, Takakura N, Otsuji A, Shirakawa S, Ueda T, Nasu K, Kyo T, Dohy H, Kamada N (Mie Univ, Tsu, Japan; Fukui Med School, Japan; Osaka Red Cross Hosp, Japan; et al)
Blood 80:470–477, 1992   4–54

Background.—In acute myeloid leukemia (AML), the 8;21 t(8;21) (q22;q22) translocation is one of the most frequent karyotypic anomalies. Characteristic cytologic and clinical features are manifested in this type of AML. Therefore, it is thought that this chromosomal abnormality transpires at a certain hematopoietic differentiation stage. The relationship between immunophenotype and karyotypic abnormality was investigated to determine whether there was a relationship between the hematopoietic stage and 8;21 translocation.

Patients and Methods.—A total of 23 adult patients with AML and t(8;21) chromosomal abnormalities (classified as M2 French-American-British), were examined. Bone marrow (BM) and heparinized peripheral blood samples were obtained, and karyotype analysis was conducted on aspired BM cells. Mononuclear cells were separated from the samples, and high-molecular-weight DNA and total RNA were extracted from the cell fractions. Southern and Northern blotting assays were performed, and CD19 and CD20 gene expression were explored via reverse transcription PCR.

Results.—Stem cell–associated antigens (CD34 and HLA-DR) and immature myeloid antigens (CD13 and CD33) revealed positive blastic cells from all patients. The more mature myeloid antigens (CD11b and CD15) were expressed by nonblastic leukemia cells, with immature phenotype loss. The positive occurrence of CD34 and HLA-DR stem cell–associated antigens in t(8;21) AML cells was significantly higher than those in other AML cells displaying granulocytic differentiation (M2 or M3). Phenotypic anomalies were also revealed in some t(8;21) AML cells. In 18 of 23 patients, frequent CD19 expression was noted in the t(8;21) AML blastic population, without additional B-cell antigens and immunoglobulin gene rearrangements. Immunocytochemistry and Northern blotting confirmed CD19 expression. The CD34 and HLA-DR were coexpressed by CD19+ blastic cells. Furthermore, among the blastic fraction, fewer CD33+ cells in t(8;21) were noted than in AML M2 or M3 minus t(8;21).

Conclusion.—Leukemic blasts of t(8;21) AML origin routinely express CD19 without altering other stem cell–associated antigens and are, therefore, more likely to maintain the properties of multipotential cells. The AML may indicate discordant maturation of these cells, resulting in anomalies such as low CD33 expression.

Expression of Myeloid-Associated and Lymphoid-Associated Cell-Surface Antigens in Acute Myeloid Leukemia of Childhood: A Pediatric Oncology Group Study

Kuerbitz SJ, Civin CI, Krischer JP, Ravindranath Y, Steuber CP, Weinstein HJ, Winick N, Ragab AH, Gresik MV, Crist WM (Johns Hopkins Oncology Ctr, Baltimore, Md; Univ of Florida, Gainesville; Wayne State Univ, Detroit; et al)
J Clin Oncol 10:1419–1429, 1992 4–55

Introduction.—At the molecular level, acute leukemias have a heterogeneity that has increasingly become apparent as methods such as monoclonal antibody staging come into use. Acute lymphoid leukemia (ALL) is now classified partially using its immunophenotype, although no classification system has been adopted to date. The outcomes of 294 patients with pediatric acute myeloid leukemia (AML) were reviewed to determine the clinical significance of the expression of the myeloid- and lymphoid-associated cell surface antigens.

Methods.—The records of 294 children with untreated AML were reviewed. Of the 294, 199 had undergone immunophenotyping for the highest-priority antibodies CD33, CD13, CD15, CD7, CD5, CD19, CD10, and HLA-DR, with the CD34 antigen predicting poor patient prognosis. Antigen expression was then associated with clinical outcome.

Results.—Of the 132 assessable patients with AML, 91% expressed at least 1 myeloid-associated antigen, with CD33, CD13, and CD15 occurring in the most patients. When tested for CD33 and/or CD13, 88% of patients expressed both, whereas those tested for CD33 and/or CD13 and/or CD15 showed a 91% expression for all 3 antigens. Of those tested, 49% expressed 1 or more of the T-lymphoid–associated antigens, whereas only 15% of the patients expressed at least 1 of the B-lymphoid antigens. The French-American-British classification significantly related with the CD14 antigen expression only. The children's response to induction chemotherapy did not correlate significantly with any myeloid-related antigen.

Conclusion.—More than 90% of the patients with childhood AML expressed at least 1 of the 5 antigens related to normal myeloid differentiation. Thus, the cell surface antigen expression in these patients usually discriminated AML from ALL.

Expression of Lymphoid-Associated Cell Surface Antigens by Childhood Acute Myeloid Leukemia Cells Lacks Prognostic Significance

Smith FO, Lampkin BC, Versteeg C, Flowers DA, Dinndorf PA, Buckley JD, Woods WG, Hammond GD, Bernstein ID (Fred Hutchinson Cancer Research Ctr, Seattle; Childrens Hosp of Cincinnati, Ohio; Univ of Southern California, Los Angeles; et al)
Blood 79:2415–2422, 1992   4–56

Background.—Blast cells from most patients with acute myeloid leukemia (AML) have antigens associated with normal myeloid development, but some also exhibit antigens associated with lymphoid development. The pesence of these antigens may predict a poor therapeutic response, but a large number of adults with lymphoid-associated antigens on their AML blasts indicated a more favorable prognosis.

Patients and Methods.—The prognostic importance of various cell surface antigens was examined in 176 patients, aged 1 month to 21 years, with previously untreated AML. The median follow-up was longer than 3 years.

Results.—Cell surface antigens associated with myeloid differentiation were found on blasts from 88% of the patients, and cells from 31% expressed antigens considered specific for lymphoid differentiation. Blasts from nearly half the patients expressed CD34, a glycoprotein found on immature myeloid and lymphoid cells. No significant correlation was found between the expression of any cell surface antigens and the outcome, whether expressed as survival, event-free survival, or death during induction.

Conclusion.—The expression of both lymphoid-associated and my-eloid-associated cell surface antigens by blasts from children with AML has no particular prognostic significance. So-called biphenotypic AML in children may not be a biologically distinctive form of leukemia.

▶ The expression of a B-cell antigen by t(8;21) cells is a surprise. The more we look, the more acute leukemias are hybrid or biphenotypic leukemias. It is not surprising that the literature is contradictory on whether biphenotypic leukemias have a poor prognosis.—P.H. Wiernik, M.D.

Relevance of *mdr*1 Gene Expression in Acute Myeloid Leukemia and Comparison of Different Diagnostic Methods
Zhou D-C, Marie J-P, Suberville A-M, Zittoun R (Univ Paris VI; Renji Hosp, Shanghai, China)
Leukemia 6:879–885, 1992   4–57

Background.—High expression of the multidrug resistance (MDR) gene *mdr*1 is described in several human cancers including acute my-eloid leukemia (AML). Nevertheless, the reported frequency of the MDR phenotype in AML varies widely. If, in fact, a high level of *mdr*1 expression correlates with a poor response to chemotherapy, prospec-tively identifying such patients could help develop strategies for over-coming or circumventing resistance.

Study Design.—A total of 126 bone marrow and peripheral blood specimens from 89 adult patients having AML in different phases was examined by RNA slot blot analysis and immunocytochemical methods.

Findings.—The slot blot analysis indicated a 43% rate of *mdr*1 expres-sion in newly diagnosed patients, whereas immunocytochemical staining with monoclonal antibody suggested a frequency of 27%. The respective rates for patients having resistant AML were 60% and 27%. Sixty-two percent of patients positive for *mdr*1–messengerRNA and 68% of those positive for P-glycoprotein eventually became resistant to chemotherapy. All 9 patients positive for both factors became clinically drug resistant, compared with 2 of 13 patients with negative findings.

Expression of the MDR gene is frequent in patients with AML, even those who are newly diagnosed and have never received chemotherapy. A direct relationship is apparent between *mdr*1 expression and clinical drug resistance in these patients.

▶ For more information, see reference 1.

Reference

1. Li Y, et al: *Med Oncol Tumor Pharmacother* 9:3–9, 1992.

A Phase III Trial Comparing Idarubicin and Daunorubicin in Combination With Cytarabine in Acute Myelogenous Leukemia: A Southeastern Cancer Study Group Study

Vogler WR, Velez-Garcia E, Weiner RS, Flaum MA, Bartolucci AA, Omura GA, Gerger MC, Banks PLC (Emory Univ, Atlanta, Ga; Univ of Puerto Rico, San Juan; Univ of Florida, Gainesville; et al)
J Clin Oncol 10:1103–1111, 1992

4–58

Introduction.—Idarubicin (IDR) was compared with daunorubicin (DNR). Each were given with cytarabine to previously untreated patients older than age 14 years with acute myeloid leukemia (AML).

Patients and Methods.—A total of 230 patients with newly diagnosed AML received an infusion of 100 mg/m² of cytarabine daily for 1 week and then were randomized to receive either 45 mg/m² of DNR or 12 mg/m² of IDR daily for 3 days. Those entering complete remission received 3 consolidation courses of cytarabine and thioguanine with either DNR or IDR. Late intensification therapy involved the same drugs as were used for induction, but cytarabine was given for 5 days and DNR or IDR for the first 2 days.

Results.—Seventy-one percent of IDR-treated patients and 58% of those given DNR had a complete response. Both median survival and the median remission duration were somewhat greater in the group given IDR. Five of 6 patients who died during late intensification therapy were IDR recipients. Nonhematologic toxicity was generally mild and similar in the 2 treatment groups.

Conclusion.—Idarubicin is more rapidly taken up by leukemic cells, probably because of greater lipid solubility. It produces more remissions than DNR at comparable levels of toxicity and may replace it for the combination treatment of AML.

▶ This is the third American study to show superiority for IDR rather than DNR in this disease.—P.H. Wiernik, M.D.

Comparative Cellular Pharmacology of Daunorubicin and Idarubicin in Human Multidrug-Resistant Leukemia Cells

Berman E, McBride M (Mem Sloan-Kettering Cancer Ctr, New York)
Blood 79:3267–3273, 1992

4–59

Background.—A recent comparison of the new anthracycline derivative idarubicin (IDR) combined with cytosine arabinoside and standard daunorubicin (DNR) plus cytosine arabinoside has shown that fewer patients treated with the IDR combination have primary refractory disease after 2 courses of induction treatment. Thus, the effects of these 2 anthracyclines in 2 leukemia cell lines displaying the multidrug resistance phenotype were studied.

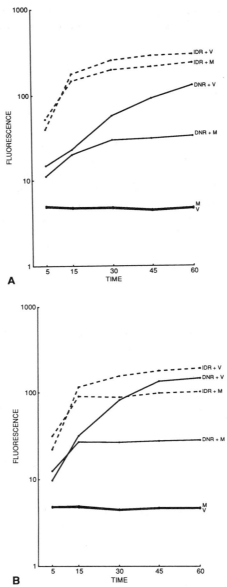

Fig 4–11.—Idarubicin (*IDR*) (*dashed line*) and DNR (*solid line*) uptake in (**A**) CEM-VBL cells and (**B**) HL-60/RV⁺ cells as measured by flow cytometric analysis after simultaneous incubation with medium (+M) alone or medium plus verapamil (+V). Note that the control experiments using medium (M) alone and verapamil (V) alone overlap. (Courtesy of Berman E, McBride M: *Blood* 79:3267–3273, 1992.)

Methods and Results.—Laser flow cytometry was used to quantitate intracelluar anthracycline content. Daunorubicin, IDR, and verapamil were studied. The vinblastine-resistant human lymphoblastic leukemia cell line CEM-VBL showed minimal DNR uptake. Simultaneous incubation with verapamil and DNR elevated intracellular DNR uptake fourfold. Idarubicin uptake was 10 times faster in these cells. Simultaneous incubation with IDR and verapamil resulted in only 1.2-fold increase of intracellular IDR. Similar findings were seen in the vincristine-resistant human myeloid leukemia cell line HL-60/RV+. For each cell line, intracellular retentions of DNR and IDR were also determined. Thirty-eight percent of the original DNR levels remained in CEM-VBL cells after a 2-hour resuspension in fresh medium, compared with 71% of the original IDR concentration. Thirty-six percent of the DNR concentrations remained in HL-60/RV+cells, compared with 51% of the IDR concentration. Intracellular DNR retention rose five- and 5.2-fold, respectively, after incubation of CEM-VBL and HV-60/RV+cells with DNR for 1 hour followed by resuspension in fresh medium plus verapamil. However, 1-hour incubation of these cells with IDR followed by resuspension in fresh medium plus verapamil resulted in only a 1.6- and 2.4-fold rise in intracellular IDR retention. Clonogenic experiments were also done to correlate intracellular anthracycline content with cytotoxicity. Daunorubicin alone minimally affected the clonogenic growth of CEM-VBL cells. The combination of DNR and verapamil inhibited growth by about 80%. Incubation of these cells with IDR alone inhibited growth by more than 95% (Fig 4–11).

Conclusion.—The clinical efficacy of IDR compared with DNR may be partly based on the differential effect of the former anthracycline on multidrug resistance cells. Because this form of drug resistance may potentially cause primary drug resistance in acute leukemia, further study of drugs that seem to circumvent this phenomenon is merited.

▶ The multidrug resistance story becomes more complicated every day, and conflicting, yet intriguing, results are reported concerning the clinical relevance of this phenotype. These results suggest a molecular basis for the superiority of IDR rather than DNR observed in 4 randomized, prospective studies to date. See reference 1.—P.H. Wiernik, M.D.

Reference

1. Michieli M, et al: *Leukemia Lymphoma* 9:255–264, 1993.

Myeloperoxidase: An Enzyme Involved in Intrinsic Vincristine Resistance in Human Myeloblastic Leukemia

Schlaifer D, Cooper MR, Attal M, Sartor AO, Trepel JB, Laurent G, Myers CE (Natl Cancer Inst, Bethesda, Md; Hôpital de Purpan, Toulouse, France)
Blood 81:482–489, 1993   4–60

Background.—Vincristine is a valuable chemotherapeutic agent for the treatment of acute lymphoid leukemia (ALL); however, acute myeloid leukemia (AML) is resistant to vincristine. The heme-centered peroxidase, horseradish peroxidase, catalyzes in vitro oxidation of *Vinca* alkaloids, abolishing their cytotoxic activity. Thus, vincristine might also be degraded by myeloperoxidase (MPO), another heme-centered peroxidase that is found in AML but not ALL. Whether vincristine's ineffectiveness in AML might result from MPO-mediated oxidative degradation of the drug was investigated.

Observations.—In a cell-free system, MPO was capable of catalyzing the oxidative breakdown of vincristine. No other enzyme tested had a similar effect. In tissue culture, vincristine broke down more rapidly in the presence of MPO-positive HL-60 cells than with an HL-60 subclone that was negative for MOP. The MPO-positive cell line was also more resistant to the cytotoxic effects of vincristine, with a positive correlation between the degree of MPO activity of the cell lines and their resistance to vincristine. Those effects occurred at clinically relevant concentrations of vincristine. Increasing the concentration of hydrogen peroxide available to the enzyme also increased the cell lines' differential resistance to vincristine.

Conclusion.—The relative inactivity of vincristine against AML appears to result in part from MPO-mediated oxidation of vincristine. Correlation of the MPO content of malignant blasts and the degradation of vincristine awaits further studies with a larger number of patients with MPO-positive and MPO-negative AML.

▶ There are conflicting data in the literature with respect to the value of vincristine in AML therapy. It may be worth revisiting the issue in patients with MO, or t(8;21) in which MPO activity is decreased or absent.—P.H. Wiernik, M.D.

Nitric Oxide Modulation of Human Leukemia Cell Differentiation and Gene Expression

Magrinat G, Mason SN, Shami PJ, Weinberg JB (Duke Univ, Durham, NC)
Blood 80:1880–1884, 1992   4–61

Background.—Nitric oxide (NO) is a free-radical gas produced by many cell types that serves as an intercellular messenger molecule in neural transmission, immune regulation, and vascular tone regulation. It is generated by endothelial cells and mononuclear phagocytes, both of which regulate hemopoietic cell differentiation in the bone marrow. The effects of NO on the differentiation of a human myeloid leukemia cell line (HL-60) and on gene expression in these cells were examined. Nitric oxide was delivered as purified gas or was released by sodium nitroprusside or 6-morpholino-sydnonimine.

Findings.—Cells exposed to NO ceased proliferating, became spread out and vacuolated, and expressed increased levels of nonspecific esterase and the monocyte marker CD14. The cells also were more capable of producing hydrogen peroxide. Treated cells had increased expression of messenger RNA for tumor necrosis factor-α and IL-1β, and decreased expression of mRNA for the proto-oncogenes c-*myc* and c-*myb*.

Conclusion.—Nitric oxide elaborated in the bone marrow may contribute to the differentiation of normal and malignant hematopoietic cells. Perhaps NO will prove useful in treating myeloid leukemia.

Clinical Implications of Decreased Retinoblastoma Protein Expression in Acute Myelogenous Leukemia
Kornblau SM, Xu H-J, del Giglio A, Hu S-X, Zhang W, Calvert L, Beran M, Estey E, Andreeff M, Trujillo J, Cork MA, Smith TL, Benedict WF, Deisseroth AB (Univ of Texas, Houston; Baylor College of Medicine, The Woodlands, Tex)
Cancer Res 52:4587–4590, 1992   4–62

Purpose.—A number of tumors show functional loss of the retinoblastoma (*RB*) gene, including some cases of acute myeloid leukemia (AML). Patients with AML were studied to determine the frequency of functional loss of the *RB* gene and whether this was correlated with a shorter overall survival.

Methods.—Levels of RB protein were measured in blast-enriched mononuclear fractions from the peripheral blood of 33 patients with newly diagnosed AML. Also studied were 10 previously treated patients, 9 of whom had a previous complete remission. Western blot assay was used to determine average levels of RB protein in the peripheral blood of each patient. In 23 patients, samples were studied at the single-cell level by immunohistochemical analysis.

Results.—Thirty percent (13) of the 43 patients had low RB protein expression. There was 100% correlation between the results of Western blot analysis and single-cell assays, suggesting that the leukemic blast cells of patients with undetectable or low RB levels had altered RB protein expression. The median survival was lower for newly diagnosed patients with low RB protein expression than for those with high RB protein expression treated by the same regimen: 39 vs. 333 days.

Conclusion.—Decreased expression of RB protein in peripheral blood myeloid leukemic cells is a common finding that may be associated with decreased survival in patients with AML. A larger prospective study is needed to confirm the prognostic significance of altered RB protein expression.

▶ Their conclusion is fascinating, but what is the explanation for the relationship between prognosis and RB protein expression?—P.H. Wiernik, M.D.

Pulmonary Leukostasis Without Hyperleukocytosis: A Clinicopathologic Study of 16 Cases
Soares FA, Landell GAM, Cardoso MCdM (Univ of São Paulo, Ribeirao Preto, SP, Brazil)
Am J Hematol 40:28–32, 1992   4–63

Introduction.—Pulmonary leukostasis is a serious complication of myeloid leukemia. It is almost always fatal. Leukemic patients with pulmonary leukostasis and a circulating leukocyte count less than 50,000/mm³ were reported.

Patients and Methods.—Sixteen subjects who died of leukemia and pulmonary leukostasis underwent autopsy. All had had a circulating leukocyte count of less than 50,000/mm³, some as late as 4 days before their death. Patient ages ranged from 2 to 61 years.

Results.—Histologic lung sections showed arteriolar involvement in 3 cases. Alveolar spetal capillaries were involved in all cases. Involvement was discrete in 4 patients, moderate in 9, and severe in 3. Clinical data on the last 4 days of life indicated that 14 of 16 with pulmonary leukostasis without hyperleukocytosis had cardiopulmonary disorders. The most prevalent symptom was dyspnea, occurring in 14 cases. Nine of 14 patients had abnormal chest radiographs, with diffuse alveolar consolidations or diffuse reticulonodular infiltrates corresponding to a radiologic diagnosis of edema or pneumonia, respectively. According to arterial blood-gas analysis, performed in 10 patients, 9 had hypoxemia and normocapnia. Acute respiratory distress was the main cause of death in 9 patients. Other causes were hemorrhagic diathesis (6) and CNS bleeding (1).

Conclusion.—Hyperleukocytosis alone cannot be the cause of pulmonary leukostasis. Other factors, such as the presence of circulating blasts and the affinity of neoplastic cells for the pulmonary endothelium, may be associated with the development of acute respiratory distress in patients with leukemia.

▶ It is important to recognize this potentially fatal problem because it responds well to low-dose whole-lung irradiation.—P.H. Wiernik, M.D.

Childhood Leukaemia Following the Chernobyl Accident: The European Childhood Leukaemia-Lymphoma Incidence Study (ECLIS)

Parkin DM, Cardis E, Masuyer E, Friedl HP, Hansluwka H, Bobev D, Ivanov E, Sinnaeve J, Augustin J, Plesko I, Storm HH, Rahu M, Karjalainen S, Bernard JL, Carli PM, L'Huillier MC, Lutz JM, Schaffer P, Schraub S, Michaelis J, Möhner M, Staneczek W, Vargha M, Crosignani P, Magnani C, Terracini B, Kriauciunas R, Coebergh JW, Langmark F, Zatonski W, Merabishvili V, Pompe-Kirn V, Barlow L, Raymond L, Black R, Stiller CA, Bennett BG (Internatl Agency for Research on Cancer, Lyon, France)
Eur J Cancer 29A:87–95, 1993   4–64

Background.—The accident at the Chernobyl nuclear power plant in April 1986 released radioactive particles into the atmosphere for 10 days. Affected areas included the eastern part of the former USSR, from Sweden south to Bulgaria, and parts of Central Europe. Most exposure was from radioactive iodine (half-life about 8 days) and caesium (half-life of 30 years). Humans were exposed internally, from ingestion of contaminated food, as well as externally. Various international organizations surveyed the long-term consequences of the Chernobyl accident. Incidence rates of childhood leukemia and lymphoma were monitored in Europe. Leukemia is 1 of the earliest cancers to show an increase in incidence after radiation exposure and provides the largest relative increase of any cancer.

Methods.—Estimates were obtained from the United Nations Scientific Committee on the Effects of Atomic Radiation for radiation doses in 20 European countries. In several countries where exposure distribution was very uneven, estimates were given for subregions. Population-based cancer registries provided data on cases of leukemia and lymphoma occurring in children younger than 15 years of age. For this preliminary analysis, incidence rates were calculated to determine whether the incidence of leukemia changed in the first 3 years after the Chernobyl accident.

Results.—There was a small increase (4.1%) in the overall incidence of leukemia in children. In the entire study population for which data were available for 1987–1988, 3,679 cases were observed. On the basis of the 1980–1985 rates, 3,533.2 cases would have been expected. The observed changes in incidence do not relate to exposure.

Conclusion.—Most studies of possible consequences of the Chernobyl accident conclude that any increase in cancer rates away from the reactor site will not be detectable against the normal incidence of cancer in the general population. On the basis of the first-year effective dose equivalent, the overall increase in the incidence of leukemia for the area covered by the European Childhood Leukaemia–Lymphoma Incidence Study study is estimated to be about .8%, with the most marked increase in Belarus (5.8%). However, at least 5 years of postaccident data will be required for a meaningful analysis. Future analyses will examine the effect of country-specific preaccident time trends in incidence on expected postaccident incidence.

▶ Unfortunately, this study may yield different results with time.—P.H. Wiernik, M.D.

Acute Myeloid Leukemia (AML) in Down's Syndrome Is Highly Responsive to Chemotherapy: Experience on Pediatric Oncology Group AML Study 8498

Ravindranath Y, Abella E, Krischer JP, Wiley J, Inoue S, Harris M, Chauvenet A, Alvarado CS, Dubowy R, Ritchey AK, Land V, Steuber CP, Weinstein H (Wayne State Univ, Detroit; Univ of Florida, Gainesville; Johns Hopkins Univ, Baltimore, Md; et al)

Blood 80:2210–2214, 1992

4–65

Introduction.—Children with Down syndrome (DS) and acute myeloid leukemia (AML) have been thought to have a poor prognosis. For a variety of reasons, however, physicians may not use intensive chemotherapy in these patients. Twelve children with DS and AML who were on Pediatric Oncology Group (POG) 8498 (protocol for newly diagnosed AML) responded well to therapy.

Patients.—The POG 8498 AML study was open from July 1984 to July 1989. Twelve of 285 assessable patients had DS. Other medical problems were present in the children with DS; 6 had congenital cardiac disease, and 3 had a history of myelodysplastic syndrome. Compared with the children without DS, those with DS and AML were predominatly male (9 of 12) and were younger at diagnosis (10 younger than 2 years of age).

Results.—All 12 children with DS had a WBC count less than $50 \times 10^3/\mu L$; 5 had French-American-British types M6 and M7. In addition to constitutional trisomy 21, 9 had an abnormal cytogenetic marker (4 involving chromosome 8). Immunologic cell surface marker studies were performed in 5 children, all of whom were positive for CD33, CD13, and/or CD11b as well as for the CD7 antigen. Chemotherapy for remission induction included daunorubicin, cytarabine (ara-C), and 6-thioguanine; high-dose ara-C with or without L-asparaginase was given early in remission. The children with DS had a better event-free survival at 4 years (100%) than those without DS (28%). When matched for age and WBC count, children with DS still maintained this advantage (100% vs. 48%).

Conclusion.—This series of 12 children represents the largest uniformly treated group of patients with DS and AML. Their response to therapy was superior to that of children without DS, despite some possibly unfavorable factors in the group with DS. Less intensive ara-C dose schedules may be possible in children with DS and AML.

Acute Nonlymphocytic Leukemia in Germ Cell Tumor Patients Treated With Etoposide-Containing Chemotherapy

Bajorin DF, Motzer RJ, Rodriguez E, Murphy B, Bosl GJ (Mem Sloan-Kettering Cancer Ctr, New York; Cornell Univ, New York)
J Natl Cancer Inst 85:60–62, 1993   4–66

Introduction.—The drug etoposide appears effective in treating germ cell tumors, but it has been associated with secondary leukemias in patients cured of these tumors, various lung cancers, and acute lymphocytic leukemia. Patients with germ cell tumors who were treated with etoposide for their primary cancer were assessed for the risk of having acute nonlymphocytic leukemia develop.

Methods.—Of the 506 patients identified with germ cell tumors who received etoposide-containing therapy, 343 participated in the study. Patients underwent induction chemotherapy only or induction treatment plus salvage therapy. A variety of combinations of etoposide plus other chemotherapeutic agents were administered. The presence of leukemia was determined morphologically by the French-American-British classification.

Results.—Among the 343 patients, 6 had acute nonlymphocytic leukemia. This condition in 2 patients was thought to be related to their therapy. A third patient with a mediastinal germ cell tumor had leukemia that was confirmed from this primary tumor using a highly specific cell marker. The other 3 patients had the leukemia simultaneously with mediastinal germ cell tumor. Of the 340 patients at risk for having leukemia develop after a complete response, 2 did so after successful tumor treatment. One of these patients had undergone etoposide induction treatment plus salvage therapy with cyclophosphamide, a noted leukemogenic agent. The other patients who had leukemia develop had received etoposide only.

Conclusion.—Patients cured of germ cell tumors by induction chemotherapy have a less than 1% incidence of secondary acute nonlymphocytic leukemia; it usually occurs in those receiving at least 2,000 mg/m² of etoposide. Although a definite risk of secondary leukemia exists with etoposide, this risk does not outweigh the drug's effectiveness against germ cell tumors.

Secondary Leukemia Associated With a Conventional Dose of Etoposide: Review of Serial Germ Cell Tumor Protocols

Nichols CR, Breeden ES, Loehrer PJ, Williams SD, Einhorn LH (Indiana Univ, Indianapolis)
J Natl Cancer Inst 85:36–40, 1993   4–67

Objective.—Epipodophyllotoxins and related agents are implicated in producing a treatment-related acute nonlymphocytic leukemia. Case reports of leukemia associated with high doses of etoposide prompted a review of patients with germ cell cancer who, in 1982–1991, entered clinical trials and received conventional doses of etoposide. A planned cumulative dose of 2,000 mg/m² or less was considered conventional.

Findings.—Of 538 patients who received cumulative doses of 1,500–2,000 mg/m² in conjunction with cisplatin and either ifosfamide or bleomycin, 348 received etoposide as part of initial chemotherapy, and 190 as part of salvage treatment. Of 337 patients who remained alive and have been followed beyond 2 years, 2 had leukemia. One of them had acute undifferentiated leukemia with a t(4;11) (q21;q23) cytogenetic abnormality 2 years after the start of etoposide-based chemotherapy. The other had acute myelomonoblastic leukemia, without chromosomal abnormality, 2.3 years after starting chemotherapy. Among several hundred other patients who received etoposide, but not in a clinical trial, were 3 who had hematologic abnormalities, including 1 with acute monoblastic leukemia and a t(11;19) (q13;p13) abnormality.

Conclusion.—Secondary leukemia occurs infrequently in patients given conventional doses of etoposide and does not alter the risk-benefit ratio of etoposide-based chemotherapy for germ cell cancer.

▶ The relationship between epipodophyllotoxins and acute myeloid leukemia is being explored further (1).—P.H. Wiernik, M.D.

Reference

1. Smith MA, et al: *J Natl Cancer Inst* 85:554–558, 1993.

Microgranular Variant of Acute Promyelocytic Leukemia in Children

Rovelli A, Biondi A, Rajnoldi AC, Conter V, Giudici G, Jankovic M, Locasciulli A, Rizzari C, Romitti L, Rossi MR, Schirò R, Tosi S, Uderzo C, Masera G (Ospedale San Gerardo, Monza, Italy; Istituti Clinici de Perfezionamento, Milan, Italy)

J Clin Oncol 10:1413–1418, 1992   4–68

Objective.—Although M3v is a recognized microgranular variant of acute promyelocytic leukemia (APL), it has rarely been reported in a pediatric series of acute nonlymphoblastic leukemia (AnLL). Previous reports of the first cases of this variant emphasized its poor prognosis. Here the clinical and biological features in 11 children with M3v were reviewed.

Patients and Methods.—Nine girls and 2 boys (median age, 8.3 years) were treated during 21 years. All had an elevated leukocyte count at onset (median 87 × 10⁹/L), with anemia of varying severity and severe thrombocytopenia. Coagulation abnormalities before treatment and hemorrhagic diathesis were present in all. All cases were diagnosed according to French-American-British criteria: bilobed or multilobular cells or cells with reniform nucleus and cytoplasm with minimal or no granulations and a few typical M3 cells in the bone marrow. A single pathologist performed all morphologic examinations, cytochemical analyses, and immunophenotyping studies. Beginning in 1984, cytogenetic and molecular analyses were done to confirm the diagnosis.

Findings.—The overall incidence of children with APL was very high: 31% of the cases of AnLL. Twenty-five percent of the cases of APL were of the M3v variant. This incidence was the same even when the analysis was restricted to cases with cytogenetic and DNA confirmation. Although the patients with M3v had an immunophenotype identical to that described for the hypergranular type, they also had an unexpected association with CD2.

Eight of 11 patients died within 10 days of the diagnosis of hemorrhagic events caused by hyperleukocytosis and disseminated intravascular coagulation (DIC). Three patients achieved complete remission after treatment with daunorubicin and cytarabine and went on to receive autologous bone marrow transplantation; 2 of them are still alive and free of disease.

Conclusion.—The M3v variant of APL may be more common in children than previously thought. The diagnosis can be made quickly with morphologic, cytochemical, and molecular studies. The course and prognosis of M3v are worse than in typical APL; as in adults, death results from marked hyperleukocytosis and severe DIC.

The "Retinoic Acid Syndrome" in Acute Promyelocytic Leukemia

Frankel SR, Eardley A, Lauwers G, Weiss M, Warrell RP Jr (Mem Sloan-Kettering Cancer Ctr, New York; Cornell Univ, New York)
Ann Intern Med 117:292–296, 1992   4–69

Background.—All-*trans* retinoic acid (tretinoin) induces complete clinical remissions in many patients with acute promyelocytic leukemia (APL). The clinical response is often accompanied by a transient increase in the peripheral leukocyte count that is well tolerated by most. However, "hyperleukocytosis" has been described in association with an unusually poor outcome. A novel complication of tretinoin treatment in patients with APL was presented.

Patients and Findings.—Thirty-five consecutive patients with a morphologic diagnosis of APL given underwent remission induction treatment at a comprehensive cancer center with tretinoin, 45 mg/m² body surface area per day. Nine of these patients had a syndrome develop consisting mainly of fever and respiratory distress. Other important signs and symptoms were weight gain, lower-extremity edema, pleural or pericardial effusions, and episodic hypotension. Symptom onset occurred 2 to 21 days after tretinoin therapy was begun. Three patients died. Postmortem assessments in 2 showed pulmonary interstitial infiltration with maturing myeloid cells. The remaining 6 patients survived, each attaining complete remission. In 6 of 9 patients, the syndrome onset was preceded by a rise in peripheral blood leukocytes to at least 20×10^9 cells/ L. After respiratory distress was established, certain interventions—leukapheresis, temporary cessation of tretinoin treatment, and cytotoxic chemotherapy in moderate doses—were not useful. However, administering high-dose corticosteroid treatment early in the course of the syndrome led to prompt symptomatic improvement and full recovery in 3 of 4 patients.

Conclusion.—In some patients, the use of tretinoin for induction of hematologic remission in APL is associated with a potentially lethal syndrome that is not always accompanied by peripheral blood leukocytosis. Recognizing the symptom complex of fever and dyspnea early and treating it promptly with corticosteroid therapy may reduce morbidity and mortality associated with the syndrome.

Clinical Pharmacology of Oral All-*trans* Retinoic Acid in Patients With Acute Promyelocytic Leukemia
Muindi JRF, Frankel SR, Huselton C, DeGrazia F, Garland WA, Young CW, Warrell RP Jr (Cornell Univ, New York; Hoffmann-La Roche Inc, Nutley, NJ)
Cancer Res 52:2138–2142, 1992   4–70

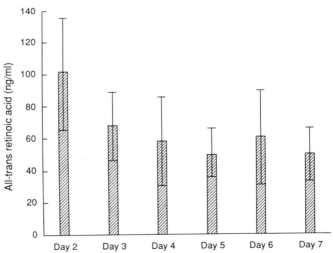

Fig 4–12.—Mean plasma concentrations of all-*trans* RA 2 hours after ingestion of morning drug dose on days 2 through 6 (*n* = 9). *Bars* indicate SEM. (Courtesy of Muindi JRF, Frankel SR, Huselton C, et al: *Cancer Res* 52:2138–2142, 1992.)

Introduction.—Many patients with acute promyelocytic leukemia (APL) achieve both leukemic cell differentiation and complete remission with all-*trans* retinoic acid (RA). Unfortunately, these remissions are usually brief and followed by relapses that are resistant to further treatment in vivo. However, in vitro, cells have been shown to remain sensitive to the cytodifferentiating effects of all-*trans* RA. The clinical pharmacology of all-*trans* RA was described.

Patients and Methods.—Thirteen patients with APL received all-*trans* RA at a constant dose of 45 mg/m²/day. A single dose was given on the first day of therapy, with 2 divided doses thereafter. Reverse-phase high-performance liquid chromatography and, if necessary, normal-phase liquid chromatography with negative chemical ionization mass spectrometry were done to measure plasma and urinary concentrations of all-*trans* RA and its metabolites.

Results.—The peak plasma all-*trans* RA level of 347 ng/mL was reached 1–2 hours after ingestion (Fig 4–12). It decayed in a monoexponential fashion, with a half-life of .8 hour. Urinary 4-oxo-all-*trans* RA, present as glucuronide conjugate, was the only metabolite detected. It made up less than 10% of the circulating drug in plasma, with its cumulative excretion accounting for less than 1% of the administered dose. No drug was found in cerebrospinal fluid. With continued administration for 2 to 6 weeks, both the plasma peak level and the area under the concentration-time curve decreased significantly. The latter finding had been previously reported to be highly correlated with clinical relapse. The major decrease appeared to occur within the first week of treatment. Along with these changes was a 10-fold increase in urinary 4-oxo-all-*trans* RA glucuronide excretion, which indicated that drug catabolism increased in association with accelerated clearance from plasma.

Conclusion.—In patients with APL, the rapid disappearacne of plasma all-*trans* RA may explain the early relapse from remissions induced by this drug. The subsequent clinical resistance may have to do with inability to sustain effective plasma concentration. Acceleration of drug catabolism by a cytochrome P-450–like enzyme system could be responsible, but other explanations are also possible. Discontinuous dosing schedules or concurrent treatment with P-450 enzyme inhibitors might improve the results of all-*trans* RA treatment in APL.

All-Transretinoic Acid Followed by Intensive Chemotherapy Gives a High Complete Remission Rate and May Prolong Remissions in Newly Diagnosed Acute Promyelocytic Leukemia: A Pilot Study on 26 Cases

Fenaux P, Castaigne S, Dombret H, Archimbaud E, Duarte M, Morel P, Lamy T, Tilly H, Guerci A, Maloisel F, Bordessoule D, Sadoun A, Tiberghien P, Fegueux N, Daniel MT, Chomienne C, Degos L (Centre Hospitalier Universitere, Lille, Paris St Louis, Lyon, France; et al)

Blood 80:2176–2181, 1992   4–71

Background.—Of patients undergoing intensive chemotherapy for acute promyelocytic leukemia (APL), 25% to 30% fail to achieve complete remission (CR). Rather than true leukemic resistance, death is caused by bleeding or sepsis during chemotherapy-induced aplasia. All-transretinoic acid (ATRA) followed by intensive chemotherapy in patients with newly diagnosed APL was investigated.

Methods.—The patients (median age, 46 years) all had a leukocyte count less than 10×10^9/L; none had the microgranular variant of APL. All but 1 of 25 patients undergoing cytogenetic analysis had a t(15;17). The study protocol consisted of ATRA, 45 mg/m²/day until complete remission was achieved, followed by an intensive course of daunorubicin (DNR) plus cytosine arabinoside (ara-C) (4 + 7 course), then three 2 + 5 courses of DNR and ara-C and maintenance chemotherapy. For patients who rapidly had hyperleukocytosis develop, the 4 + 7 course was given on an emergency basis to prevent leukostasis.

Results.—The CR rate was 96%, with 14 patients achieving CR with ATRA alone. Another 11 patients achieved CR after addition of the 4 + 11 course on day 20 to 30 of treatment; 9 patients had a rapid increase in leukocytes, 1 patient was resistant to ATRA, and 1 had organomegaly. The 1 patient who did not respond died of sepsis on day 6. Side effects other than hyperleukocytosis were moderate.

Allografting was done after the 4 + 7 course in 3 patients, and 4 patients did not receive the 4 + 7 courses but went on to the 2 + 5 and maintenance courses; the rest followed the scheduled protocol. Three patients had relapses after 8 to 15 months, and 2 died in CR after 6 and 17 months, respectively. At a median of 21 months, the other patients remained in CR. The 18-month actuarial disease-free interval (DFI) was 87% and the event-free survival (EFS) was 77%. In a previous trial of chemotherapy alone in newly diagnosed APL, the CR rate was 76% and the 18-month DFI and EFS were 59% and 48%, respectively, the latter 2 differences being significant (Fig 4–13).

Conclusion.—Chemotherapy after ATRA may be superior to chemotherapy only in the treatment of newly diagnosed APL. The addition of ATRA produces a slight increase in the CR rate and a more important decrease in the relapse rate. A randomized, multicenter trial of these treatments is being conducted.

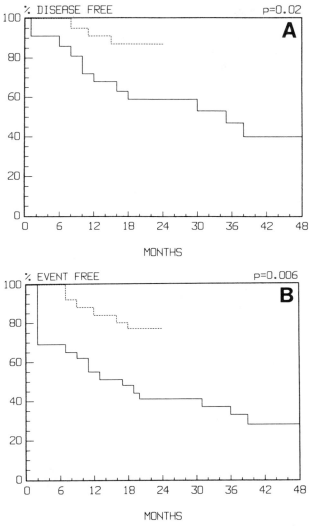

Fig 4–13.—Comparisons between ATRA followed by intensive chemotherapy and our previous APL 84 trial with chemotherapy alone. **A,** actuarial disease-free interval. **B,** actuarial EFS. *Dashed line,* ATRA plus chemotherapy; *solid line,* APL 84. (Courtesy of Fenaux P, Castaigne S, Dombret H, et al: *Blood* 80:2176–2181, 1992.)

Combined Therapy With All-*trans*-Retinoic Acid and High-Dose Chemotherapy in Patients With Hyperleukocytic Acute Promyelocytic Leukemia and Severe Visceral Hemorrhage

Dombret H, Sutton L, Duarte M, Daniel MT, Leblond V, Castaigne S, Degos L
(Hôpital Saint-Louis, Paris; Hôpital Pitié-Salpétrière, Paris)
Leukemia 6:1237–1242, 1992   4–72

Introduction.—Acute promyelocytic leukemia (APL), which constitutes about 10% of all adult acute nonlymphocytic leukemias, frequently is accompanied by disseminated intravascular coagulation (DIC) and death from bleeding early in the course of illness. Fatal hemorrhage is especially likely to occur when severe DIC, a high peripheral-blood blast-cell count, and visceral hemorrhage are present at diagnosis.

Treatment.—Three patients with APL who had severe visceral bleeding and DIC at the time of diagnosis received chemotherapy and all-*trans*-retinoic acid (ATRA) at the same time. All the patients were hyperleukocytic. One had cerebral hemorrhage, and 2 had acute respiratory failure that was probably secondary to leukemic infiltration of the lungs and pulmonary hemorrhage. Treatment with ATRA, 45 mg/m² daily, was begun on the first or second day of chemotherapy and withdrawn after complete remission was achieved.

Outcome.—All 3 patients entered complete remission. The patients with respiratory failure required intensive care briefly, and 1 of them needed mechanical ventilation. The patient with cerebral bleeding did not worsen during treatment. Differentiating granular cells appeared in the peripheral blood after 5 to 12 days of cytotoxic therapy.

Conclusion.—Combined treatment with standard chemotherapeutic agents in high dosage and ATRA appears to be an effective approach to patients with hyperleukocytic APL.

▶ These are important articles (Abstracts 4–68 through 4–72) about an acute leukemia that has suddenly become extremely interesting because of the discovery of the activity of ATRA against it. The current intergroup study coordinated by the Eastern Cooperative Oncology Group includes children and adults with APL. Therefore, any difference in prognosis between microgranular and other APL variants (as suggested by the Rovelli et al. study [Abstract 4–68]) shoud emerge on both the ATRA induction therapy arm and the standard chemotherapy induction arm. The "retinoic acid syndrome" described by Frankel et al. (Abstract 4–69) is an important contribution, but it has not been seen with the same frequency and severity in the first 50 patients on the ATRA arm of the intergroup study as reported in this paper. The report on the clinical pharmacology of ATRA (Abstract 4–70) is important and provocative, but it remains to be proven that early relapse or resistance to ATRA is related to its peculiar pharmacology. The studies of Fenaux et al. (Abstract 4–71) and of Dombret el al. (Abstract 4–72) suggest that induction with ATRA followed by postremission chemotherapy is optimum therapy for

APL. The intergroup study tests that observation and also tests whether the reverse sequence has merit. It further tests whether any postremission therapy other than high-dose ara-C consolidation is necessary after either induction therapy.—P.H. Wiernik, M.D.

Phase II Clinical Trial of Carboplatin in Relapsed and Refractory Leukemia

Vogler WR, Harrington DP, Winton EF, Lazarus HM, Bennett JM, Cassileth PA, Oken MM (Emory Univ, Atlanta, Ga; Dana-Farber Cancer Inst, Boston; Case Western Reserve Univ, Cleveland, Ohio; et al)
Leukemia 6:1072–1075, 1992   4–73

Objective.—Carboplatin has antileukemic action, especially when it is administered by continuous intravenous infusion. The effectiveness of a dosage of 315 mg/m²/day for 5 days, given by continuous intravenous infusion, for patients with relapsed and refractory leukemia was assessed.

Patients and Methods.—The subjects were 46 adults, 36 with acute myelogenous leukemia (AML) and 10 with acute lymphoblastic leukemia (ALL). All had a relapse after their first or second remission or had failed no more than 2 attempts at induction. If the bone marrow showed persistent leukemia at day 14, a second course of carboplatin was given. The second course was delayed until marrow recovery was documented if the marrow was hypoplastic. A second course was given for patients with residual leukemia, and an additional course was given as consolidation for those who achieved complete remission (CR).

Results.—There was a 17% CR rate, including 6 patients with AML and 2 with ALL. Two of 9 patients with primary refractory disease achieved CR, 1 in each disease group. After exclusion of 18 patients who were unevaluable because of protocol violations, refusing further therapy, or death before day 14, the CR rate was 29%. Two induction courses were needed to achieve CR in all but 2 patients. Seventeen patients had greater than grade 2 renal toxicity, which was associated with the concomitant use of nephrotoxic antibiotics. Renal failure was a major contributor to death in 2 patients. Eleven patients were ototoxic; only 3 reached grade 3. Of the 18 patients who died during the study, 14 died of infection, 2 of infection and hemorrhage, 1 of hemorrhage while aplastic, and 1 of other causes.

Conclusion.—Given by continuous infusion, carboplatin appears to be an active compound in the treatment of relapsed and refractory acute leukemia. Because of the cumulative toxicity and prolonged marrow aplasia that occur with carboplatin treatment, a smaller dose at a less frequent interval may be beneficial.

▶ Carboplatin clearly has activity in AML, unlike cisplatin. Although there is apparently little or no activity in ALL, responses have been observed in blast crisis of chronic myeloid leukemia. Carboplatin deserves further study in AML and chronic myeloid leukemia blast crisis.—P.H. Wiernik, M.D.

2-Chlorodeoxyadenosine Produces a High Rate of Complete Hematologic Remission in Relapsed Acute Myeloid Leukemia

Santana VM, Mirro J Jr, Kearns C, Schell MJ, Crom W, Blakley RL (St Jude Children's Research Hosp, Memphis, Tenn; Univ of Tennessee, Memphis)
J Clin Oncol 10:364–370, 1992   4-74

Introduction.—The purine analogue 2-chlorodeoxyadenosine (2-CDA) has exhibited activity against human leukemic cell lines. It appears to rapidly inhibit DNA synthesis in proliferating cells and to produce DNA strand breaks in nonproliferating cells. The efficacy of 2-CDA in children and young adults with acute leukemia in first or subsequent hematologic relapse was determined.

Patients and Methods.—Of 24 patients (median age, 11 years) who entered the study, 17 had acute myeloid leukemia, and 7 had acute lymphoid leukemia. The drug was given by continuous infusion at a rate of 8.9 mg/m² daily for 5 days. If blast cells remained 10 days after treatment, a second course was administered.

Results.—Eight of 17 patients with acute myeloid leukemia had a complete hematologic response and 2 others had a partial response. Only 1 patient with lymphoid leukemia responded. Six patients remain in complete remission a median of 7 months after marrow transplantation. Febrile episodes associated with neutropenia complicated 38% of treatment courses, but there were no fatal infectious complications.

Conclusion.—These results suggest that 2-CDA is an effective drug for use in treating acute myeloid leukemia. It lacks the serious nonhematologic complications that occur with other agents.

▶ Despite the good results observed in pediatric acute myeloid leukemia, 2-CDA has been inactive in several studies of adult acute myeloid leukemia. This discrepancy requires explanation.—P.H. Wiernik, M.D.

Fludarabine Potentiates Metabolism of Cytarabine in Patients With Acute Myelogenous Leukemia During Therapy

Gandhi V, Estey E, Keating MJ, Plunkett W (Univ of Texas, Houston)
J Clin Oncol 11:116–124, 1993   4-75

Objective.—In the chemotherapy of acute myelogenous leukemia (AML), giving fludarabine infusion before cytarabine (ara-C) might increase accumulation of the active metabolite ara-C triphosphate (ara-CTP) in leukemic cells.

Methods.—Five patients with AML were given 1 g/m² of ara-C by 2-hour intravenous infusion, followed 20 hours later by 30 mg/m² of fludarabine for 30 minutes; ara-C was given in the same dose at 24 hours. Another 5 patients were given ara-C infusion of 3 g/m² during 6 hours. The pharmacokinetics of ara-CTP in circulating AML cells was investigated in all patients.

Results.—After fludarabine infusion, the area under the curve of ara-CTP increased by a median of 1.8 times, with no effect on median plasma ara-C concentrations; levels of arabinosyluracil, the deamination product of ara-C; or rate of ara-CTP elimination from circulating blasts. There was, however a median twofold increase in the rate of ara-CTP accumulation by AML cells, peaking within 1 hour of the end of fludarabine infusion. When those cells were incubated with arabinosyl-2-fluoroadenine before ara-C, the ara-CTP accumulation rate increased a median of 1.7-fold. The rate of ara-CTP accumulation was potentiated longer than 2 hours but not as long as 6 hours.

Conclusion.—In patients with AML, giving fludarabine infusion before ara-C can augment the rate of synthesis of ara-CTP. Maximal potentiation of ara-CTP synthesis is noted for as long as 4 hours in most patients. This regimen should be considered for use along with other antileukemic drugs.

▶ This is a major discovery of genuine interest. However, a high incidence of unusual infections such as *Pneumocystis* and cytomegalovirus may require modification of the regimen for optimal results.—P.H. Wiernik, M.D.

Late Intensification With POMP Chemotherapy Prolongs Survival in Acute Myelogenous Leukemia: Results of a Southwest Oncology Group Study of Rubidazone Versus Adriamycin for Remission Induction, Prophylactic Intrathecal Therapy, Late Intensification, and Levamisole Maintenance

Morrison FS, Kopecky KJ, Head DR, Athens JW, Balcerzak SP, Gumbart C, Dabich L, Costanzi JJ, Coltman CA, Saiki JH, Hussein KK, Fabian CJ, Appelbaum FR (Univ of Mississippi, University; Southwest Oncology Group Statistical Ctr; St Jude Children's Research Hosp, Memphis, Tenn; et al)
Leukemia 6:708–714, 1992   4–76

Purpose.—Between August 1978 and September 1982 patients with newly diagnosed acute myeloid leukemia (AML) were examined to answer 4 specific questions about AML therapy: Is rubidazone or Adriamycin better for induction of remission? Is there a role for prophylactic intrathecal therapy? How does late intensification of therapy with mercaptopurine, vincristine, methotrexate, prednisone (POMP) affect outcome? Does levamisole maintenance influence survival?

Results.—Of 642 patients, 611 were evaluated. Among these, 329 achieved complete remission (CR). There was no difference in the CR rate for those receiving rubidazone and those receiving Adriamycin. Prophylactic intrathecal therapy with cytosine arabinoside had no effect on the incidence of CNS disease or survival. After 9 months of CR, patients were randomized to continue maintenance or late intensification with POMP. Those patients who received late intensification had better survival and disease-free survival. After 1 year of CR, patients were randomized to receive levamisole or no further treatment. There was no effect of levamisole therapy on survival.

Discussion.—Although no difference was found between induction therapy with rubidazone or with Adriamycin, this point has become of limited significance as neither agent is currently used for the treatment of AML. The minor effect of CNS prophylaxis in patients with AML using current regimens was confirmed, as was the usefulness of late intensification therapy with POMP. As intensive consolidation therapy has become commonplace, the usefulness of late intensification therapy in this setting should also be evaluated. No beneficial effect of levamisole after late intensification was found. Inclusion of levamisole during chemotherapy may still have a beneficial effect.

▶ This is the third or fourth study that shows no value for levamisole in postremission therapy of AML.—P.H. Wiernik, M.D.

Long-Term Outcome of High-Dose Cytarabine-Based Consolidation Chemotherapy for Adults With Acute Myelogenous Leukemia
Schiller G, Gajewski J, Territo M, Nimer S, Lee M, Belin T, Champlin R (Univ of California, Los Angeles; MD Anderson Cancer Ctr, Houston)
Blood 80:2977–2982, 1992   4–77

Objective.—The long-term effects of high-dose cytarabine-anthracycline consolidation chemotherapy without maintenance treatment were examined in 227 adults with newly diagnosed acute myeloid leukemia. The median follow-up from the time of remission induction is nearly 5 years.

Treatment.—Induction therapy was with daunorubicin combined with cytarabine. Complete remission was achieved in 151 patients and 123 patients who were not assigned to allogeneic bone marrow transplantation were eligible for high-dose cytarabine-based consolidation. Two to 3 courses were administered, starting a median of 1 month after achieving complete remission. Doses of cytarabine as high as 3 g/m² were combined with daunorubicin, mitoxantrone, or etoposide.

Results.—Forty patients remained alive at the last follow-up, 28 of them in continued remission. The median duration of remission for all patients was 12.8 months, and the actuarial leukemia-free survival rate at

5 years is 26%. Male and older patients had a worse outlook than the others. Patients aged 45 years and younger at complete remission had a 5-year leukemia-free survival of 35%, compared with 18% for older patients. There were 9 treatment-related deaths, and 5 other patients had serious neurotoxic effects.

Conclusion.—Cytarabine-based consolidation therapy appears to be beneficial for younger patients with acute myelogenous leukemia. High-dose cytarabine is not likely, however, to improve the outlook for older patients.

▶ Some have suggested that those studies that conclude that idarubicin is more active than daunorubicin in the induction therapy of acute myeloid leukemia are not valid because too small a daunorubicin dose was used in the control arm. In this study, cytarabine plus daunorubicin at a dosage of 60 mg/m² daily for 3 days was used, and the complete response rate was 67%. This result is not better than the results reported from around the world with daunorubicin at a 25% lower dosage.—P.H. Wiernik, M.D.

Varying Intensity of Postremission Therapy in Acute Myeloid Leukemia

Cassileth PA, Lynch E, Hines JD, Oken MM, Mazza JJ, Bennett JM, McGlave PB, Edelstein M, Harrington DP, O'Connell MJ (Univ of Pennsylvania, Philadelphia; Dana-Farber Cancer Inst, Boston; Case Western Reserve Univ, Cleveland, Ohio; et al)
Blood 79:1924–1930, 1992   4–78

Background.—Induction chemotherapy in patients with acute myeloid leukemia (AML) produces complete remission (CR) in most patients.

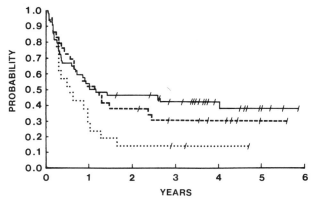

Fig 4–14.—Event-free survival for patients younger than age 41 years. *Solid line* indicates alloBMT (*n* = 54); *dashed line* indicates consolidation therapy (*n* = 29); *dotted line* indicates maintenance therapy (*n* = 21). (Courtesy of Cassileth PA, Lynch E, Hines JD, et al: *Blood* 79:1924–1930, 1992.)

Without postremission therapy, patients rapidly relapse because of the regrowth of occult residual leukemia cells. The Eastern Cooperative Oncology Group determined whether increasing the intensity of postremission treatment in AML would improve outcomes.

Methods.—Data on 449 evaluable patients were analyzed. After uniform induction therapy, 54 patients younger than age 41 years in CR and with a histocompatible sibling underwent allogeneic bone marrow transplantation (alloBMT). By random assignment, 83 other patients received 2 years of continuous outpatient maintenance treatment with cytarabine and 6-thioguanine, and 87 received a single course of inpatient consolidation treatment consisting of 6 days of high-dose cytarabine and 3 days of amsacrine. The median follow-up was 4 years.

Findings.—The 4-year event-free survival (EFS) was 27% for the consolidation therapy and 16% for maintenance therapy. Event-free survival was 28% and 15%, respectively, in patients younger than age 60 years. When outcomes for patients receiving alloBMT were compared with those in patients younger than age 41 years who received consolidation or maintenance therapy, the 4-year EFS was 42%, 30%, and 14%, respectively (Fig 4–14). Patients undergoing alloBMT had a significantly better EFS than patients having maintenance therapy but did not differ significantly from those having consolidation treatment. Among patients younger than age 41 years, the 4-year survival after alloBMT and after consolidation therapy was comparable; both were significantly better than maintenance therapy. Mortality rates were 0% for maintenance therapy, 21% for consolidation therapy, and 36% for alloBMT. Consolidation treatment was associated with an especially high death rate (57%) among patients aged older than 60 years.

Conclusion.—One course of consolidation treatment or alloBMT after initial CR produces better outcomes in patients with AML than lengthy maintenance therapy. Event-free survival and survival associated with alloBMT and consolidation therapy do not differ; however, further research is needed before it can be concluded that these 2 treatments are equivalent. The toxicity of combined high-dose cytarabine and amsacrine is unacceptable, particularly in older patients. Alternative approaches to consolidation therapy (e.g., high-dose cytarabine alone) need to be studied.

▶ This is a major study that addresses the most important current clinical AML question: How can we prolong the disease-free state after successful induction therapy? The results strongly suggest that intensive therapy is needed to achieve optimal remission duration and survival results with agents that are available today, but the question of the relative merits of consolidation therapy vs. marrow transplantation remains open. A current intergroup study coordinated by the Eastern Cooperative Oncology Group seeks to answer that question.—P.H. Wiernik, M.D.

Treatment of Newly Diagnosed Acute Myelogenous Leukemia With Granulocyte-Macrophage Colony-Stimulating Factor (GM-CSF) Before and During Continuous-Infusion High-Dose ara-C + Daunorubicin: Comparison to Patients Treated Without GM-CSF

Estey E, Thall PF, Kantarjian H, O'Brien S, Koller CA, Beran M, Gutterman J, Deisseroth A, Keating M (Univ of Texas, Houston)
Blood 79:2246–2255, 1992   4–79

Introduction.—The GM-CSF has been used effectively to sensitize leukemic blast cells to cytotoxic chemotherapy. The GM-CSF in 56 newly diagnosed cases of acute myeloid leukemia was evaluated, and the results were compared with those obtained in 176 similar patients given comparable cytarabine (ara-C) therapy without GM-CSF.

Patients and Methods.—Study patients received 20 or 125 µg/m² of GM-CSF daily, subcutaneously, for as long as 8 days or until complications developed. The treatment accompanied chemotherapy with ara-C and daunorubicin. The comparison patients received ara-C on the same schedule, alone or with amsacrine or mitoxantrone.

Results.—Both the chance of complete remission and the probability of survival were lower in patients given GM-CSF in addition to chemotherapy (Fig 4–15). The adverse effects of GM-CSF treatment did not appear to reflect an imbalance in patient characteristics and was not a

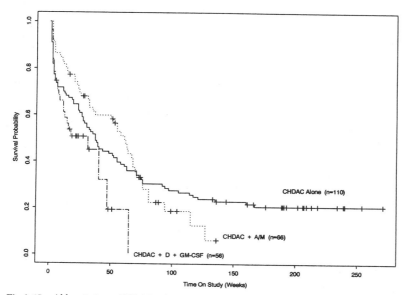

Fig 4–15.—*Abbreviations:* CHDAC, chemotherapy with daunorubicin and ara-C. A/M, amsacrine or mitoxantrone. Kaplan-Meir survival plots for patients treated. (Courtesy of Estey E, Thall PF, Kantarjian H, et al: *Blood* 79:2246–2255, 1992.)

result of acute toxicity. Patients who failed to enter complete remission tended to have persistent leukemia, not prolonged marrow aplasia.

Conclusion.—It appears best to be cautious when considering the use of GM-CSF to sensitize myeloid leukemia cells to chemotherapy with daunorubicin and ara-C. Different results might be obtained with other CSFs that target different hematopoietic progenitors.

▶ This important article shows that certain schedules of GM-CSF may actually be harmful. In practice, growth factors should only be used in schedules in which they have been *demonstrated* to be helpful. One cannot assume anything.—P.H. Wiernik, M.D.

Risk Factors for High-Dose Cytarabine Neurotoxicity: An Analysis of a Cancer and Leukemia Group B Trial in Patients With Acute Myeloid Leukemia

Rubin EH, Andersen JW, Berg DT, Schiffer CA, Mayer RJ, Stone RM (Harvard Med School, Boston; Univ of Maryland; Cancer and Leukemia Group B, Lebanon, NH)
J Clin Oncol 10:948–953, 1992

4–80

Background.—A variety of high-dose cytarabine (HIDAC) neurotoxicity risk factors have been suggested. Because of the lack of consensus, the Cancer and Leukemia Group B (CALGB) recently reviewed HIDAC-induced neurotoxicity occurrences and identified HIDAC neurotoxicity-related risk factors. Pretreatment aspects of postremission of patients with acute myeloid leukemia (AML) treated with HIDAC were analyzed.

Patients and Methods.—A CALGB protocol, designed to determine the optimal dose of cytarabine (ara-C) for postremission AML treatment, was used. A total of 176 patients received at least 1 HIDAC course, consisting of 3 g/m² ara-C. On days 1, 3, and 5, this treatment was infused during 3 hours at 12-hour intervals. The pretreatment features of 170 patients were accessible for risk evaluation.

Results.—Neurotoxicity was noted in 18 patients (10%). Associations between neurotoxicity incidence and elevated serum creatinine, age, and alkaline phosphatase (AP) were demonstrated via univariate analysis. Multivariate analysis revealed that these variables were independent risk components. A risk model was subsequently assembled based on these findings. Parameters used included creatinine $\geq$ 1.2 mg/dL, age $\geq$ 40 years, and AP $\geq$ 3 times normal. Neurotoxicity was found in 17 of 46 patients with 2 or more of these model parameters (37%), compared with 1 of 124 who had either 1 or none. The model sensitivity was 94%; specificity was 81%.

Conclusion.—Patients with 2 or more of the model criteria may be expected to have HIDAC-related neurotoxicity. However, another group of patients comparably treated with HIDAC must be considered before this model can be confirmed.

Severe Myelosuppression Resulting From Concurrent Administration of Granulocyte Colony-Stimulating Factor and Cytotoxic Chemotherapy

Meropol NJ, Miller LL, Korn EL, Braitman LE, MacDermott ML, Schuchter LM (Hosp of the Univ of Pennsylvania, Philadelphia; Natl Cancer Inst, Bethesda, Md; Univ of Pennsylvania, Philadelphia)
J Natl Cancer Inst 84:1201–1203, 1992   4–81

Introduction.—The G-CSF is administered after the completion of chemotherapy to decrease the incidence of chemotherapy-induced febrile neutropenia. This use of G-CSF also appears to reduce the incidence of oral mucositis. This hypothesis was tested by administering G-CSF concurrently in patients treated with fluorouracil (5-FU) and low-dose leucovorin (LV), a regimen commonly causing mucositis but not associated with severe myelosuppression.

Patients and Methods.—Eleven patients, ranging in age from 33 to 72 years, had metastatic cancer. Six patients had received no prior treatment, 1 had undergone radiotherapy, and 3 had been treated with both chemotherapy and radiotherapy. Fluorouracil plus LV was administered by an intravenous bolus on the first 5 days of each 28-day cycle. The G-CSF was administered on days 1 through 14 of the first cycle in a dose of 5 μg/kg body weight per day by subcutaneous injection.

Results.—One patient died of a cerebrovascular accident on day 5 of the first cycle of therapy, leaving 10 patients evaluable for hematologic toxic effects. Four of the first 5 patients treated with G-CSF concurrently with 5-FU and LV had grade 4 neutropenia during the second week of therapy. In response to the high incidence of severe neutropenia in previously untreated patients, the trial was amended to begin G-CSF administration 24 hours after the last dose of 5-FU. None of the 5 patients enrolled after the protocol amendment experienced neutropenia.

Conclusion.—Concurrent administration of G-CSF with chemotherapy appears to have caused the observed increase in toxicity. Future trials should be designed with early stopping rules because of the potential for myelotoxicity when a growth factor and a cytotoxic agent are given together.

▶ This is an important, but limited, observation suggesting that the initial concerns with regard to the concurrent use of cytokines and chemotherapy were probably well founded. Here, it appears that G-CSF in the setting of 5-FU and LV caused relatively severe myelotoxicity. Presumptively, this is because of an induction of cycling of progenitor cells that then become more susceptible to the action of the chemotherapeutic agent.—P.J. Quesenberry, M.D.

ACUTE LYMPHOCYTIC LEUKEMIA

Prognostic Significance of Karyotype at Diagnosis in Childhood Acute Lymphoblastic Anemia
van der Plas DC, Hählen K, Hagemeijer A (Erasmus Univ, Rotterdam, The Netherlands; Univ Hosp Rotterdam, The Netherlands)
Leukemia 6:176–184, 1992   4–82

Introduction.—During the past 15 years, various discoveries have provided new tools for diagnosis and follow-up of childhood acute lymphoblastic leukemia (ALL). The chromosome number of leukemic cells at diagnosis is of prognostic significance, and several mechanisms have been molecularly shown to be responsible for ALL. A total of 135 patients were reviewed to determine the value of cytogenetic investigations at diagnosis for predicting treatment outcome in childhood ALL.

Methods.—The study group included 155 children younger than the age of 15 who had ALL diagnosed between January 1, 1980 and November 1, 1990. Ten children with very high-risk features were treated differently and excluded from the study. Cytogenetic analysis, performed on bone marrow aspirates and usually on peripheral blood, was successful in 135 patients. Patients were classified as high risk (mediastinal enlargement and/or WBC count $\geq 50 \times 10^9/L$) or standard risk. Event-free survival (EFS) was calculated for each patient and EFS curves constructed for ploidy of the karotype and for patients with a normal karotype.

Results.—An abnormal karotype was identified in 101 of 135 patients. Structural chromosomal rearrangements were detected in 71 (53%) patients (71% of the cytogenetically abnormal cases). For all categories, the EFS was shorter in the high-risk group than in the standard-risk group. Hyperdiploidy, frequent in the standard-risk group, was a favorable prognostic feature. Except for the pseudodiploid subgroup, survival curves for each ploidy subgroup were different for patients in the clinically high- and standard-risk groups. In both groups, patients with a normal karotype had a relatively poor EFS. Children with abnormalities involving the short arm of chromosome 12 in combination with pre-B or common ALL phenotype had an increased risk for CNS relapse.

Conclusion.—The ploidy of the karotype appears to be of prognostic importance in childhood ALL. Patients in subgroups known to have a poor outcome may benefit from alternative approaches to therapy and more aggressive treatment regimens.

Cytogenetic Analysis in Relapsed Childhood Acute Lymphoblastic Leukemia
Heerema NA, Palmer CG, Weetman R, Bertolone S (Indiana Univ, Indianap-

olis; Univ of Louisville and Kosair Children's Hosp, KY)
Leukemia 6:185–192, 1992

4–83

Introduction.—Little is known about the nature of cytogenetic abnormalities present at the time of a relapse of childhood acute lymphoblastic leukemia (ALL) or about their relationship to the karyotypic findings at the time of diagnosis. Marrow samples from 51 consecutive children with ALL were obtained at the time of relapse.

Results.—Ten of 50 evaluable patients had normal metaphases at the time of relapse. Twelve other patients were hyperdiploid with more than 50 chromosomes, and 3 were hyperdiploid with 47 to 50 chromosomes. Three patients were hypodiploid with 45 chromosomes. Twenty-one patients had pseudodiploid clones at relapse; most of them had gains and losses of chromosomes and multiple structural abnormalities. Karyotypic evolution was a frequent finding. Rearrangements involving chromosome 1 were common, especially in patients with more than 50 chromosomes. In those with 50 or fewer chromosomes, structural aberrations often were unbalanced, resulting in a loss of genetic material.

Conclusion.—The chromosomal abnormalities found in childhood ALL appear to reflect biologically different underlying events. Distinct biological processes seemingly are involved not only at the outset, but also during evolution of the disease.

Trisomy 21 As the Sole Acquired Chromosomal Abnormality in Children With Acute Lymphoblastic Leukemia

Raimondi SC, Pui C-H, Head D, Behm F, Privitera E, Roberson PK, Rivera GK, Williams DL (St Jude Children's Research Hosp; Univ of Tennessee, Memphis)

Leukemia 6:171–175, 1992

4–84

Background.—Chromosome 21 frequently is involved in trisomies and tetrasomies associated with hyperdiploid acute lymphoblastic leukemia (ALL), but only isolated cases are described in which trisomy 21 is the only acquired numerical chromosome abnormality. Trisomy 21 is characteristic of patients with Down syndrome, who are at increased risk of having leukemia develop. In addition, mosaicism of trisomy 21 is often seen in infants with transient leukemoid reaction.

Patients.—Cytogenetic findings were reviewed in 922 consecutive children with newly diagnosed ALL. Of 601 patients whose marrow metaphases could be analyzed for cytogenetic abnormality, 11 had trisomy 21 as the sole chromosomal aberration.

Observations.—One of the 11 patients had a duplication of the 47, XX,+21 line, indicating clonal evolution. In all but 1, 8% to 77% of the marrow cells had a normal karyotype. None of 5 patients who supplied stimulated peripheral blood samples during remission had evidence of mosaicism. None of 11 study patients had findings of Down syndrome. In all, the leukemic cell immunophenotype was typical of B-cell precursors. All the patients entered complete remission, and hematologic remission has continued for as long as 6½ years. Only 2 patients had relapsed, and both were in the second complete remission at the last follow-up.

Conclusion.—Among children with ALL, those with trisomy 21 as the only acquired chromosomal anomaly appear to have a good outlook.

▶ The chromosome 12 abnormalities and their relationship to CNS leukemia reported by van der Plas et al. (Abstract 4–82) are of interest. I am not aware of any such association in adults with ALL. The suggestion that trisomy 21 may be associated with a good prognosis in childhood ALL (Abstract 4–84) is consistent with the observation of Ravindranath et al. (Abstract 4–65) that AML in patients with Down syndrome is highly responsive to treatment.—P.H. Wiernik, M.D.

Clinical Significance of the BCR-ABL Fusion Gene in Adult Acute Lymphoblastic Leukemia: A Cancer and Leukemia Group B Study (8762)
Westbrook CA, Hooberman AL, Spino C, Dodge RK, Larson RA, Davey F, Wurster-Hill DH, Sobol RE, Schiffer C, Bloomfield CD (Univ of Chicago; CALGB Statistical Office, Durham, NC; State Univ of New York, Syracuse; et al)
Blood 80:2983–2990, 1992   4–85

Background.—The Philadelphia chromosome, and its molecular counterpart, the BCR-ABL fusion gene, is universally present in chronic myelogenous leukemia and also is rarely present in childhood acute lymphoblastic leukemia (ALL), where it is a prognostic marker. The influence of this gene on adult ALL is uncertain. To clarify the role of the BCR-ABL gene, 56 untreated adult patients received intensive multidrug chemotherapy including daunorubicin.

Methods.—Patients were examined for molecular evidence of a BCR-ABL gene by using the Southern blot and pulsed-field gel hybridization methods. The findings were compared with cytogenetic evidence of a Philadelphia chromosome.

Results.—The BCR-ABL gene was detected by molecular methods in 30% of patients, but only 23% had cytogenetic evidence of the Philadelphia chromosome. A large majority of patients (76%) exhibited the p190 gene subtype resembling childhood ALL. The presence of the BCR-ABL gene did not influence the chance of achieving complete remission, but early relapses were more frequent in gene-positive patients, especially those who were positive for the B-cell surface antigen and the common ALL antigen.

Conclusion.—The BCR-ABL fusion gene is a prominent finding in adult ALL. Patients with this gene tend to relapse early and may, therefore, benefit from early intensification of treatment, possibly by bone marrow transplantation.

▶ The Eastern Cooperative Oncology Group of Great Britain, in their joint adult ALL study that has just been initiated, will have an opportunity to study the association of the BCR-ABL fusion gene with response rate, response duration, and survival after chemotherapy alone, autologous bone marrow transplant, and allogeneic bone marrow transplant.—P.H. Wiernik, M.D.

Prognostic Significance of Elevated Serum β2-Microglobulin Levels in Adult Acute Lymphocytic Leukemia
Kantarjian HM, Smith T, Estey E, Polyzos A, O'Brien S, Pierce S, Beran M, Feldman E, Keating MJ (MD Anderson Cancer Ctr, Houston)
Am J Med 93:599–604, 1992   4–86

Objective.—In patients with certain lymphoproliferative disorders, such as multiple myeloma and lymphoma, elevated serum beta₂-microglobulin (β_2M) levels carry a poor prognosis. However, there are few data on the prognostic significance of β_2M levels in patients with acute lymphocytic leukemia (ALL).

Patients and Methods.—A total of 159 adult patients with newly diagnosed ALL were studied to analyze the association between serum β_2M levels at diagnosis and pretreatment characteristics and prognosis. At di-

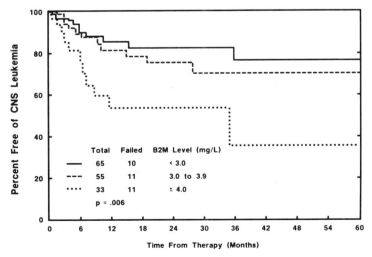

Fig 4–16.—Development of CNS leukemia by pretreatment serum β_2M levels. (Courtesy of Kantarjian HM, Smith T, Estey E, et al: *Am J Med* 93:599-604, 1992.)

agnosis, all patients had measurement of β_2M levels in fresh peripheral blood samples using the Pharmacia β_2 Micro radioimmunoassay. Multivariate analysis was conducted to assess the independent prognostic value of serum β_2M.

Findings.—The complete response rate was 61% in patients with β_2M levels of 4 mg/L or more, compared with 80% in other patients. Those with elevated β_2M levels also had decreased survival and were more likely to have CNS leukemia develop (Fig 4–16). Older patients; those with elevated creatinine, bilirubin, and alkaline phosphatase levels; those with low albumin levels; and those with B-cell disease were all more likely to have high β_2M levels. After adjustment for the pretreatment creatinine level and age, β_2M was found to be an independent prognostic variable. There also appeared to be an association between elevated β_2M levels and a worse incidence of CNS disease in high-risk patients.

Conclusion.—The serum β_2M level is an important prognostic indicator in adult ALL and should be measured as part of the pretreatment evaluation. The monitoring of the serum β_2M level could provide important leads for the design of future treatments for patients with resistant disease. The importance of serum β_2M in childhood ALL needs to be studied.

▶ This is a very interesting observation. New studies of adult ALL should include measurements of β_2M.—P.H. Wiernik, M.D.

Favorable Outcome of B-Cell Acute Lymphoblastic Leukemia in Childhood: A Report of Three Consecutive Studies of the BFM Group
Reiter A, Schrappe M, Ludwig W-D, Lampert F, Harbott J, Henze G, Niemeyer CM, Gadner H, Müller-Weihrich S, Ritter J, Odenwald E, Riehm H (Medizinische Hochschule Hannover, Germany; Free Univ of Berlin; Justus-Liebig-Univ, Giessen, Germany; et al)
Blood 80:2471–2478, 1992   4–87

Introduction.—A decade ago, the BFM group introduced a new approach to treating B-cell acute lymphoblastic leukemia (B-ALL). A cytoreductive prephase with prednisone and cyclophosphamide was followed by eight 5-day courses of chemotherapy. Fractionated cyclophosphamide, methotrexate (MTX), and intrathecal MTX were given with each course, and cytosine arabinoside/teniposide was alternated with doxorubicin. Treatment strategies, patient characteristics, and outcome in B-ALL were studied in the 3 BFM groups.

Patients and Methods.—Of 87 patients, 22 were enrolled in study ALL-BFM-81, 24 in ALL-BFM-83, and 41 in ALL-BFM-86. In the ALL-BFM-83 study, CNS treatment was intensified by adding dexamethasone, and MTX/cytosine arabinoside was given intraventricularly. Six courses of treatment were given rather than 8. In the ALL-BFM 86 study,

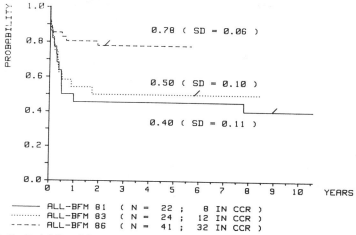

Fig 4–17.—Probability of duration of the event-free survival for B-ALL patients. *Slash* indicates last patient entering each study. P = .014 (study 81: study 86); P = .025 (study 83: study 86). (Courtesy of Reiter A, Schrappe M, Ludwig W-D, et al: *Blood* 80:2471–2478, 1992.)

MTX was given at high doses (5 g/m² in 24 hours) and also intrathecally along with cytosine arabinoside and prednisolone. Doses of cytosine arabinoside and teniposide were increased, and cyclophosphamide was partly replaced by ifosfamide. Vincristine was added. The CNS irradiation was used in ALL-BFM-81 and -83 but was omitted in ALL-BFM-86.

Results.—The estimated 5-year event-free survival rate was highest in study ALL-BFM-86 (Fig 4–17). All but 5 of 24 relapses occurred during or shortly after treatment. No isolated CNS relapses occurred in ALL-BFM-83, in contrast to ALL-BFM-81, but marrow relapse was more frequent. In ALL-BFM-86, there were no isolated marrow relapses and only 1 CNS relapse occurred. The only significant predictor of outcome was the presence of residual disease after the first 2 courses of treatment. Toxicity was considerable; 4 patients definitely died of treatment-related complications.

Conclusion.—Intensive, brief-pulse treatment given within 4 months is a highly effective approach to B-ALL. In addition to fractionated cyclophosphamide/ifosfamide therapy, an infusion of high-dose MTX and intrathecal treatment will help prevent both systemic and CNS relapses.

▶ B-cell ALL should no longer be excluded from studies on the basis that this phenotype has a poor prognosis. This is true for adult ALL as well, and it should be noted that such patients were excluded from the Linker study (Abstract 4–100).—P.H. Wiernik, M.D.

Treatment of Occult or Late Overt Testicular Relapse in Children With Acute Lymphoblastic Leukemia: A Pediatric Oncology Group Study

Wofford MM, Smith SD, Shuster JJ, Johnson W, Buchanan GR, Wharam MD, Ritchey AK, Rosen D, Haggard ME, Golembe BL, Rivera GK (Bowman-Gray School of Med, Winston-Salem, NC; Univ of Chicago; Univ of Florida, Gainesville; et al)

J Clin Oncol 10:624–630, 1992   4–88

Introduction. —Patients in whom testicular leukemia develops after the completion of primary therapy for acute lymphoblastic leukemia (ALL) have an improved disease-free survival rate compared with that in boys who relapse during initial therapy. Teniposide (VM-26) and doxorubicin were initiated in 80 boys with ALL who experienced an isolated testicular relapse. The outcome and toxicity associated with the Pediatric Oncology Group (POG) 8304 protocol was described.

Methods. —The POG 8304 2-arm protocol included reinduction chemotherapy, testicular irradiation, and CNS prophylaxis. Continuation therapy consisted of 6-mercaptopurine/methotrexate and vincristine/cyclophosphamide. The patients were randomized to receive pulses of either VM-26 and cytarabine or doxorubicin/prednisone.

Results. —Fifty-five of the boys with ALL had isolated microscopic testicular leukemia, and 25 had a late isolated overt testicular relapse. Univariate analysis showed that age older than 10 years, WBC greater than 50,000/µL at time of diagnosis, and black race were significantly poor prognostic factors. The overall 4-year event-free survival rate was 53% ± 8% among boys with occult testicular relapse compared with 84% ± 10% for boys with late overt testicular relapse. Neither arm of the continuation therapy was significantly superior.

Conclusion. —The treatment approach for isolated testicular leukemia, including reinduction chemotherapy, testicular irradiation, CNS prophylaxis, continuation therapy, and late intensification, secured a prolonged second remission in many patients with occult or late overt testicular leukemia. The POG 8304 protocol offers effective and relatively nontoxic therapy with a high curative potential.

Superior Treatment Results in Females With High-Risk Acute Lymphoblastic Leukemia in Childhood

Lanning M, Garwicz S, Hertz H, Jonmundsson G, Kreuger A, Lie SO, Moe PJ, Salmi TT, Schröder H, Siimes MA, Wesenberg F, Yssing M, Åhström L, Gustafsson G (Nordic Society of Pediatric Hematology and Oncology (NOPHO), Finland, Sweden, Denmark, Iceland, and Norway)

Acta Paediatr 81:66–68, 1992   4–89

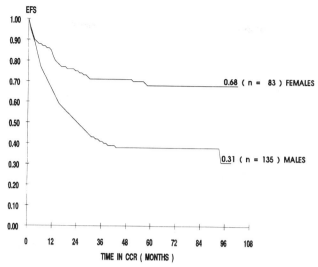

Fig 4–18.—Event-free survival (*EFS*) in high-risk ALL with regard to sex (*P* < .001). (Courtesy of Lanning M, Garwicz S, Hertz H, et al: *Acta Paediatr* 81:66–68, 1992.)

Background.—Substantial progress has been made in the treatment of children with acute lymphoblastic leukemia (ALL), much of it as a result of risk-adjusted treatment. Total WBC count and age at diagnosis are well-defined major risk factors; there is controversy, however, as to the prognostic importance of gender. In children with ALL, the male sender was suggested to be a negative prognostic factor.

Patients and Methods.—The study included 808 children, aged 1–15 years, with a diagnosis of non–B-cell ALL during a 5-year period. The children were drawn from 5 Nordic countries with a combined population of 4.5 million children. Based on risk criteria at diagnosis, the children were classified as being at standard risk, 41% of the boys and 49% of the girls; intermediate risk, 27% of the boys and 29% of the girls; and high risk, 32% of the boys and 22% of the girls. The treatment was standard for most children within the risk groups. The cure rate was assessed for event-free survival (EFS).

Results.—A remission was obtained in 95% of the patients, with no differences between the sexes. At 102 months, the EFS was .47 for the boys and .62 for the girls, with no differences in the EFS between sexes in either the standard-risk or intermediate-risk groups. However, for the high-risk group, the EFS was .68 for the girls vs. .31 for the boys (Fig 4–18). On Cox multivariate analysis, the significant prognostic factors for all children were WBC count, gender, age, and thrombocyte count.

Conclusion.—Intensified treatment of pediatric ALL according to prognostic factors results in equal EFS for girls with ALL in all risk groups. For boys in the high-risk group, however, intensified treatment does not appear to be of benefit. These boys may need even more intensive treatment than girls with the same high-risk prognostic factors.

▶ Similar results were found in the Schiller et al. (Abstract 4–77) adult AML study.—P.H. Wiernik, M.D.

Long-Term Survivors of Leukemia Treated in Infancy: Factors Associated With Neuropsychologic Status

Mulhern RK, Kovnar E, Langston J, Carter M, Fairclough D, Leigh L, Kun LE (St Jude Children's Research Hosp, Memphis, Tenn; Univ of Tennessee, Memphis)

J Clin Oncol 10:1095–1102, 1992

4–90

Objective.—The prognosis and risk of late toxicity are worse in infants and very young children with acute lymphoblastic leukemia (ALL) than in their older counterparts. There is particular concern about the effects of cranial radiation therapy (CRT). Survival and functional outcome in infants treated for ALL has only been assessed in 1 small cohort. The functional and neuropsychological statuses of 26 long-term survivors of ALL diagnosed in the first 2 years of life were compared with those of 26 children who were previously treated for Wilms' tumor.

Methods.—All children had completed treatment at least 2 years earlier; the ALL group was diagnosed at a mean of 1.5 years and the Wilms' tumor group at 1.2 years. Both were reevaluated at about 12 years of age. In the ALL group, 6 children had received no CRT, 5 had received 18 Gy of CRT, 7 had received 20 Gy of CRT, and 5 had received 24 Gy of CRT. Another 3 children who sustained CNS relapse received CRT doses of 24, 40, and 44 Gy, respectively. Neuropsychological testing was performed in both the ALL and Wilms' tumor groups; diagnostic imaging studies were also done in the ALL group.

Findings.—Objective measures of global function showed no significant differences between the ALL and Wilms' tumor groups. However, the mean intelligence quotient (IQ) was lower in the ALL group, 87 vs. 96. The ALL group also had a poorer performance on 4 of 6 measures of visual and auditory memory, less advanced arithmetic skills, and a higher frequency of special education intervention. The ALL group showed an inverse correlation of IQ and auditory memory performance with time since the completion of therapy and total CRT dose.

Conclusion.—Patients treated for ALL in infancy appear to have intellectual, academic, and neurologic sequelae that can be directly attributed to the intensity of their CNS therapy. These findings support the practice of omitting CRT except for children at risk of CNS relapse. The authors also present evidence that, in such cases, it is better to delay CRT until the child is older.

Impact of Three Methods of Treatment Intensification on Acute Lymphoblastic Leukemia in Children: Long-Term Results of St Jude Total Therapy Study X

Pui C-H, Simone JV, Hancock ML, Evans WE, Williams DL, Bowman WP, Dahl GV, Dodge RK, Ochs J, Abromowitch M, Rivera GK (St Jude Children's Research Hosp, Memphis, Tenn; Univ of Tennessee, Memphis)

Leukemia 6:150–157, 1992   4–91

Background.—Early intensification therapy is useful in pediatric acute lymphoblastic leukemia (ALL), whereas prolonged intensification is useful in high-risk ALL. Different methods of intensification were examined in subgroups of pediatric patients with ALL who were followed for an average of 9 years.

Patients.—There were 427 pediatric patients with ALL divided into 2 groups. The high-risk group had greatly increased leukocyte counts, T-cell ALL, a mediastinal mass, or initial CNS leukemia. The standard-risk group had none of these prognostic indicators.

Treatment.—In the standard-risk trial, 154 of 309 patients in complete remission were randomly assigned to receive high-dose methotrexate (HDMTX) during the first 72 weeks of standard continuation therapy, whereas the remaining patients received cranial irradiation and standard continuation therapy. In the high-risk trial, patients received periodic pulses of teniposide/cytarabine with a standard antileukemic regimen and delayed cranial irradiation.

Results.—In the standard-risk trial, after an average of 9 years of follow-up, significantly higher proportions of those patients who received HDMTX have maintained complete remission, hematologic remission, and testicular remission. However, a lower proportion of this group has maintained CNS remission. In the high-risk trial, about 36% are predicted to be event-free survivors at 9 years. The total number of long-term survivors was 68%.

Conclusion.—Postremission therapy that includes HDMTX is effective for standard-risk pediatric patients with ALL. The long-term survival rate of 68% will be useful for comparison with later trials of new treatment regimens.

▶ Is it not time to replace prophylactic cranial irradiation with systemic HDMTX and/or cytarabine in all children?—P.H. Wiernik, M.D.

Intensive Chemotherapy With Mitoxantrone and High-Dose Cytosine Arabinoside Followed by Granulocyte-Macrophage Colony-Stimulating Factor in the Treatment of Patients With Acute Lymphocytic Leukemia

Kantarjian HM, Estey EH, O'Brien S, Anaissie E, Beran M, Rios MB, Keating MJ, Gutterman J (Univ of Texas, Houston)
Blood 79:876–881, 1992   4–92

Introduction.—Chemotherapeutic agents with different mechanisms of actions used in intensification regimens have improved the prognosis of patients with acute lymphocytic leukemia (ALL). When tested in the salvage setting, regimens containing high-dose cytosine arabinoside (ara-C) resulted in significant morbidity and mortality related to myelosuppression. The value of GM-CSF in reducing the myelosuppression that followed mitoxantrone and high-dose ara-C therapy in adult patients with ALL was examined.

Patients and Methods.—The study group included 34 patients with refractory ALL treated between May 1989 and April 1991. Therapy with GM-CSF was started 24 hours after chemotherapy was completed, with patients receiving 125 μg/m² of body surface during 4 hours until the granulocyte level recovered to $2 \times 10^3/\mu L$. The results of this regimen were compared with those reported in 29 patients treated between March 1985 and April 1989 with identical chemotherapy and supportive care but without GM-CSF.

Results.—Complete response (CR) rates were the same (38%) in both the treatment and historical control groups. Patients who received GM-CSF had a lower induction mortality (6% vs. 21%) and a higher incidence of resistant disease (56% vs. 34%). The 2 groups did not differ significantly in CR duration or overall survival. The recovery of the granulocyte counts more than 500/μL was significantly faster in the GM-CSF group, but febrile episodes and documented infections occurred at rates similar to those of the control group.

Conclusion.—The use of GM-CSF after intensive chemotherapy in adult patients with refractory ALL significantly decreased the duration of granulocytopenia, lowered the induction mortality, and prolonged short-term survival. Long-term prognosis, however, was not improved. Therapy with GM-CSF may prove beneficial when added to chemotherapy in earlier stages or as part of maintenance intensification in remission.

▶ This group of investigators continues to teach us that we have much more to learn about growth factors before we fully understand the clinical implications of their use. In certain circumstances, their use in acute leukemia may be dangerous.—P.H. Wiernik, M.D.

Effective Immunochemotherapy of CALLA+Cμ+ Human Pre-B Acute Lymphoblastic Leukemia in Mice With Severe Combined Immunodeficiency Using B43 (Anti-CD19) Pokeweed Antiviral Protein Immunotoxin Plus Cyclophosphamide

Uckun FM, Chelstrom LM, Finnegan D, Tuel-Ahlgren L, Manivel C, Irvin JD, Myers DE, Gunther R (Univ of Minnesota, Minneapolis; Southwest Texas State Univ, San Marco)
Blood 79:3116–3129, 1992

4–93

Objective.—A very aggressive subclone of the human CALLA+Cμ+ pre-B acute lymphoblastic leukemia (ALL) cell line NALM-6, designated NALM-6-UM1, produces fatal disseminated leukemia in CB.17 mice having severe combined immunodeficiency. This murine model of human pre-B ALL was used to compare the antileukemic effects of B43 (anti-CD19)-pokeweed antiviral protein (PAP) immunotoxin and cyclophosphamide (CPA), administered individually and in combination.

Findings.—Combined treatment with B43-PAP plus CPA was superior to either agent alone, markedly improving the event-free survival of mice with the severe combined immunodeficiency challenged with NALM-6-UM1 pre-B ALL cells. From 90% to 100% of mice given the combined treatment achieved long-term survival after a challenge with 10^6 leukemia cells. Combined treatment was especially beneficial to mice challenged with 5×10^6 leukemia cells. Long-term survivors lacked molecular evidence of occult leukemia in the bone marrow, spleen, liver, or brain.

Conclusion.—This is the first demonstration of in vivo antileukemic efficacy for combined immunochemotherapy using anti-CD19 immunotoxin plus CPA against the aggressive human pre-B ALL cell line in mice with severe combined immunodeficiency.

▶ Uckun and colleagues have previously shown that a 3-day treatment with nontoxic doses of B43 (anti-CD19) PAP immunotoxin improved event-free survival in mice with severe combined immunodeficiency challenged with the lymphoblastic leukemia cell line NALM-6(1). The present studies extend these observations and show superior survival when the immunotoxins are combined with cyclophosphamide. This is obviously pointing to future clinical trials with these agents in lymphoid malignancies. The B-43 immunotoxin has entered phase 1 dose escalation studies in relapsed pre-B and pre-B patients with ALL, and word of mouth has it that clinical responses have been seen. Further information in this area is awaited with intense interest.—P.J. Quesenberry, M.D.

Reference

1. Uckun FM, et al: *Blood* 79:2201, 1992.

Transplantation of Bone Marrow Cells From Transgenic Mice Expressing the Human *MDR*1 Gene Results in Long-Term Protection Against the Myelosuppressive Effect of Chemotherapy in Mice

Mickisch GH, Aksentijevich I, Schoenlein PV, Goldstein LJ, Galski H, Stahle C, Sachs DH, Pastan I, Gottesman MM (Natl Cancer Inst, Bethesda, Md)
Blood 79:1087–1093, 1992   4–94

Introduction.—Many human cancers that at first respond to chemotherapy later become unresponsive. Dose escalation sometimes is not possible because of cytotoxic effects on sensitive tissues such as the bone marrow. Another possible approach is to transplant bone marrow cells containing physiologic amounts of a multidrug resistance (MDR1) complementary DNA (cDNA).

Methods.—In this study, bone marrow cells from transgenic mice expressing *MDR*1 cDNA were transplanted to lethally irradiated mice. Subsequently, various chemotherapeutic agents were administered in doses that rapidly reduced white cell numbers by at least 50% in unprotected animals. The drugs given included doxorubicin, daunomycin, taxol, vinblastine, vincristine, etoposide, and actinomycin D.

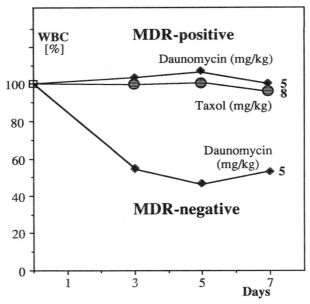

Fig 4–19.—Time course of WBCs after chemotherapy 258 days after bone marrow transplantation. Results were expressed as percentage of WBCs on day 5 as compared with WBCs on day 0 (before treatment). (Courtesy of Mickisch GH, Aksentijevich I, Schoenlein PV, et al: *Blood* 79:1087–1093, 1992.)

Results.—Southern blot analysis demonstrated MDR1 DNA in splenic and bone marrow specimens from recipient animals 6 weeks to 10 months after transplantation. Expression of MDR1 messenger RNA was observed in marrow samples subjected to slot blot analysis. Transplanted animals were resistant to administration of daunomycin and taxol (Fig 4–19). Chemoprotection was reversed by adding chemosensitizers such as cyclosporine A and R-verapamil to chemotherapy.

Conclusion.—These findings suggest a role for the MDR1 gene treatment in patients who require cancer chemotherapy.

▶ This contribution, along with the recent publication of Sorrentino et al. (1), presents impressive evidence that the *MDR*1 gene can be transferred in marrow stem cells to animals and result in resistance to chemotherapeutic agents that are pumped by the P170 MDR protein. Recent evidence that the *MDR* gene is expressed in relatively primitive stem cells does not preclude this approach, as there are major quantitative differences, and the insertion of the *MDR* gene into hematopoietic cells has led to enhanced resistance to the effects of drugs pumped by the P-glycoprotein. Transfer of the *MDR* gene into hematopoietic stem cells is now the target of a number of clinical investigators to enhance the resistance of bone marrow to a variety of P170-pumped chemotherapeutic agents such as doxorubicin, daunomycin, taxol, vinblastine, vincristine, etoposide, and actinomycin-D, thus allowing for repetitive high-dose therapy in patients with metastatic cancer.—P.J. Quesenberry, M.D.

Reference

1. Sorrentino et al: *Science* 1992.

Bone Marrow Transplantation

Use of Recombinant Human Granulocyte-Macrophage Colony-Stimulating Factor in Patients With Lymphoid Malignancies Transplanted With Unpurged or Adjusted-Dose Mafosfamide-Purged Autologous Marrow
Carlo-Stella C, Mangoni L, Almici C, Cottafavi L, Meloni G, Mandelli F, Rizzoli V (Univ of Parma, Italy; "La Sapienza" Univ, Rome)
Blood 80:2412–2418, 1992   4–95

Rationale.—Purging of bone marrow increases neutropenia-related morbidity after autologous bone marrow transplantation. Recombinant human GM-CSF has been shown to enhance neutrophil recovery after this procedure, but the results when purged marrow was used have been controversial.

Methods.—The effectiveness of rhGM-CSF was examined in 15 patients with lymphoid malignancy who underwent marrow transplantation when in complete remission. Five received unpurged bone marrow, but in 10 instances, the marrow was purged with mafosafamide to remove the GM-CFU compartment while sparing many primitive adherent blast CFUs. Treatment with rhGM-CSF began within 24 hours of transplantation and was continued for a week after the absolute neutrophil count reached 500×10^6/L.

Results.—Neutrophil recovery took place at similar rates whether or not purged marrow was used. Granulocyte recovery, however, took about twice as long after receiving purged marrow. The number of blast CFUs infused correlated significantly with the time needed for neutrophils to recover. There was no toxicity directly ascribed to the administration of rhGM-CSF.

Conclusion.—The administration of rhGM-CSF effectively hastens neutrophil recovery after bone marrow transplantation when the transplant contains few GM-CFUs. The use of chemically purged bone marrow now is safer and may be possible in a larger number of patients.

▶ This is an interesting study suggesting that GM-CSF may partially compensate for the defective repopulation seen after many purging approaches. This study has the general problems of historical controls, different purging techniques, no 1 chemotherapeutic regimen, and mixed patients somewhat unevenly distributed. However, I like the dose adjustment to biological parameters (50% CFUs). Something like this adjustment should be extended to all chemotherapy because our current practice with regard to determining dose is totally empiric without a sound scientific base, i.e., milligrams per kilogram or per square meter.

It should be noted that the overall role of GM-CSF in marrow transplantation remains uncertain, although this is the indication for which the Food and Drug Administration approved its use. In a relatively large series reported at the American Society of Hematology meetings in Anaheim, California, a survival advantage for GM-CSF and graft failure was implied (1). However, the historical control group in this study was essentially all acute leukemias, whereas the test group had a significant percentage of lymphomas and other diseases. When the presenter was questioned on this, it was acknowledged that if the leukemics were compared with the leukemics, there was no difference in survival (1). Finally, it should be noted that toxicity in this setting is obviously very difficult to evaluate. A number of symptoms occurred, and it is not clear why the death with congestive cardiomyopathy might not be a GM-CSF toxicity.—P.J. Quesenberry, M.D.

Reference

1. The American Society of Hematology, 1992.

Dynamic Assessment of Quality of Life After Autologous Bone Marrow Transplantation

Chao NJ, Tierney DK, Bloom JR, Long GD, Barr TA, Stallbaum BA, Wong RM, Negrin RS, Horning SJ, Blume KG (Stanford Univ, Calif; Univ of California, Berkeley)

Blood 80:825–830, 1992   4–96

Introduction.—Progress in cancer therapy has effected various gains in the lives of the patients surviving the disease. Bone marrow transplantation (BMT) has aided this progress, but the long-term overall psychological, functional, and physical outcome of this treatment remains unknown. A questionnaire assessing the well-being and quality-of-life parameters was given to patients with cancer who underwent autologous BMT, and the results were studied.

Patients and Methods.—A total of 102 patients undergoing an autologous BMT for lymphomas or nonlymphoblastic leukemia who had at least a 1-year follow-up were included. Of these patients, 58 (26 women and 32 men with a median age at transplantation of 36 years) survived 1 year after the BMT and completed the questionnaire. The quality-of-life assessment tool included 10 distinct dimensions among 14 questions. The questionnaire reliability was tested by randomly selecting 20 patients who received the test 2 times, 90 and 365 days after the BMT.

Results.—The majority of patients maintained their appetite, sleep patterns, health status (measured by frequency of colds), and medication use, whereas 45% and 27% either maintained or lost weight after the transplant. Sexual activity and body image remained high in more than two thirds of the patients. Improvements occurred in the self-rated quality-of-life ratings. Significant differences occurred between patients who rated their appetite and sleep as poor or good at 90 days after BMT. Patients who worked full-time or who had higher body-image ratings also had significantly higher quality-of-life scores.

Conclusion.—Most patients in this survey considered their quality of life above average, which suggests that the majority of these patients can expect a reasonable return to normal living 1 year after the BMT.

Improvement in Outcome for Children Receiving Allogeneic Bone Marrow Transplantation in First Remission of Acute Myeloid Leukemia: A Report From the Groupe d'Etude des Greffes de Moelle Osseuse

Michel G, Gluckman E, Blaise D, Esperou-Bourdeau H, Vernant JP, Kuentz M, Bordigoni P, Milpied N, Rubie H, Thuret I, Troussard X, Frappaz D, Herve P, Plouvier E, Gratecos N, Bernaudin F, Lioure B, Bergeron C, Jouet JP, Gardembas-Pain M, Belanger C, Gouvernet J, Perrimond H, Maraninchi D (Hôpital d'Enfants La Timone, Marseille, France; Hôpital St Louis, Paris; Hôpital Henri Mondor, Creteil, France; et al)
J Clin Oncol 10:1865–1869, 1992   4–97

Introduction.—About 60% of children with acute myeloid leukemia (AML) who undergo allogeneic bone marrow transplantation (BMT) during their first complete remission (CR) will obtain long-term disease-free survival. As many as 20% of patients will have recurrent disease, with the rest of treatment failures resulting from transplant-related mortality. The results of HLA-identical BMT in 74 children with AML treated in their first CR were evaluated.

Patients and Methods.—The patients were treated at 13 French centers during an 11.5-year period. There were 43 boys and 31 girls (median age, 10 years). Fifty-four patients received total body irradiation as their conditioning regimen; the rest received busulfan and cyclophosphamide. Thirty-eight patients received graft-vs.-host disease (GVHD) prophylaxis with cyclosporine (CycloA) plus methotrexate (MTX); 18 received CycloA only; 17 received MTX only; and 1 received T-cell depletion only. The mean time from diagnosis to transplantation was 167 days.

Outcomes.—There were 16 deaths from transplant-related complications. At a median follow-up of 46 months, 46 patients were alive and in continuous CR; 12 relapsed within a median of 8 months. The probability of event-free survival (EFS) increased from 43% in children treated from 1979 to 1982 to 82% in those treated from 1987 to 1990, whereas transplant-related mortality decreased from 36% to 3%. A short interval from diagnosis to transplantation, the absence of significant acute GVHD, and the absence of chronic GVHD were all associated with better EFS on univariate analysis; on multivariate analysis, the significant factors were undergoing transplantation in the most recent period and the absence of acute GVHD.

Conclusion.—Mainly because of reductions in treatment-related mortality, the results of BMT for children with AML in their first CR appear to have improved significantly in the last few years. The very good EFS figures reported in this study will have to be confirmed; there is still the possibility of late relapses or transplant-related complications. Still, early allogeneic BMT is a promising form of consolidation therapy for children with an HLA-matched sibling.

▶ A similar improved outcome has been reported in the United States as well.—P.H. Wiernik, M.D.

Allogeneic Marrow Transplantation During Untreated First Relapse of Acute Myeloid Leukemia

Clift RA, Buckner CD, Appelbaum FR, Schoch G, Petersen FB, Bensinger WI, Sanders J, Sullivan KM, Storb R, Singer J, Hansen JA, Thomas ED (Fred Hutchinson Cancer Research Ctr, Seattle; VA Med Ctr, Seattle; Univ of Washington, Seattle)
J Clin Oncol 10:1723–1729, 1992
4–98

Background.—Allogeneic bone marrow transplantation (ABMT) from HLA-identical siblings is commonly done for patients with acute myeloid leukemia (AML) in first remission. Typically, it is accomplished with a regimen of cyclophosphamide (CY) and total body irradiation (TBI) or busulfan (BU) and CY. The Seattle experience with BMT for AML during untreated first relapse was reviewed.

Patients and Methods.—The study included 126 patients, and several preoperative regimens were used. Regimen 1, given to 29 patients, consisted of CY, 120 mg/kg, and 15.75 Gy of fractionated TBI, with methotrexate (MTX) given intermittently during 102 days to prevent graft-vs.-host disease (GVHD). In regimen 2, given to 22 patients, the same CY and TBI treatment was combined with MTX and cyclosporine (CSP) for prevention of GVHD. Seventeen other transplant regimens were used for the remaining 75 patients.

Findings.—Overall, the 5-year probability of relapse-free survival was 23%; of relapse, 57%; and of nonrelapse mortality, 44%. The relapse with regimen 1 was 26%, significantly less than for regimen 2, with a relapse rate of 70%, or of any other regimen, with a relapse rate of 76%. Sixty-seven percent of regimen 1 patients had acute GVHD, compared with 22% of regimen 2 patients and 41% of patients on other regimens. Regimen 1 patients also had increased nonrelapse mortality. However, regimen 1 patients had a significantly higher 3-year relapse-free survival (38%) than those on regimen 2 (18%) or those on any other regimen (20%).

Conclusion.—Patients who received the CY and TBI treatment had a lower incidence of relapse and a better survival after GVHD prophylaxis with MTX alone than after a combination of MTX and CSP, even though patients who received the former regimen had a significantly higher incidence of acute GVHD. Future studies of the optimal timing of ABMT in the treatment of patients with AML are justified.

Allogeneic Bone Marrow Transplantation for Acute Myeloid Leukemia in First Remission: A Randomized Trial of a Busulfan-Cytoxan Versus Cytoxan-Total Body Irradiation as Preparative Regimen: A Report From the Groupe d'Etudes de la Greffe de Moelle Osseuse

Blaise D, for the Group d'Etude de la Greffe de Moelle Osseuse (Institut Paoli Calmettes, Marseille, France)
Blood 79:2578–2582, 1992   4–99

Introduction.—The results of allogeneic marrow transplantation, as early consolidation of initial complete remission, were examined in 101 patients with acute myeloid leukemia.

Patients and Methods.—The patients all were older than 14 years of age (median age, 32). All patients received 60 mg/kg of Cytoxan (CY) intravenously on 2 successive days. Fifty-one patients (BUSCY) first received a total dose of 16 mg/kg of busulfan (BUS) orally in 4 days. The other 50 patients (CYTBI) received total body irradiation after CY treatment. Most of them had fractionated therapy to a median dose of 12 Gy. Methotrexate and cyclosporine were used for post-transplant immunosuppression; some patients also received an anti-P55 monoclonal antibody.

Results.—The likelihood of relapse was 14% in the CYTBI group and 34% in the BUSCY group. Survival was greater in the irradiated patients (Fig 4–20). Differences in outcome between the 2 treatment groups were most evident in patients given transplants within 4 months. The conditioning regimen and chronic graft-vs.-host disease were the only factors that independently influenced the risk of relapse.

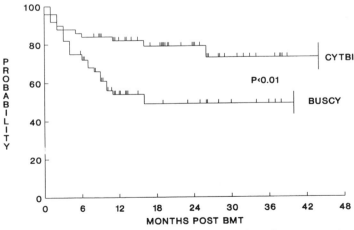

Fig 4–20.—Actuarial probability of disease-free survival. The *tick marks* represent patients without relapse. (Courtesy of Blaise D, for The Group d'Etude de la Greffe de Moelle Osseuse: *Blood* 79:2578–2582, 1992.)

Conclusion.—Cytoxan therapy and total body irradiation are an effective conditioning regimen for marrow transplantation in patients with acute myeloid leukemia.

Autologous Bone Marrow Transplantation for Acute Myeloid Leukemia Using Busulfan Plus Etoposide as a Preparative Regimen
Linker CA, Ries CA, Damon LE, Rugo HS, Wolf JL (Univ of California, San Francisco; Alta Bates Hosp, Berkeley, Calif)
Blood 81:311–318, 1993   4-100

Introduction.—In allogeneic bone marrow transplantation (BMT) for acute myelogenous leukemia (AML), intensive preparative regimens have been found to sometimes significantly reduce the relapse rate, but these gains are offset by increased treatment-related mortality. With autologous BMT, however, intensive preparative regimens might be more practical and gains in disease control might not be countered by increases in graft-vs.-host disease and treatment-related mortality. A preparative regimen of high-dose busulfan and etoposide was used for the treatment of patients with AML with autologous BMT in remission.

Patients and Methods.—The subjects were 58 patients with AML, none older than 60 years of age. Thirty-two were treated in their first remission and 21 in their second or third remission. Five patients had primary refractory AML that did not respond to high-dose cytosine arabinoside, but they did go into remission with aggressive salvage therapy. All patients received busulfan, 1 mg/kg every 6 hours for 4 days, given 7–4 days before BMT. The total busulfan dose was thus 16 mg/kg. On the third day before BMT, patients received etoposide, 60 mg/kg by intravenous infusion during 6–10 hours. Before transplantation, the autologous bone marrow was treated with 4-hydroperoxycyclophosphamide, 100 μg/mL.

Results.—Patients were followed for a median of 22 months. In the first-remission group, there was 1 treatment-related death and 5 patients had relapsed disease. The actuarial relapse rate was 22% and the 3-year disease-free survival was 76%. Results were especially good for the 15 patients with the favorable French-American-British (FAB) subtypes M3 or M4 EO, with no relapses during a median 30-month follow-up. In comparison, patients with less favorable FAB subtypes had a 3-year actuarial relapse rate of 48%. In the subsequent-remission group, there were 5 treatment-related deaths and 4 patients relapsed, with an actuarial relapse rate of 25% and a 3-year disease-free survival of 56%. All but 1 of the patients with primary refractory AML died during treatment.

Conclusion.—Promising results have been obtained with aggressive preparative therapy and autologous purged BMT for adult patients with AML. With confirmation of these results, autologous BMT could become the treatment of choice for patients in their first remission. The preparative regimen described here is a highly toxic one, requiring meticulous supportive care to avoid a high death rate.

Busulfan/Etoposide: Initial Experience With a New Preparatory Regimen for Autologous Bone Marrow Transplantation in Patients With Acute Nonlymphoblastic Leukemia
Chao NJ, Stein AS, Long GD, Negrin RS, Amylon MD, Wong RM, Forman SJ, Blume KG (Stanford Univ, Calif; City of Hope Natl Med Ctr, Duarte, Calif)
Blood 81:319–323, 1993   4–101

Objective.—Most patients with acute nonlymphoblastic leukemia (ANLL) will achieve a complete remission with intensive chemotherapy. However, these remissions do not last long, and most patients will have a relapse of their underlying disease. Autologous bone marrow transplantation (BMT) might improve relapse-free survival in ANLL. The combination of busulfan and etoposide (formerly used as a preparatory regimen for second allogeneic BMT) was used in an attempt to improve antitumor efficacy.

Patients and Methods.—Fifty patients with ANLL were treated with autologous BMT. All but 2 were adults (median age, 40 years). Two patients had biphenotypic acute leukemia. All patients received the combination of busulfan, 16 mg/kg, and etoposide, 60 mg/kg, as a preparative regimen. The initial 20 patients received unpurged marrow; the next 28 received marrow purged with 4-hydroperoxycyclophosphamide (4-HC), 60 μg/mL. For the 2 patients with biphenotypic acute leukemia, the marrow was purged with both H-HC and etoposide, 5 μg/mL. The transplant was done during the first complete remission (CR) in 34 patients, during the second CR in 12, and during a relapse in 4. Patients received a median of .7 × 10^8 mononuclear cells an average of 1 month after harvest.

Results.—An absolute neutrophil count of 500/μL or greater was achieved at a median of 26 days. An untransfused platelet count of 20,000/μL or greater was achieved at a median of 56 days, and a sustained hematocrit value of 30% or greater was achieved at a median of 50 days. Twenty-six patients continue in CR at a median follow-up of 31 months. Actuarial disease-free survival is 57% in patients receiving purged marrow, with a relapse rate of 28%. For those receiving unpurged marrow, disease-free survival is 32% and the relapse rate is 62%. The most serious extramedullary toxic effects were hepatic and cutaneous, including mucositis.

Conclusion.—Many patients with ANLL can achieve disease-free survival with the combination of busulfan and etoposide followed by autologous BMT. Treatment is most successful when purged marrow is used, but the preparative regimen carries significant skin and liver toxicity.

Randomized studies are needed to determine whether this treatment offers a significant improvement in disease-free survival.

▶ This transplant chemotherapy regimen has attracted widespread attention recently, and the results reported in these 2 studies (Abstracts 4–100 and 4–101) show why. One caveat, however, is that 4-HC is no longer available. It will be important to demonstrate that the results with this regimen are similar when nonpurged marrow is used. It will also be important to pursue the study of etoposide and alkyl-lysophospholipid (Vogler et al. [Abstract 4–58]) as purging agents.—P.H. Wiernik, M.D.

Sequential Cycles of High-Dose Carboplatin Administered With Recombinant Human Granulocyte-Macrophage Colony-Stimulating Factor and Repeated Infusions of Autologous Peripheral-Blood Progenitor Cells: A Novel and Effective Method for Delivering Multiple Courses of Dose-Intensive Therapy
Shea TC, Mason JR, Storniolo AM, Newton B, Breslin M, Mullen M, Ward DM, Miller L, Christian M, Taetle R (Univ of California at San Diego; Univ of Arizona, Tucson; Natl Cancer Inst, Bethesda, Md)
J Clin Oncol 10:464–473, 1992   4–102

Introduction.—Administration of high-dose chemotherapy along with autologous hematopoietic stem-cell reinfusion has yielded substantial cure rates in patients with a variety of cancers. If the concurrent use of hematopoietic growth factors and autologous blood progenitor cell support could limit the risk of hemorrhage, those chemotherapeutic agents with myelosuppression as their dose-limiting toxicity would be excellent candidates for repeated administration. The effect of giving GM-CSF, with and without peripheral blood progenitor cells (PBPCs), on the toxicity associated with multiple cycles of high-dose carboplatin was assessed.

Patients and Methods.—The subjects were 18 patients younger than 65 years of age with a variety of incurable solid tumors. They received a total of 40 cycles of carboplatin (1,200 mg/m²), administered by continuous infusion during 96 hours. A daily 4-hour intravenous infusion of recombinant human *Escherichia coli*–derived GM-CSF, 5 or 10 μg/kg/day was given with each course. No PBPCs were given for the first 20 courses (treatment A), which resulted in severe neutropenia and thrombocytopenia. Therefore, the next 20 courses were given with PBPCs and oral antibiotic prophylaxis (treatment B).

Results.—The addition of PBPCs reduced neutropenia from 11 to 8 days, thrombocytopenia from 12 to 5 days, the number of RBC transfusions from 6 to 3, the number of platelet transfusions from 10 to 4, the hospital days from 13 to 3, and the days of intravenous antibiotics from 12 to 2. In addition, treatment B increased weekly carboplatin dose intensity from 206 to 285 mg/m² and the total dose from 2,287 to 3,600 mg/m². The overall response rate was 70%. Of 16 evaluable patients, 8 achieved a partial and 3 a complete remission.

Conclusion.—The GM-CSF and PBPC combination described allows delivery of multiple cycles of high-dose carboplatin chemotherapy. This combination may be a useful model for future trials of high-dose chemotherapy to improve treatment of common solid tumors. Such treatment could improve the results achieved with single courses of dose-intensive therapy, which yield high response rates but only modest improvements in long-term survival and cure rates.

▶ This is an interesting approach to escalating drug therapy using both peripheral stem cells and GM-CSF. Unfortunately, there are no data on whether this approach leads to increased effectiveness of chemotherapy, i.e., increased survival or cure rates. This is a major deficiency in most of the current studies on growth factor action in the cancer setting. This is analogous to studies in the cardiovascular area in which a long time and a lot of money were spent in studying various modes of administration of tissue plasminogen activator on the mistaken assumption that it was, in fact, superior to urokinase rather than continuing direct comparisons of these 2 agents.

It is important to understand that most of the improved parameters presented in these types of studies represent self-fulfilling prophecies of any agent raising white counts irrespective of true patient benefit. Certainly, if hospital stays are adjusted on the actual level of the white count, they will be shortened and, thus, an apparent cost benefit obtained. It is interesting here that pheresis/storage costs equaled approximately 9 days of hospitalization for a patient with febrile neutropenia. Therefore, cost-effectiveness remains in question.—P.J. Quesenberry, M.D.

Progress Report From the International Bone Marrow Transplant Registry
Horowitz MM, for the Advisory Committee of the International Bone Marrow Transplant Registry (Med College of Wisconsin, Milwaukee)
Bone Marrow Transplant 10:113–122, 1992   4–103

Background.—The International Bone Marrow Transplant Registry (IBMTR) receives reports of approximately 200 new cases of bone marrow transplant (BMT) annually from 219 transplant centers worldwide, with about 20 new teams joining each year. The registry now has data on more than 15,000 cases. The current state of BMT is reviewed, the results of recent IBMTR investigations are summarized, and upcoming investigations are described.

Recent studies.—The most recent survey shows a continuing increase in the use of allogeneic BMT, partly resulting from an increase in the use of unrelated donors. A study of alternative related donor transplants found that T-cell depletion increased graft failure and decreased acute

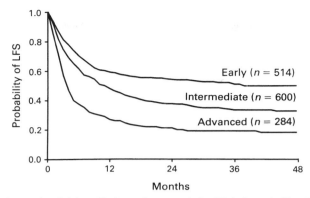

Fig 4–21.—Actuarial probability of leukemia-free survival after HLA-identical sibling BMTs for ALL, 1985-1990. $P < .0001$. (Courtesy of Horowitz MM, for the Advisory Committee of the International Bone Marrow Transplant Registry: *Bone Marrow Transplant* 10:113-122, 1992.)

graft-vs.-host disease (GVHD) but did not improve leukemia-free survival. A study of graft-vs.-leukemia reactions suggested an antileukemia effect, independent of GVHD, that is altered by T-cell depletion. Another study identified acute GVHD as the main risk factor for chronic GVHD; in patients with no or stage I acute GVHD, risk factors were age older than 20 years, use of non–T cell–depleted marrow, and alloimmune female donors for male recipients. A technology assessment study identified 17 controllable treatment variables and their associations with clinical end points; another study found that the risks of mortality and treatment failure were higher in centers doing 5 or less transplants annually. T-cell depletion was found to decrease acute and chronic GVHD but to increase graft failure in HLA-identical BMT for leukemia. The IBMTR also created an empirical data base to study chemotherapy vs.

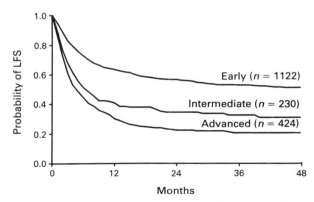

Fig 4–22.—Actuarial probability of leukemia-free survival after HLA-identical sibling BMTs for acute myeloid leukemia, 1985-1990. $P < .0001$. (Courtesy of Horowitz MM, for the Advisory Committee of the International Bone Marrow Transplant Registry: *Bone Marrow Transplant* 10:113-122, 1992.)

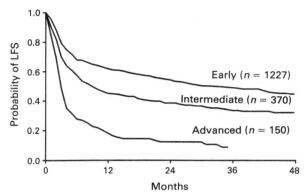

Fig 4–23.—Actuarial probability of leukemia-free survival after HLA-identical sibling BMTs for chronic myelogenous leukemia, 1985-1990. P < .0001. (Courtesy of Horowitz MM, for the Advisory Committee of the International Bone Marrow Transplant Registry: *Bone Marrow Transplant* 10:113-122, 1992.)

BMT in adult acute lymphoblastic leukemia (ALL) and investigated the use of transplantation in patients with severe aplastic anemia.

Current Status.—Current 4-year actuarial probability of leukemia-free survival in recipients of first-remission HLA-identical sibling BMT for ALL is 50% (Fig 4–21); for patients with acute myeloid leukemia, it is 51% (Fig 4–22); and for patients with chronic myelogenous leukemia, it is 45% (Fig 4–23). In all 3 diseases, the disease state at transplant is highly correlated with outcome. The outcome data for patients with severe aplastic anemia suggest that patients younger than 30 years of age do significantly better than older patients (Fig 4–24).

Summary.—The recent research findings of the IBMTR and the current state of BMT for various indications are summarized. It also lists 19

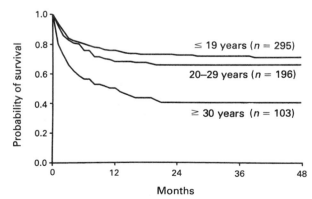

Fig 4–24.—Actuarial probability of survival after HLA-identical sibling BMTs for severe aplastic anemia by age of patient, 1985-1990. P < .0001. (Courtesy of Horowitz MM, for the Advisory Committee of the International Bone Marrow Transplant Registry: *Bone Marrow Transplant* 10:113-122, 1992.)

new studies that are underway. The success of this registry reflects its members' desire to accelerate progress in patient care.

▶ The data from this analysis suggest that allogeneic transplant results in first remission are essentially identical for patients with ALL or acute myeloid leukemia.—P.H. Wiernik, M.D.

Neuropsychologic Impairment in Adult Bone Marrow Transplant Candidates

Andrykowski MA, Schmitt FA, Gregg ME, Brady MJ, Lamb DG, Henslee-Downey PJ (Sanders-Brown Ctr on Aging, Lexington, Ky; Univ of Kentucky, Lexington)
Cancer 70:2288–2297, 1992   4–104

Purpose.—Adults and children undergoing bone marrow transplantation (BMT) reportedly have evidence of long-term cognitive impairment. This is usually attributed to pretransplant conditioning regimens; it is unknown how much of the impairment results from BMT itself. The presence, nature, and factors related to neuropsychological impairment in adult recipients of BMT were evaluated.

Methods.—The patients (mean age, 36 years) were all undergoing medical evaluation for BMT for a malignant condition. The mean time since diagnosis was 25 months, and three fourths of the patients had leukemia. Patients had received a mean of 1.4 courses of cytotoxic therapy, with 39 having chemotherapy alone and the rest having irradiation in addition. A history of CNS disease was present in 16% of patients, all of whom had received treatment for it. Before pre-BMT conditioning, all patients underwent a battery of standardized neuropsychological tests designed to assess a range of abilities and functions, as well as the Brief Profile of Mood States.

Findings.—Eighteen percent of patients were deemed to be neuropsychologically impaired, i.e., they scored in the impaired range on at least one third of the test indexes completed. The neuropsychological performance was significantly associated with a history of cranial irradiation or CNS disease treated with intrathecal chemotherapy. Impairments were more likely to be seen on tests reflecting memory or higher cognitive processing. For individual patients, as the number of disease and treatment risk factors for cognitive impairment increased, so did the risk of impairment.

Conclusion.—Neuropsychological impairment appears to be common among adult patients being evaluated for BMT. The effects of this impairment on the patient's ability to make decisions about undergoing BMT or taking part in research protocols and on the ability to perform self-care behaviors after BMT are unknown. More research is needed on the presence of long-term neuropsychological impairment in adult patients with cancer.

▶ It is amazing that, faced with such a monumental decision, patients do not routinely become insane.—P.H. Wiernik, M.D.

Exercise Assessment of Cardiac Function in Children and Young Adults Before and After Bone Marrow Transplantation
Larsen RL, Barber G, Heise CT, August CS (Children's Hosp, Philadelphia; Univ of Pennsylvania, Philadelphia)
Pediatrics 89:722–729, 1992   4–105

Objective.—Because of the cardiotoxic chemotherapy or irradiation (or both) that they receive, bone marrow recipients run the risk of cardiac toxic effects, which usually occur within a few weeks of transplantation. Cardiac status before transplantation or long afterward has been largely unstudied. Cardiopulmonary exercise testing was performed before and after bone marrow transplantation (BMT) to determine whether such testing could reveal cardiac dysfunction that could not be detected or predicted by echocardiography.

Patients and Methods.—Cycle ergometry, with measurement of oxygen consumption, cardiac output, and ventilatory anaerobic threshold, was performed in 20 young patients preceding BMT and in another 31 young patients after BMT. The mean survival in the latter group was 3.9 years. None of the patients had any symptoms of cardiac dysfunction. The exercise data were compared with those of 70 healthy controls. Patients also underwent echocardiography to assess left ventricular size and shortening fraction at rest.

Findings.—Both before and after BMT, the patients had reduced exercise times, maximal oxygen consumptions, and ventilatory anaerobic thresholds. They also showed severe reductions in cardiac reserve, as reflected by the cardiac output response to exercise. The pretransplant and post-transplant groups showed no significant differences. Cardiac performance was significantly better in patients undergoing transplantation for aplastic anemia, who had less intensive pretransplant therapy. Echocardiographic abnormalities were noted in only 4 patients.

Conclusion.—This study reveals serious limitations in the exercise performance among patients scheduled for BMT, probably as a result of cardiotoxic conventional cancer therapy, as well as in long-term survivors of BMT. Although this study cannot define the effect of BMT itself on cardiac function, it does show that exercise testing is a sensitive technique for assessing patients at risk for cardiac dysfunction from potentially cardiotoxic agents.

Risk Factors for Hepatic Veno-Occlusive Disease After High-Dose Busulfan-Containing Regimens Followed by Autologous Bone Marrow Transplantation: A Study in 136 Children

Méresse V, Hartmann O, Vassal G, Benhamou E, Valteau-Couanet D, Brugieres L, Lemerle J (Institut Gustave-Roussy, Villejuif, France)
Bone Marrow Transplant 10:135–141, 1992   4–106

Background.—Hepatic veno-occlusive disease (HVOD), a toxic side effect of cytoreductive therapy given before bone marrow transplantation (BMT), is associated with a variety of agents, particularly high-dose alkylating agents. The HVOD predisposing risk factors in patients treated with high-dose busulfan (BU), thought to be one of the most hepatotoxic alkylating agents, were analyzed.

Patients and Methods.—A total of 136 autografted children participated. Each had undergone a conditioning regimen of high-dose BU before autologous BMT. All post-BMT hepatic complications were examined and classified as HVOD and non-HVOD, according to McDonald's criteria. Evolutionary variables for HVOD included timing of onset, duration and final outcome, hepatic/renal failure, coagulation changes, bleeding indications, and number of RBC transfusions. Post-transplant HVOD risk factors analyzed were nature of underlying disease; gender; age; number of drugs, courses, and total duration of standard chemotherapy; tumor status at BMT; bone marrow graft ex vivo treatment; number of alkylating agents; dose of BU and its position within the drug combination; and ketoconazole administration.

Results.—Compared with other conditioning regimens, this series had an especially high incidence of HVOD (22%). However, in 26 patients, the outcome was promising (87%). Of 4 deaths (13%), 1 was caused by HVOD. None of the factors examined were predictive of patient outcome, although risk factors for HVOD occurrence were identified. These included total BU in excess of 16 mg/kg, using 3 rather than 2 alkylating agents, BU given first rather than second in conditioning regimens using 3 alkylating agents, and accompanying ketoconazole treatment.

Conclusion.—The study results confirm that BU hepatotoxicity is dose dependent. Further BU monitoring in children may aid in reducing the incidence of HVOD.

Prevention of Hepatic Veno-Occlusive Disease After Bone Marrow Transplantation by Continuous Infusion of Low-Dose Heparin: A Prospective, Rendomized Trial

Attal M, Huguet F, Rubie H, Huynh A, Charlet J-P, Payen J-L, Voigt J-J, Brousset P, Selves J, Muller C, Pris J, Laurent G (Chu Toulose, France)
Blood 79:2834–2840, 1992   4–107

Background.—Veno-occlusive liver disease (VOD), a narrowing or fibrous obliteration of terminal hepatic venules and small lobular veins, is a predominant regimen-related complication after bone marrow transplantation (BMT). The pathogenesis of VOD is thought to be caused by endothelial injury, which leads to coagulation factor deposition within the terminal hepatic venules. The safety and efficacy of VOD prophylaxis with heparin after BMT was assessed.

Patients and Methods.—A prospective randomized study was performed on 161 patients undergoing allogenic (77), autologous (82), or syngeneic (2) BMT. Of these, 81 received continuous prophylactic heparin infusion (100 units/kg/day) beginning 8 days preoperatively and continuing until 30 days after surgery. The remaining 80 patients served as controls. All patients were well matched regarding age, gender, underlying disease, graft type, preoperative routine, pre-BMT hepatitis B and cytomegalovirus serology, and pre-BMT serum glutamate oxaloacetate transaminase and bilirubin values.

Results.—In the heparin group, VOD was noted in only 2 of 81 patients (2.5%), compared with 11 of 80 patients (13.7%) in the control group. After allogenic BMT, VOD did not occur in any of the 39 heparin-group patients. However, 7 of 38 control-group patients did have VOD develop. The prophylactic effect was obtained without added bleeding risk. In fact, the low-dose heparin used in this study did not prolong partial thromboplastin time, and no RBC or platelet increases were required.

Conclusion.—Heparin prophylaxis was effective in VOD prevention after BMT. Therefore, it is recommended that this treatment be included in early mortality prevention programs after BMT.

▶ These are important articles in that 1 clearly identifies those at risk for a potentially fatal complication (Abstract 4–106) and the other (Abstract 4–107) suggests that the complication may be prevented. The high-risk patients identified by Méresse et al. should be prospectively studied with prophylactic heparinization as described by Attal et al.—P.H. Wiernik, M.D.

Host-Specific Interleukin-2–Secreting Donor T-Cell Precursors as Predictors of Acute Graft-Versus-Host Disease in Bone Marrow Transplantation Between HLA-Identical Siblings

Theobald M, Nierle T, Bunjes D, Arnold R, Heimpel H (Univ Hosp Ulm, Germany)
N Engl J Med 327:1613–1617, 1992   4–108

Background.—Acute graft-vs.-host disease (GVHD) remains a major cause of morbidity and mortality in HLA-identical bone marrow transplant recipients, despite advances in immunosuppressive therapy. It has been suggested that lymphokine-secreting donor T cells specific for minor histocompatibility antigens may help to determine which patients will have acute GVHD.

Patients and Methods.—The subjects were 16 consecutive recipients of non–T-cell–depleted bone marrow grafts who survived at least 100 days after transplantation. They and their HLA-identical sibling donors were retrospectively evaluated for the presence of host-specific IL-2–secreting donor T-cell precursors before transplantation. Those findings were correlated with the development of acute GVHD after transplantation.

Findings.—Host-specific T-cell precursors were present in high frequencies—1/100,000 or more—in 8 donors whose siblings later had grade II or III GVHD. The other 8 donors had low frequencies of host-specific T-cell precursors, and their siblings had grade O or I acute GVHD. Four donors had been previously sensitized by pregnancy; in 2 of those cases, high frequencies of host-specific T-cell precursors preceded the development of grade II acute GVHD in their sibling recipients.

Conclusion.—In HLA-identical bone marrow transplantation, there appears to be a significant correlation between a high pretransplant frequency of host-specific IL-2–secreting donor T-cell precursors and the development of severe acute GVHD. Neither the donor T-cell response nor the development of acute GVHD seems to be related to other factors, such as patient age or sex mismatch. This finding may be useful in identifying patients at risk for serious problems with acute GVHD, who may then be assigned to alternative immunosuppressive regimens.

IL-2 Reduces Graft-Versus-Host Disease and Preserves a Graft-Versus-Leukemia Effect by Selectively Inhibiting CD4+ T Cell Activity
Sykes M, Abraham VS, Harty MW, Pearson DA (Harvard Med School, Boston; Natl Cancer Inst, Bethesda, Md)
J Immunol 150:197–205, 1993   4–109

Background.—Severe graft-vs.-host disease (GVHD) remains a major problem in allogeneic marrow transplantation, but its increased occurrence has been offset by lower rates of leukemic relapse, suggesting that a greater graft-vs.-leukemia (GVL) effect might be possible with wider HLA mismatches. In a fully major histocompatibility mismatched murine model of marrow transplantation, administration of a short course of high-dose IL-2 markedly reduced GVHD without compromising engraftment or the GVL effect of allogeneic T cells. Mice have been used to learn the mechanism by which GVHD and GVL are dissociated in this model.

Findings.—Severe GVHD required the presence of CD4+ T cells. When CD4+ T cells were administered without CD8+ cells, IL-2 diminished the degree of GVHD. The GVL effect, in contrast, was mediated by CD8+ T cells only, and this activity was not inhibited by administration of IL-2.

Conclusion.—The dissociation of GVHD and the GVL effect in this murine model can be ascribed to selective inhibition of CD4+ T-cell activity by IL-2. Interleukin-2 may actually augment the GVL effect, and it may help preserve the engraftment-promoting effect of allogeneic T cells.

▶ Two major intergroup studies of IL-2 in acute myeloid leukemia are on the drawing board. One is a study of purged, autologous bone marrow transplantation (ABMT) with or without IL-2 in second complete remission and is based on results reported by Fefer in which ABMT plus IL-2 appeared to be better treatment than ABMT alone with respect to disease-free survival. The other study is for older patients in second complete remission who are not transplant candidates. It will be a randomization between IL-2 and low-dose cytarabine. That study is based on observations from a German study and from Einstein that IL-2 may prolong second complete remission in acute myeloid leukemia. An Eastern Cooperative Oncology Group study recently demonstrated that low-dose cytarabine was significantly better than no postremission treatment for acute myeloid leukemia in second remission.—P.H. Wiernik, M.D.

Thalidomide for the Treatment of Chronic Graft-Versus-Host Disease
Vogelsang GB, Farmer ER, Hess AD, Altamonte V, Beschorner WE, Jabs DA, Corio RL, Levin LS, Colvin OM, Wingard JR, Santos GW (Johns Hopkins Univ, Baltimore, Md)
N Engl J Med 326:1055–1058, 1992   4–110

Introduction.—Allogeneic bone marrow transplantation is used to treat hematologic cancer, aplastic anemia, and inherited immunodeficiencies. The main complication in patients surviving longer than 100 days is chronic graft-vs.-host disease (GVHD).

Patients and Methods.—To determine whether thalidomide is effective against GVHD, 23 patients with chronic GVHD refractory to conventional therapy and 21 with "high-risk" chronic GVHD were studied. Doses of thalidomide were given to produce a plasma level of 5 μg/mL 2 hours after administration. Treatment was continued 3 and 6 months after a complete and partial response, respectively.

Results.—Overall, the actuarial survival rate was 64%. The survival rate was 76% for patients undergoing salvage therapy for refractory GVHD and 48% for those with high-risk GVHD. A complete response was achieved in 14 patients; 12 had a partial response, and 18 had no response. There were only minor side effects, most notably sedation, present in almost all patients.

Conclusion.—Thalidomide appears to be safe and effective for the treatment of chronic GVHD. Research comparing this treatment with prednisone in patients with newly diagnosed chronic GVHD is now needed to establish the relative efficacy of thalidomide.

▶ The activity of thalidomide in this setting is a major observation.—P.H. Wiernik, M.D.

Successful Foscarnet Therapy for Acyclovir-Resistant Mucocutaneous Infection With Herpes Simplex Virus in a Recipient of Allogeneic BMT

Verdonck LF, Cornelissen JJ, Smit J, Lepoutre J, de Gast GC, Dekker AW, Rozenberg-Arska M (Univ Hosp Utrecht, The Netherlands; Natl Inst of Public Health and Environmental Protection, Bilthoven, The Netherlands)
Bone Marrow Transplant 11:177–179, 1993   4–111

Introduction.—Many bone marrow transplant (BMT) recipients have recurrent herpes simplex virus (HSV) infections, which usually are treated by the administration of acyclovir. A patient with severe HSV-1 infection that did not respond to oral or intravenous acyclovir, but cleared up after a 16-day course of foscarnet, was evaluated.

Methods.—The HSV antigens for screening for resistance to acyclovir were tested with enzyme-linked immunosorbent assay in which Vero cell monolayers underwent incubation with several HSV strains in the presence of various levels of either acyclovir or foscarnet.

Case Report.—Man, 41, had an allogeneic BMT to treat chronic myelogenous leukemia, receiving acyclovir prophylaxis. He had severe graft-vs.-host disease develop on day 16 but did not respond to high-dose prednisone or acyclovir. At day 70, foscarnet was given intravenously 3 times a day. After 14 days of foscarnet treatment, the skin lesions healed totally. After resuming acyclovir prophylaxis starting on day 90, the patient relapsed on day 288. Another 14-day course of foscarnet, 200 mg/kg, produced a complete response.

Results.—The in vitro tests showed that the HSV isolate was resistant to acyclovir but was sensitive to the antiviral drug foscarnet. The patient required a second course of foscarnet after another relapse of the acyclovir-resistant HSV infection to fully clear lesions.

Conclusion.—The HSV-1 infections increasingly show acyclovir resistance in immunocompromised patients. If BMT recipients demonstrate recurrent or persistent HSV infections, any viral isolates should undergo testing for susceptibility to various antiviral drugs.

Donor Leucocyte Infusions After Chemotherapy for Patients Relapsing With Acute Leukaemia Following Allogeneic BMT

Szer J, Grigg AP, Phillips GL, Sheridan WP (Alfred Hosp, Prahran, Australia; Royal Melbourne Hosp, Melbourne, Australia; Vancouver Gen Hosp, BC, Canada)

Bone Marrow Transplant 11:109–111, 1993   4–112

Introduction.—Patients with acute myeloid leukemia (AML) readily respond to allogeneic bone marrow transplantation (BMT), which had a lower relapse rate than chemotherapy or autologous or syngeneic BMT. However, patients who relapse soon after the allogeneic BMT have only a small chance of survival because other available therapies are not effective. The effect of donor peripheral blood leukocyte fusion in 4 patients with AML who had relapse after allogeneic BMT were evaluated.

Patients and Methods.—Four patients with AML underwent BMT for an HLA-identical sibling donor, but all relapsed within 6 months of the transplant. Three of 4 received cytosine arabinoside (ara-C) and amsacrine (amsa), whereas the remaining patient underwent chemotherapy for 6 months. All 4 received infusions of leukocytes harvested by repeated leukapheresis from the initial bone marrow donor.

Results.—Two patients did not achieve complete remission after ara-C and amsa treatment, and both died of progressive leukemia. Three patients had graft-vs.-host disease (GVHD) develop and needed immunosuppressive therapy. One patient had a complete remission 4 weeks after chemotherapy and appeared well more than 400 days later. This individual had biopsy-demonstrated grade III GVHD that responded to various pharmacotherapies. She continues to require constant corticosteroid treatment.

Conclusion.—Salvage chemotherapy followed by the infusion of leukocytes from the original donor may benefit some patients who have an AML relapse soon after allogeneic BMT. This treatment method appears to help individuals with a minimal leukemic burden from the chemotherapy, while being immunosuppressive enough to promote donor cell engraftment.

▶ Those of us who were heavily involved in granulocyte transfusions had the clear impression that such transfusions were associated with improved remission induction rates and remission duration. Unfortunately, such data have never been published to my knowledge.—P.H. Wiernik, M.D.

Additional Reading

HODGKIN'S DISEASE

Boivin JF, Hutchinson GB, Lubin JH, et al: Coronary artery disease mortality in patients treated for Hodgkin's disease. *Cancer* 69:1241–1247, 1992.

Dürkop H, Latza U, Hummel M, et al: Molecular cloning and expression of a new member of the nerve growth factor receptor family that is characteristic for Hodgkin's disease. *Cell* 68:421–427, 1992.

Gospodarowicz MK, Sutcliffe SB, Clark RM, et al: Analysis of supradiaphragmatic clinical stage I and II Hodgkin's disease treated with radiation alone. *Int J Radiat Oncol Biol Phys* 22:859–865, 1992.

Gruss HJ, Brach MA, Drexler HG, et al: Expression of cytokine genes, cytokine receptor genes, and transcription factors in cultured Hodgkin and Reed-Sternberg cells. *Cancer Res* 52:3353–3360, 1992.

Hessol NA, Katz MH, Liu YJ, et al: Increased incidence of Hodgkin disease in homosexual men with HIV infection. *Ann Intern Med* 117:309–311, 1992.

Janov AJ, Anderson J, Cella DF, et al: Pregnancy outcome in survivors of advanced Hodgkin disease. *Cancer* 70:688–692, 1992.

Longo DL, Duffey PL, Young RC, et al: Conventional-dose salvage combination chemotherapy in patients relapsing with Hodgkin's disease after combination chemotherapy: the low probability for cure. *J Clin Oncol* 10:210–218, 1992.

Muller CP, Trilling B, Steinke B: The prognostic significance of total serum cholesterol in patients with Hodgkin's disease. *Cancer* 69:1042–1046, 1992.

O'Brien MER, Pinkerton CR, Kingston J, et al: "VEEP" in children with Hodgkin's disease—a regimen to decrease late sequelae. *Br J Cancer* 65:756–760, 1992.

Shimoda K, Okamura S, Harada N, et al: Granulocyte colony-stimulating factor receptors on human acute leukemia: biphenotypic leukemic cells possess granulocyte colony-stimulating factor receptors. *Cancer Res* 52:3052–3055, 1992.

Uckun FM, Mitchell JB, Obuz V, et al: Radiation and heat sensitivity of human t-lineage acute lymphoblastic leukemia (ALL) and acute myeloblastic leukemia (AML) clones displaying multiple drug resistance (MDR). *Int J Radiat Oncol Biol Phys* 23:115–125, 1992.

Yahalom J, Ryu J, Straus DJ, et al: Impact of adjuvant radiation on the patterns and rate of relapse in advanced-stage Hodgkin's disease treated with alternating chemotherapy combinations. *J Clin Oncol* 9:2193–2201, 1991.

Young JW, Papadopoulos EB, Cunningham I, et al: T-cell–depleted allogenic bone marrow transplantation in adults with acute nonlymphocytic leukemia in first remission. *Blood* 79:3390–3387, 1992.

MARROW TRANSPLANTATION

Biggs JC, Horowitz MM, Gale RP, et al: Bone marrow transplants may cure patients with acute leukemia never achieving remission with chemotherapy. *Blood* 80:1090–1093, 1992.

Fried RH, Murakami CS, Fisher LD, et al: Ursodeoxycholic acid treatment of refractory chronic graft-versus-host disease of the liver. *Ann Intern Med* 116:624–629, 1992.

Jenkins RB, Le Beau MM, Kraker WJ, et al: Fluorescence in situ hybridization: a sensitive method for trisomy 8 detection in bone marrow specimens. *Blood* 79:3307–3315, 1992.

Johnson BD, Truitt RL: A decrease in graft-vs.-host disease without loss of graft-vs.-leukemia reactivity after MHC-matched bone marrow transplantation by selective depletion of donor NK cells by in vivo. *Transplantation* 54:104–112, 1992.

Nemunaitis J, Anasetti C, Storb R, et al: Phase II trial of recombinant human granulocyte-macrophage colony-stimulating factor in patients undergoing allogenic bone marrow transplantation from unrelated donors. *Blood* 79:2572–2577, 1992.

MISCELLANEOUS

Baker DK, Relling MV, Pui Ch, et al: Increased teniposide clearance with concomitant anticonvulsant therapy. *J Clin Oncol* 10:311–315, 1992.
Giralt M, Rubio D, Cortés MT, et al: Alpha interferon in the management of essential thrombocythemia. *Eur J Cancer* 27:72S–74S, 1991.

NON-HODGKIN'S LYMPHOMA

Gordon LI, Harrington D, Andersen J, et al: Comparison of a second-generation combination chemotherapeutic regimen (m-BACOD) with a standard regimen (CHOP) for advanced diffuse non-Hodgkin's lymphoma. *N Engl J Med* 327:1342–1349, 1992.
Ladanyi M, Offit K, Parsa NZ, et al: Follicular lymphoma with t(8;14) (q24;q32): a distinct clinical and molecular subset of t(8;14)-bearing lymphomas. *Blood* 79:2124–2130, 1992.
Price CGA, Rohatiner AZS, Steward W, et al: Interferon alfa-2b in addition to chlorambucil in the treatment of follicular lymphoma: preliminary results of a randomized trial in progress. *Eur J Cancer* 27:34S–36S, 1991.

MULTIPLE MYELOMA

Björkholm M: Melphalan/prednisone versus melphalan/prednisone plus human alpha interferon therapy in patients with multiple myeloma, stages II and III. *Eur J Cancer* 27:51S–52S, 1991.
Paglieroni T, Caggiano V, MacKenzie M: Abnormalities in immune regulation precede the development of multiple myeloma. *Am J Hematol* 40:51–55, 1992.

CHRONIC LEUKEMIAS

Anastasi J, Le Beau MM, Vardiman JW, et al: Detection of trisomy 12 in chronic lymphocytic leukemia by fluorescence in situ hybridization to interphase cells: a simple and sensitive method. *Blood* 79:1796–1801, 1992.
Estey EH, Kurzrock R, Kantarjian HM, et al: Treatment of hairy cell leukemia with 2-chlorodeoxyadenosine (2-CdA). *Blood* 79:882–887, 1992.
Felicetto F, Rametta V, Mele G, et al: Recombinant interferon-α2A as maintenance treatment for patients with advanced stage chronic lymphocytic leukemia responding to chemotherapy. *Am J Hematol* 41:45–49, 1992.
Gandhi V, Kemena A, Keating MJ, et al: Fludarabine infusion potentiates arabinosylcytosine metabolism in lymphocytes of patients with chronic lymphocytic leukemia. *Cancer Res* 52:897–903, 1992.
Gratwohl A, Herman J, Biezen A, et al: No advantage for patients who receive splenic irradiation before bone marrow transplantation for chronic myeloid leukaemia: results of a prospective randomized study. *Bone Marrow Transplant* 10:147–152, 1992.
Herrmann F, Helfrich SG, Linderman A, et al: Elevated circulating levels of tumor necrosis factor predict unresponsiveness to treatment with interferon alfa-2b in chronic myelogenous leukemia. *J Clin Oncol* 10:631–634, 1992.
Juliusson G, Liliemark J: Rapid recovery from cytopenia in hairy cell leukemia after treatment with 2-chloro-2′-deoxyadenosine (CdA): relation to opportunistic infections. *Blood* 79:888–894, 1992.

Lee MS, Kantarjian H, Talpaz M, et al: Detection of minimal residual disease by polymerase chain reaction in Philadelphia chromosome–positive chronic myelogenous leukemia following interferon therapy. *Blood* 79:1920–1923, 1992.

Thompson JD, Brodsky I, Yunis J: Molecular quantification of residual disease in chronic myelogenous leukemia after bone marrow transplantation. *Blood* 79:1629–1635, 1992.

MYELODYSPLASIA

Andreeff M, Stone R, Michaeli J, et al: Hexamethylene bisacetamide in myelodysplastic syndrome and acute myelogenous leukemia: a phase II clinical trial with a differentiation-inducing agent. *Blood* 80:2604–2609, 1992.

Maschek H, Georgii A, Kaloutsi V, et al: Myelofibrosis in primary myelodysplastic syndromes: a retrospective study of 352 patients. *Eur J Haematol* 48:208–214, 1992.

Park CH, Kimler BF, Bodensteiner D, et al: In vitro growth modulation by L-ascorbic acid of colony-forming cells from bone marrow of patients with myelodysplastic syndromes. *Cancer Res* 52:4458–4466, 1992.

ACUTE LEUKEMIAS

Barrett AJ, Horowitz MM, Ash RC, et al: Bone marrow transplantation for Philadelphia chromosome–positive acute lymphoblastic leukemia. *Blood* 79:3067–3070, 1992.

Behm FG, Raimondi SC, Schell MJ, et al: Lack of CD45 antigen on blast cells in childhood acute lymphoblastic leukemia is associated with chromosomal hyperdiploidy and other favorable prognostic features. *Blood* 79:1011–1016, 1992.

Broudy VC, Smith FO, Lin N, et al: Blast from patients with acute myelogenous leukemia express functional receptors for stem cell factor. *Blood* 80:60–67, 1992.

Cornic M, Delva L, Guidez F, et al: Induction of retinoic acid–binding protein in normal and malignant human myeloid cells by retinoic acid in acute promyelocytic leukemia patients. *Cancer Res* 52:3329–3334, 1992.

Cuneo A, Michaux JL, Ferrant A, et al: Correlation of cytogenetic pattern and clinicobiological features in adult acute myeloid leukemia expressing lymphoid markers. *Blood* 79:720–727, 1992.

Curtis RE, Boice JD, Stovall M, et al: Risk of leukemia after chemotherapy and radiation treatment for breast cancer. *N Engl J Med* 326:1745–1751, 1992.

Diverio D, Lo Coco F, D'Adamo F, et al: Identification of DNA rearrangements at the retinoic acid receptor-α (RAR-α) locus in all patients with acute promyelocytic leukemia (APL) and mapping of APL breakpoints within the RAR-α second intron. *Blood* 79:3331–3336, 1992.

Elliot S, Taylor K, White S, et al: Proof of differentiative mode of action of all-*trans* retinoic acid in acute promyelocytic leukemia using x-linked clonal analysis. *Blood* 79:1916–1919, 1992.

Gerard EL, Ferry JA, Amrein PC, et al: Compositional changes in vertebral bone marrow during treatment for acute leukemia: assessment with quantitative chemical shift imaging. *Radiology* 183:39–46, 1992.

Koike T, Tatewaki W, Aoki A, et al: Brief report: severe symptoms of hyperhistaminemia after the treatment of acute promyelocytic leukemia with tretinoin (all-*trans*-retinoic acid). *N Engl J Med* 327:385–387, 1992.

Kreissman SG, Gelber RD, Cohen HJ, et al: Incidence of secondary acute myelogenous leukemia after treatment of childhood acute lymphoblastic leukemia. *Cancer* 70:2208–2213, 1992.

Lotz M, Moats T, Villiger PM: Leukemia inhibitory factor is expressed in cartilage and synovium and can contribute to the pathogenesis of arthritis. *J Clin Invest* 90:888–896, 1992.

Michieli M, Damiani D, Geromin A, et al: Overexpression of multidrug resistance-associated p170-glycoprotein in acute non-lymphocytic leukemia. *Eur J Haematol* 48:87–92, 1992.

Moskowitz C, Dutcher JP, Wiernik PH: Association of thyroid disease with acute leukemia. *Am J Hematol* 39:102–107, 1992.

Pui CH, Carroll AJ, Raimondi SC, et al: Isochromosomes in childhood acute lymphoblastic leukemia: a collaborative study of 83 cases. *Blood* 79:2384–2391, 1992.

Shaffer DW, Burris HA, O'Rourke TJ: Testicular relapse in adult acute myelogenous leukemia. *Cancer* 70:1541–1544, 1992.

Wagner JE, Broxmeyer HE, Byrd RL, et al: Transplantation of umbilical cord blood after myeloablative therapy: analysis of engraftment. *Blood* 79:1874–1881, 1992.

Zahm SH, Weisenburger DD, Babbitt PA, et al: Use of hair coloring products and the risk of lymphoma, multiple myeloma, and chronic lymphocytic leukemia. *Am J Public Health* 82:990–998, 1992.

5 Transfusion Medicine

Introduction

One of my strongest motivations for editing a section for the YEAR BOOK OF HEMATOLOGY is the rigorous process forced on me, whereby I must inspect all of the transfusion literature for the year and select the highlights for your review. Each Section Editor is committed to select a target number of articles in a given year, with the selections made in increments as the literature appears. It has always been my purpose to select those articles of potential interest to the clinical hematologist, but the Editor's target has been a stretch in some years, if only articles of clinical relevance are featured. When I began to review the entirety of this year's selections, however, the wealth of clinically relevant articles or papers from the basic sciences, with important implications for patient care issues, was very impressive. If the transfusion literature continues to expand, I may need to request a larger allowance from the Editor in coming years.

In keeping with my practice of previous years, I have divided the "Transfusion Medicine" chapter into a number of distinct sections. In recognition of the growing number of excellent articles discussing autologous transfusion, I have given that topic its own section. Perhaps some of our surgical colleagues might pick up this volume while meandering through the bookstore and find this additional emphasis sufficiently stimulating to learn some transfusion medicine and hematology.

In the "Blood Component Collection and Preparation" section, I have selected an intriguing article about platelet storage and transfusion reactions (Abstracts 5–1) that may occur by a previously undescribed molecular mechanism. The potential problems with leukocyte depletion on bacterial contamination of stored red cells are highlighted with emphasis on *Yersinia enterocolitica* (Abstract 5–2). Another microbe, *Helicobacter pylori*, is presented (Abstract 5–3) because of its implications for peptic ulcer disease and the ancient medical lore about ABO types and gastric diseases. Two other articles relevant to leukocyte depletion issues (Abstracts 5–4 and 5–5) discuss animal models for platelet refractoriness and measurement of circulating white cells after transfusions. The implications of methods of virologic donor screening for HIV (Abstract 5–6), hepatitis C virus (Abstract 5–7), and cytomegalovirus (Abstract 5–8) complete this growing section; I made a conscious decision to include them in the donor-screening section rather than the section on "Adverse Effects" to reassure the reader of the proactive intent of blood centers to implement new technologies to make transfusions safer.

The "Red Blood Cell Immunology" section presents the latest in the evolution of our understanding of the molecular basis for Rh blood group polymorphisms (Abstract 5-9). A reassuring article (Abstract 5-10) about the safety of transfusions for the majority of patients with warm autoimmune hemolytic anemia comes next; most medically indicated transfusions are not hindered by the positive direct antiglobulin test. Two articles expand our knowledge of characteristics of alloimmune hemolysis (Abstracts 5-11 and 5-12), a particular interest of mine. A final citation describing the development of an alloantibody in a transfused infant (Abstract 5-13) may provoke some reconsideration of our current pretransfusion testing protocols.

The section on "Platelet Immunology and Transfusion" features the potential clinical use of GP-140 (Abstract 5-14), a factor studied by platelet molecular biologists, to assess the adequacy of platelet storage. The mysteries of platelet alloimmunization and the study of practical methods to deal with this vexing problem are prominently featured with 2 articles (Abstracts 5-15 and 5-16).

The articles in the "Autologous Transfusion" section hopefully will balance the advocacy of the strong proponents of maximizing autologous blood use and the critics who are beginning to question the cost-benefit ratio of some of our practices. Rather than relying on opinions and anecdotes, both sides of these arguments are producing data from which to defend their practices. Autologous practices are being extended to hemodilution and intraoperative blood salvage with several articles (Abstracts 5-20 through 5-23) featuring these perioperative techniques.

Quantitative data bases to analyze transfusion practices are presented in "Adult Transfusion Practices." Several articles (Abstracts 5-25, 5-26, and 5-27) examining in vitro parameters of oxygen delivery describe innovations to transfusion that could make our behavior more rational. Another article by Dr. Mohr and his colleagues from Israel (Abstract 5-28) has me convinced that our standard notions about platelet preparation in the blood center and transfusion practices on the ward may be erroneous. Hemoglobin-based blood substitutes, a topic of broad interest to patients and their stockbrokers, are also presented with clinical and developmental viewpoints (Abstracts 5-30 and 5-31). Finally, 2 excellent studies (Abstracts 5-32 and 5-33) suggest the limitations of plasma exchange and the potential benefits of other therapies such as intravenous gamma-globulin to avoid the invasive nature of plasma exchange.

An article on obstetric blood transfusion (Abstract 5-35) is included in the "Pediatric Transfusion Practice" section; one never knows whether to classify obstetric cases as adult or pediatric. An interesting article about Glanzmann's thrombasthenia and the implications of this qualitative platelet disorder on perinatal practice may have missed your attention previously (Abstract 5–36). The measurement and prevalence of inhibitors for patients with hemophilia has become a hot topic in view of the introduction of recombinant factor concentrates and the reports of higher rates of inhibitor detection. Although the final article in this section (Abstract 5–38) discusses autologous transfusions, it appears in the pediatric section to direct the attention of specialists in pediatric hematology.

The "Transplantation" section is short on quantity but not on quality. Donor-specific transfusions are addressed (Abstract 5–39) with a simplified protocol. The topic of ABO-unmatched liver transplantation caused by the production of isohemagglutinins from passenger lymphocytes is presented (Abstract 5–40); patients with the acute onset of serious hemolysis after transplants are often mistakenly considered to have idiopathic warm autoimmune hemolytic anemia even by experienced hematologists.

The chapter ends with the section on the "Adverse Effects of Transfusion." A number of studies describing the evolution of the AIDS epidemic in hemophilia are featured. A provocative article (Abstract 5–42) on reactivation of viruses by leukocytes contaminating blood components may lead eventually to widespread leukocyte depletion of all blood components. Articles quantitating the risks of hepatitis C (Abstract 5–44), HIV (Abstract 5–41), and HTLV (Abstract 5–43) from a multicenter prospective evaluation are cited. An article (Abstract 5–45) suggesting that hepatitis C may not shorten the life span of infected transfusion recipients sheds a different light on the hepatitis C story. Three articles on transfusion graft-vs.-host disease (Abstracts 5–47 through 5–49) are presented in view of heightened interest in this topic and its applicability to clinical hematologists who must decide which of their patients should receive irradiated blood components. The section closes with a series of articles (Abstracts 5–51 through 5–55) on transfusion immunomodulation. This year's representative selections are more rigorous in their methodology and more persuasive that these phenomena may be real, and they begin to lay a foundation of transfusion practices to avoid their occurrence.

Because transfusion medicine is a multifaceted discipline with many overlaps in other areas of clinical hematology, the reader is advised to scan the other excellent chapters in this book for a comprehensive picture of transfusion medicine and its multiple connections in hematology.

Paul M. Ness, M.D.

Blood Component Collection and Preparation

Stored Blood Components Contain Agents That Prime the Neutrophil NADPH Oxidase Through the Platelet-Activating-Factor Receptor

Silliman CC, Thurman GW, Ambruso DR (Univ of Colorado, Denver; Belle Bonfils Mem Blood Ctr, Denver)
Vox Sang 63:133–136, 1992   5-1

Background.—The production of toxic oxygen metabolites is initiated by polymorphonuclear neutrophils (PMNs) via reduced nicotinamide adenine dinucleotide phosphate (NADPH) oxidase stimulation. This results in the reduction of oxygen to a superoxide anion, known as the respiratory burst. Several agents can prime PMN NADPH oxidase activity, which can subsequently create adverse effects in patients with traumatic and thermal injuries. Experiments performed on stored blood components to determine whether they contain PMN-priming factors that could result in harmful hemotherapy complications were detailed.

Methods.—Three units each of outdated whole blood, packed RBCs separated from whole blood, and platelet concentrates were obtained. Fresh plasma isolated from platelets within 30 minutes of collection, outdated fresh frozen plasma stored for 1 year, and citrate-phosphate-dextrose-adenine-1 (CPDA-1) preservative served as controls. The neutrophils were isolated and incubated in 40 µM of either WEB 2170 (a specific platelet-activating factor [PAF] receptor antagonist) or a buffer control for 5 minues at 37°C. Isolated plasma from whole blood, packed RBCs, platelet concentrates, fresh frozen plasma, and fresh plasma, with CPDA-1 and buffer acting as controls, was added to the incubation solution. The PMNs were incubated for 10 minutes at 37°C. The same sequence was used in separate experiments, but 2 µM of PAF was used in the priming incubation, rather than plasma. Formyl-Met-Leu-Phe (fMLP) was then added to each well to initiate the respiratory burst. Assays were repeated on 3 different occasions for each component.

Results.—Outdated whole blood, packed RBCs, and platelet concentrates contained a priming agent that augmented the PMN NADPH oxidase activity in response to fMLP by 2.1 to 2.8 times. The WEB 2170 virtually inhibited this priming activity entirely. No priming activity was noted in frozen plasma or fresh frozen plasma. Neutrophils incubated with 2 µM of PAF increased the PMN oxidase activity by 5 to 6 times in response to 1 µM of fMLP. When pretreated with WEB 2170, this activity was inhibited by nearly 80%.

Conclusion.—Outdated whole blood, packed RBCs, and platelet concentrates are capable of priming the PMN NADPH oxidase, with PAF or PAF-like compounds serving as the probable agonists.

▶ A biological activity in stored blood components that resembles PAF was described. This factor appears in stored cellular blood components and may cause transfusion reactions in some recipients, most likely by priming the action of granulocytes. Further investigations were presented by this group at the 1992 American Society of Hematology meetings, suggesting that complete reports on this evolving story will be available soon.—P.M. Ness, M.D.

Prevention of *Yersinia enterocolitica* Growth in Red-Blood-Cell Concentrates

Pietersz RNI, Reesink HW, Pauw W, Dekker WJA, Buisman L (Red Cross Blood Bank, Amsterdam; Slotervaart Hosp, Amsterdam)

Lancet 340:755–756, 1992   5–2

Objective. —The risk of *Yersinia enterocolitica* contamination of blood products is a concern. Although many methods can be used to prevent contamination and delay growth of bacteria in blood products, little use has been made of the bactericidal activity of donor blood. The effects of holding whole blood at 22°C for 20 hours and then removing leukocytes on *Y. enterocolitica* growth were assessed.

Methods. —Thirty pools of 3 bags of blood were inoculated with 2×10^1 to 3×10^4 CFUs/ml of *Y. enterocolitica*. In each pool, 1 bag was stored for 6 hours at 4°C before processing to RBC concentrate; the other 2 bags were held at 22°C for 20 hours before being processed to buffy-coat-depleted RBC (BCd-RBC). Filtration leukocyte depletion (Ld-RBC) was then performed on 1 of these bags. The bags were stored at 4°C for 5 weeks, during which samples were taken for culture.

Results. —At all time points, removal of *Y. enterocolitica* was better in Ld-RBC than in BCd-RBC or RBC. Growth was seen after the shortest storage times in RBC bags, followed by BCd-RBC and then Ld-RBC bags.

Conclusion. —Whole blood should be held at 22°C overnight before processing to allow leukocytes to carry out phagocytosis and killing, after which leukocytes should be removed by filtration. Giving leukocyte-depleted blood products will also reduce HLA immunization and prevent cytomegalovirus and HTLV transmission.

▶ A number of isolated cases of transfusion-related sepsis have been attributed to the organism *Y. enterocolitica*. The clinical picture is usually septic shock with early death of the recipient. Because the organism grows preferentially in the cold and can metabolize citrate, refrigeration of blood components favors its growth. Most infected donor units come from donors with transient bacteremia associated with asymptomatic gastrointestinal disease. A number of approaches have been suggested to eliminate this problem, including shortening the storage period for red cell components, which was not recommended by the Food and Drug Administration in view of the rarity of these occurrences. Current discussions of using more leukocyte-depleted blood components have raised other questions about whether early leukocyte depletion by filters could remove white cells that protect the unit from growth of these organisms. Although data vary, this report favors a prolonged storage period before leukocyte depletion to maximize the efficiency of donor white cells. Other reports suggest that delayed leukocyte depletion may lead to fragmentation of the white cells and make some leukocyte-depleted components less likely to reduce antigen sensitization. A series of articles and an accompanying editorial in the September 1992 issue of *Transfusion* discussed these issues and suggested that a prolonged waiting period may not be necessary. The reader can expect a continuing series of technologic and clinical reports as well as advertising promotions in this evolving area of prestorage leukocyte depletion and its risks and benefits.—P.M. Ness, M.D.

Influence of Age and *Helicobacter pylori* Infection on Serum Pepsinogens in Healthy Blood Transfusion Donors
Veenendaal RA, Biemond I, Peña AS, van Duijn W, Kreuning J, Lamers CBHW (Leiden Univ Hosp, The Netherlands)
Gut 33:452–455, 1992   5–3

Background.—Pepsinogen A and pepsinogen C increase with aging in healthy individuals. These pepsinogens are increased in chronic superficial gastritis caused by *Helicobacter pylori* infection. Whether *H. pylori* is responsible for the age-related increase of pepsinogens A and C was investigated.

Methods and Findings.—Serum samples were obtained from 122 male and 69 female blood donors for examination. The subjects' maximum age was 59 years. Serum pepsinogen A and C concentrations were significantly higher in *H. pylori*–positive donors than in *H. pylori*–negative donors. The serum pepsinogen A:C ratio was significantly reduced because of a relatively greater increase in serum pepsinogen C in *H. pylori*-positive donors. In an analysis of variance, pepsinogen A and C levels differed significantly among different age groups when all donors and *H. pylori*–positive donors were considered. The mean pepsinogen levels were highest in the oldest subjects. However, in *H. pylori*–negative donors, there was no such age-related difference in pepsinogen A and C. In positive donors, there was a weak positive, significant correlation between pepsinogen A and C and age. No such correlation was observed in the *H. pylori*–negative donors.

Conclusion.—The age-related elevation in serum pepsinogens A and C found in healthy populations appears to be caused by an increasing prevalence of *H. pylori* infection. Therefore, serum pepsinogen A and C levels in patients should be related to the presence or absence of such infection.

▶ This article demonstrates that serum pepsinogens are increased in blood donors with previous *H. pylori* infection regardless of their increasing age. It would be of interest to know if a history of infection with this organism can also explain previous reports of increased incidence of ulcer in group O individuals and gastric carcinoma in group A individuals. My limited review of this topic suggests that there is no explanation to be afforded on the question of ABO blood group and disease associations by the developing information on this organism and its relationship to peptic ulcer disease.—P.M. Ness, M.D.

An Animal Model of Allogeneic Donor Platelet Refractoriness: The Effect of the Time of Leukodepletion
Blajchman MA, Bardossy L, Carmen RA, Goldman M, Heddle NM, Singal DP (McMaster Univ, Hamilton, Ont, Canada; Canadian Red Cross Society Blood Transfusion Service, Hamilton, Ont; Cutter Biological, Berkeley, Calif)
Blood 79:1371–1375, 1992   5–4

Background.—About half of the persons receiving multiple transfusions become refractory to random donor platelets. Patients receiving leukocyte-depleted blood products may be less likely to become refractory to random donor platelets than recipients of non–leukocyte-depleted products. Leukocyte depletion can be done just after a unit of whole blood is collected and before its storage or just before the transfusion of a blood product to a recipient, after storage. The best time for leukocyte depletion has not been determined.

Methods.—An animal model of allogeneic platelet refractoriness was developed, and the effects of prestorage and poststorage leukocyte depletion on the frequency of refractoriness to allogeneic donor platelets were compared. Two strains of rabbits were used. California Black rabbits served as blood donors, and New Zealand White rabbits served as recipients.

Results.—After 8 weekly infusions of non–leukocyte-depleted allogeneic fresh blood, the allogeneic platelet refractory rate was 91.2%. Prestorage leukocyte depletion of donor blood was associated with an allogeneic platelet survival rate significantly higher than that of poststorage leukocyte depletion. The refractory rate to allogeneic platelets after prestorage leukocyte depletion was 33.3%, significantly lower than the 66.7% rate after poststorage leukocyte depletion. Cell-free plasma products appeared to be capable of inducing refractoriness to allogeneic donor platelets. The stored plasma had a greater likelihood of inducing such refractoriness than fresh plasma did.

Conclusion.—Prestorage leukocyte depletion of allogeneic donor blood may be associated with a lower frequency of refractoriness and better allogeneic platelet survival than poststorage leukocyte depletion. However, as this study involved an animal model, further research is needed to determine whether prestorage leukocyte depletion is superior to poststorage leukocyte depletion in humans also.

▶ A number of clinical investigations suggest that prestorage leukocyte depletion may delay or prevent sensitization of platelet transfusion recipients to HLA antigens. Because most transfusion recipients are clinically complex and clear-cut prospective studies of transfusion effects are difficult to perform in such patients with hematologic malignancies, these studies with a rabbit model were undertaken. These studies were also able to investigate the timing of the leukocyte depletion and provide some initial information that prestorage leukocyte depletion may be better than poststorage leukocyte depletion in preventing subsequent alloimmunization. Of particular interest was the use of plasma from which white cells had been removed, which suggests that residual white cell fragments from cells that disintegrate on storage can also promote alloimmunization as opposed to plasma from rapidly leukocyte-depleted blood.—P.M. Ness, M.D.

Detection of Circulating Donor White Blood Cells in Patients Receiving Multiple Transfusions
Adams PT, Davenport RD, Reardon DA, Roth MS (Univ of Michigan, Ann Arbor)
Blood 80:551–555, 1992   5-5

Objective.—Many of the morbidities arising from routine administration of blood products are thought to result from incidental transfusion of "donor" lymphocytes. There are few data on the ability of these incidentally transfused WBCs to survive in the circulation of immunocompetent hosts. A new Y chromosome–specific PCR was used to detect circulating transfused male WBCs after transfusion into female patients.

Methods.—The study sample comprised 20 female patients who were undergoing open heart surgery or liver transplantation. They received an average of 9 units of packed RBCs, 5 of them from male donors, and 12 units of platelets, 6 of them from male donors. The DNA was extracted from the patients' whole blood or peripheral blood buffy coats after transfusion. The PCR was done using oligonucleotides designed to amplify a segment within the repetitive Y chromosome DYZ1 locus.

Findings.—For an average of 2 days after transplantation, 15 of the recipients showed PCR evidence of circulating male WBCs. These patients were more likely than those without evidence of circulating WBCs to have received larger quantities of platelets and of male platelets.

Conclusion.—Using DYZ1 PCR analysis, small numbers of circulating male WBCs in female patients have been found. In most women receiving multiple transfusions, the circulating donor WBCs persisted for a mean of 2 days. By detecting persisting or proliferating WBCs, this PCR technique may add to our understanding of common transfusion-related morbidities.

▶ A number of adverse effects of transfusion have been blamed on the persistent circulation of donor white cells; these reactions include alloimmunization, immunomodulation, graft-vs.-host disease, and viral transmission. This article described a method by which white cells from male donors can be detected in the circulation of transfused females with the use of a PCR-based technique. The method may help to explain the role of these white cells in instigating these adverse reactions and to develop methods to suppress them.—P.M. Ness, M.D.

Risk of HIV Infection From Transfusion With Blood Negative for HIV Antibody in a West African City
Savarit D, De Cock KM, Schutz R, Konate S, Lackritz E, Bondurand A (Ctr Natl de Transfusion Sanguine, Abidjan, Côte d'Ivoire; Ctrs for Disease Control, Atlanta, Ga)
BMJ 305:498–501, 1992   5–6

Background.—The HIV-1 and -2 infection risks from screened blood unit transfusions in a high-prevalance West African area were estimated.

Methods.—A total of 10,907 units of blood were collected and measured. Of these, 5,076 units were from first-time donors (46.5%), and 5,831 were from repeat donors (53.5%). All blood was screened with HIV-1 and -2 whole virus enzyme-linked immunosorbent assay (ELISA), and blood that was reactive at the first screening test was discarded. Repeat donors who seroconverted were identified, and HIV infection incidence in first and repeat donors was estimated. False-negative results were determined using an assumed test sensitivity level of 99%.

Results.—Prevalence of HIV was 11% overall in first-time donors and 2.1% in repeat donors. Further testing was undertaken on 476 (69.9%) of the 681 specimens with positive ELISA results: all were reactive (73.1% to HIV, 14.7% to HIV-2, and 12.2% to both). A total of 29 HIV antibody-positive donors were identified; each had given earlier seronegative blood units. Of these, 27 had HIV-1, 1 had HIV-2 and 1 had both. In 26 of the seroconverters, the assumed seroconversion date was within 8 weeks of the seronegative donation. Therefore, the minimum rate of potentially HIV-infected blood taken from repeat donors was 26 in 5,831 (4.5 in 1,000). In repeat donors, the estimated infection incidence was 1.2% to 2.5%. Estimated false-negative units in first-time donors was 1.1 in 1,000 and .2 in 1,000 from repeat donors, because of laboratory insensitivity. The rate of potentially infected units from first-time and repeat donors, seroconversions, and errors was approximated at 5.4 to 10.6 in 1,000.

Conclusion.—In areas of increased HIV prevalence, the risk of contracting HIV from a single unit of blood is considerable. To reduce this risk, donors with a low incidence of HIV infection should be selected. Additionally, transfusions should be avoided in all but those who positively require them.

▶ Although American blood banks, physicians, and their patients have had to deal with a multitude of problems resulting from the effects of the AIDS epidemic on transfusion therapy, the American battle with this disease is puny compared with the enormous problems encountered in the Third World as described in this article from Africa. This article should make interesting reading for physicians dealing with the AIDS problem in more developed countries. Careful epidemiologic investigations of the African situation or similar high-risk areas in Asia, such as Thailand, can also provide valuable insights into the problems of donor screening and an invaluable resource of blood samples that may be infectious but are in the window period before detectable seroconversion.—P.M. Ness, M.D.

Increased Detection of Hepatitis C Virus (HCV)-Infected Blood Donors by a Multiple-Antigen HCV Enzyme Immunoassay
Kleinman S, Alter H, Busch M, Holland P, Tegtmeier G, Nelles M, Lee S, Page E, Wilber J, Polito A (American Red Cross Blood Services, Los Angeles; NIH, Bethesda, Md; Irwin Mem Blood Ctrs, San Francisco; et al)
Transfusion 32:805–813, 1992   5–7

Introduction.—First-generation enzyme immunoassays (EIAs-1) for anti–hepatis C virus (HCV) are effective but not optimally sensitive. De-

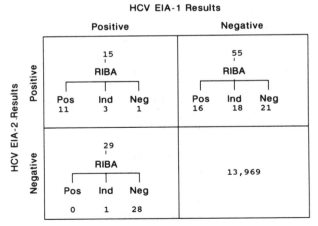

Fig 5–1.—*Abbreviations: Pos,* positive; *Ind,* indeterminate; *Neg,* negative. Correlation of HCV EIA-1 and EIA-2 results with recombinant immunoblot assay (*RIBA*) findings in the total blood donor study population. (Courtesy of Kleinman S, Alter H, Busch M, et al: *Transfusion* 32:805–813, 1992.)

tection of antibody is delayed, and no anti-HCV–reactive donor is identified in as many as one fourth of the cases of transfusion-related HVC. A second-generation assay (EIA-2) incorporates new antigens from the core and nonstructural regions of HCV.

Methods.—The EIA-2 for HCV antibody was evaluated in parallel with the EIA-1 in a series of 14,088 blood donors and also in 25 cases of transfusion-associated HVC where both donor and recipient samples were available. A recombinant immunoblot assay using 4 HCV antigens was also carried out.

Findings.—The EIA-2 detected HCV-infected blood donors more sensitively than did the EIA-1, locating infection in an additional 1 in 1,000 EIA-1–negative donors. The EIA-2 was as specific as the EIA-1, but the 2 assays detect different populations of false-positive donors. The EIA-2 detected infection in donors whose recombinant immunoblot assays were indeterminate 5 times more often than the EIA-1. The results of the 3 assays are compared in Figure 5–1. The EIA-2 also was more sensitive in the transfused patients with HCV, although it failed to detect a seropositive donor in 16%.

Conclusion.—Use of the EIA-2 for anti-HCV will make blood transfusions safer and will not significantly increase donor deferrals from false-positive reactions.

▶ In 1990, blood centers introduced HCV screening with EIAs-1 that were produced from recombinant proteins from the evolving spectrum of proteins available from the HCV. These initial assays were limited in sensitivity and were subject to a high rate of false-positive tests among low-risk populations of blood donors. A subsequent HCV immunoassay was introduced that incorporated new antigens from the core and coat of the virus. This article demonstrated that the blood supply was made safer by this test because more positive donors can be detected. An additional benefit is the more rapid detection of a donor who has recently seroconverted. Fewer false-positive donors are now identified, making the onerous task of explaining a false-positive test result to a noninfected blood donor rather a less common responsibility.—P.M. Ness, M.D.

Failure to Detect Human Cytomegalovirus DNA in Peripheral Blood Leukocytes of Healthy Blood Donors by the Polymerase Chain Reaction
Bitsch A, Kirchner H, Dupke R, Bein G (Univ of Lübeck, Germany)
Transfusion 32:612–617, 1992   5–8

Introduction.—In immunocompromised patients, transfusion of blood from donors with latent human cytomegalovirus (CMV) can result in transmission of the virus. Identification of which blood component harbors infectious virus and can transfer it to the patient cannot be achieved with serologic tests; some sensitive method of detecting the virus itself is needed. Using the PCR, CMV DNA has been found in all seropositive and most seronegative blood donors, but these findings have not been confirmed. Therefore, an extremely sensitive and specific PCR for the detection of CMV DNA in peripheral blood leukocytes was developed.

Methods and Findings.—The PCR was developed with strict precautions against PCR product carryover. Using this technique, none of the 116 samples from volunteer blood donors was found to be positive for CMV DNA. However, when used to study renal transplant patients early in the course of active CMV infection, the PCR detected CMV DNA in 10 of 10 cases. In plasmid studies, DNA had to be extracted and purified before amplification to avoid false-negative results.

Conclusion.—Current PCR techniques are probably unable to detect the CMV genome copy number in peripheral blood leukocytes of healthy subjects. Therefore, it is not sufficient for screening blood donors for CMV. Development of an appropriate in situ PCR assay would be the only way to determine how many WBCs in blood components are latently infected.

▶ In the 1993 YEAR BOOK OF HEMATOLOGY, I cited an article using PCR technology that implied that almost any unit of donor blood tested had evidence of previous CMV infection (1). The current article from Bitsch et al. suggests that CMV is not so ubiquitous; when strict adherence to PCR protocols limiting carryover and contamination were used, CMV DNA could not be detected in blood donors although CMV DNA could be detected in patients with active CMV disease. Thus, the authors suggest that PCR is less sensitive than serology for detecting previous CMV infection and is of limited use in transfusion medicine. These data suggest to me, however, that PCR could be of use in identifying truly infectious donors rather than eliminating a large number of previously infected but currently noninfectious donors that are most likely to be identified by the serologic methods used in blood centers.—P.M. Ness, M.D.

Reference

1. Bevan IS, et al: *Br J Haematol* 78:94–99, 1991.

Red Blood Cell Immunology

Multiple Rh Messenger RNA Isoforms Are Produced by Alternative Splicing

Le Van Kim C, Chérif-Zahar B, Raynal V, Mouro I, Lopez M, Cartron J-P, Colin Y (Inst Natl de Transfusion Sanguine, Paris)
Blood 80:1074–1078, 1992   5–9

Background.—Recent findings are consistent with a 2-locus model of Rh inheritance, with 1 of the 2 genes of the RH locus encoding the RhD protein and the other encoding the RhC/c and E/e polypeptides. It is unknown how these genes control the production of Rh antigens and how many polypeptides are needed to account for the great diversity of Rh antigens. Several Rh complementary DNA (cDNA) clones derived from alternative splicing of the gene encoding Cc and Ee antigens were characterized.

Observations.—Sequence analysis of specimens from a human bone marrow cDNA library and PCR amplification of human bone marrow and erythroblast messenger RNAs (mRNAs) identified 3 Rh-related cDNAs. Compared with the Rh polypeptide encoded by the previously described cDNA clone, these cDNAs potentially encoded a family of Rh protein isoforms with several unexpected structural properties. There were several peptide deletions, the predicted alteration of Rh protein topology within the cell membrane, variations in the number and surface exposition of cysteine residues, and generation of new C-terminal polypeptide segments caused by frameshift mutations. Thus, 4 Rh mRNAs corresponding to different splicing isoforms transcribed from the same Rh gene are now described. All of these mRNAs exist in the same erythroid cell lineage. At least 3 of the RNA species existed in reticulocytes from donors with different commonly expressed Rh phenotypes, as shown by PCR experiments.

Conclusion.—Two genes at the RH locus may direct the synthesis of a number of protein species, possibly coinciding with the different Rh antigenic variants. The molecular basis of RH locus expression in various genetic conditions may be understood by characterization of these multiple mRNA structures and their deduced encoded proteins.

▶ Our understanding of the inheritance of the complicated Rh antigens continues to grow as a result of studies from Cartron in France and Agre in the United States. The current article suggests that 2 Rh genes encode Rh proteins: 1 for the D antigen and a second gene for the Rh C/c and E/e polypeptides. This basic conformation can be used to explain the variety of Rh phenotypes seen in transfusion practice. The continuing mystery of why this protein complex is so antigenic remains to be elucidated.—P.M. Ness, M.D.

Red Blood Cell Transfusion in Warm-Type Autoimmune Haemolytic Anaemia

Salama A, Berghöfer H, Mueller-Eckhardt C (Justus Liebig Univ, Giessen, Germany)
Lancet 340:1515–1517, 1992   5–10

Introduction.—In patients with warm-type autoimmune hemolytic anemia (AIHA), blood transfusion is generally regarded as dangerous because of the potential for intensifying hemolysis and the presumed high incidence of alloimmunization. Some findings about transfusion in patients with classic AIHA, however, do not support the recommendation to avoid red cell transfusions.

Patients and Methods.—A total of 79 patients with detectable warm autoantibodies and transitory or persistent hemolytic anemia received at least 2 blood transfusions. Five of the patients were children. All patients were reevaluated at least twice within 6 months after transfusion.

Findings.—The reason for blood transfusion was decompensated AIHA in 53 patients, all of whom had detectable autoantibodies against RBCs. There were no cases of transfusion-related alloimmunization in this group, nor any definite increase in hemolysis. This was so even when free serum autoantibodies made the cells serologically incompatible. In the other 26 patients, there were no direct signs of AIHA at the outset, with both direct and indirect antiglobulin tests being negative. Transfusion was given for anemia of other causes, most commonly chronic lymphocytic leukemia. Transfusion was followed by development of alloantibodies as well as autoantibodies in 23 of these patients, whereas the other 3 had autoantibodies alone.

Conclusion.—This study finds no reason to avoid transfusion therapy for the correction of anemia in patients with AIHA. Patients with AIHA appear to have a lower incidence of alloimmunization and adverse hemolytic transfusion reaction than other patients receiving multiple transfusions. Until other types of therapy become effective, transfusions should be given even though the transfused red cells survive for only a few days.

▶ Most hematologists are reluctant to transfuse patients with warm AIHA even when their anemia becomes symptomatic. These patients have positive direct antiglobulin tests that can cause serologic laboratory complexity that makes the detection and identification of alloantibodies difficult. Although autoantibodies in this disease cause the immune hemolysis, adverse transfusion reactions would be more likely from alloantibodies that are difficult to detect. The common impression among hematologists and blood bank serologists is that a high proportion of these patients have underlying alloantibodies, based on studies largely collected in reference serology laboratories. This study from a clinical institution suggests that alloimmunization in patients with autoimmune hemolysis is relatively uncommon and that patients meeting the clinical criteria justifying transfusions can be safely transfused.—P.M. Ness, M.D.

Cytokine Production in IgG-Mediated Red Cell Incompatibility

Davenport RD, Burdick M, Moore SA, Kunkel SL (Univ of Michigan, Ann Arbor)
Transfusion 33:19–24, 1993

Introduction.—For reasons that are not clear, transfusing incompatible RBCs may lead to fever and systemic symptoms. Certain cytokines may be involved in these transfusion reactions. The production of ILβ, IL-6, IL-8, and tumor necrosis factor (TNF) by monocytes in response to anti-D–sensitized red cells was examined to simulate IgG-dependent hemolytic transfusion reactions.

Results.—All the interleukins were detected in culture supernates at 4–6 hours, and their levels increased for as long as 24 hours. Levels of TNF peaked at 6 hours. The presence of IL-1β, IL-8, and TNF was confirmed immunocytochemically in monocytes phagocytozing RBCs. Both production of IL-8 and phagocytosis were inhibited by monomeric IgG. Neutralizing antibodies to IL-1β and TNF failed to inhibit the production of IL-8.

Conclusion.—Production of inflammatory cytokines by phagocytic cells may explain the symptoms of IgG-mediated hemolytic transfusion reactions.

▶ Although the clinical effects of transfusion of incompatible red cells have been characterized to include fever, renal failure, and the potential for disseminated intravascular coagulation, the mechanisms by which these clinical effects are produced are largely unexplained. Most settings in which alloimmune hemolysis occurs are untoward transfusion complications that would not be amenable to prospective study; in many cases in which delayed immune hemolysis would be expected to occur, the clinical symptomatology is minimal. For these reasons, an in vitro system was developed to investigate factors that may explain the symptoms of transfusion reactions that occur because of IgG-mediated immune hemolysis. The results demonstrated that a number of cytokines and interleukins are produced in vitro when these reactions occur. These results may ultimately be useful in cases in which immune hemolysis is unavoidable, such as the transplantation of group O organs into group A recipients with immune hemolysis resulting from antibodies produced by lymphocytes associated with the donor organ. These reactions could potentially be treated or prevented based on further studies along these lines.—P.M. Ness, M.D.

Hemolysis of Transfused Group O Red Blood Cells in Minor ABO-Incompatible Unrelated-Donor Bone Marrow Transplants in Patients Receiving Cyclosporine Without Posttransplant Methotrexate
Gajewski JL, Petz LD, Calhoun L, O'Rourke S, Landaw EM, Lyddane NR, Hunt LA, Schiller GJ, Ho WG, Champlin RE (Univ of California at Los Angeles)
Blood 79:3076–3085, 1992   5–12

Background.—In allogeneic bone marrow transplantation between a minor ABO-incompatible donor and a recipient, hemolysis usually occurs 1 to 2 weeks post-transplant. This may result from destruction of incompatible erythrocytes by donor-derived anti-A and/or anti-B antibody produced from "passenger" immunocompetent donor lymphocytes. Prompted by an experience with this type of hemolysis resulting in extraordinary transfusion requirements of group O erythrocytes, whether the proposed mechanism could account for this excessive hemolysis was determined.

Methods.—The experience consisted of 7 minor ABO-incompatible unrelated-donor bone marrow transplant recipients treated during 31 months. All had a strongly reactive donor-derived ABO blood group antibody in association with excessive erythrocyte transfusion requirement and laboratory evidence of hemolysis. All received cyclosporine without post-transplant methotrexate. The first 3 patients in the index group required 26 units of group O erythrocytes each. This amount, which greatly exceeded the recipient's volume of incompatible erythrocytes, suggested that transfused group O erythrocytes were being lysed as well. The remaining 4 patients had pretransplant erythrocyte exchange transfusion with group O erythrocytes; although this decreased the severity of hemolysis, it did not prevent it. On analysis of variance, transfusion requirements were affected by the donor-recipient relationship being unrelated and the use of post-transplant methotrexate, with an interaction between these 2 factors.

Conclusion.—Minor ABO-incompatible bone marrow transplantation may result in immune-mediated hemolysis, particularly in those receiving marrow from unrelated donors. Hemolysis may include bystander-transfused group O erythrocytes as well as group A or group B erythrocytes. This is a serious complication that might be prevented by post-transplant methotrexate treatment; further study is needed to determine the mechanism of hemolysis.

▶ ABO-incompatible bone marrow is frequently used when the donor represents the best HLA match available. In this setting, a syndrome of immune hemolysis frequently occurs because of the production of alloantibody from lymphocytes of the bone marrow donor that is incompatible with the red cells of the recipient. Although the hemolysis is usually short-lived and not of major consequence, occasional cases of severe hemolysis requiring major blood transfusions or hemodialysis have been described. This series from UCLA is of interest for 2 reasons. First, the authors suggest that the immune-mediated hemolysis can be prevented in some cases by post-transplant methotrexate therapy. Second, using this clinical picture, the authors clearly demonstrated that the immune hemolysis in some cases results in destruction of compatible as well as serologically incompatible red cells, a phenomenon that has been called bystander hemolysis. This phenomenon probably occurs in other settings such as delayed hemolytic transfusion reactions but has been difficult to demonstrate convincingly. The mechanism of this bystander hemolysis is unknown.—P.M. Ness, M.D.

Presence of the Red Cell Alloantibody Anti-E in an 11-Week-Old Infant

DePalma L, Criss VR, Roseff SD, Luban NLC (Children's Natl Med Ctr; George Washington Univ, Washington, DC)
Transfusion 32:177–179, 1992   5–13

Background.—Red blood cell alloantibody formation in infants younger than 4 months of age is thought to be extremely rare. The development of alloantibody-E in an 11-week-old boy who received multiple transfusions for necrotizing enterocolitis was studied.

Case Report.—Infant, 1 month, was hospitalized with moderate respiratory distress. He had been a full-term infant, weighing 9 lb 6 oz at birth. His parents had noticed his difficulty breathing and poor eating several days before the hospital admission. The infant was found to have several congenital cardiac abnormalities. He was typed as group B, D+. Necrotizing enterocolitis developed, which delayed cardiac surgery. Surgical resection of a segment of necrotic bowel was done. Septic shock and acute renal failure then developed, and the infant needed ultrafiltration and hemodialysis for nearly 3 weeks. Ventilatory support was required for several weeks. He had sustained metabolic acidosis with daily spiking fevers. Thirty-one RBC transfusions were delivered, consisting of group B, D+ or group O, D+ washed or unwashed RBCs. Eleven transfusions of fresh frozen plasma and 39 units of random-donor platelets were needed for increased prothrombin and partial thromboplastin times and thrombocytopenia. The transfusions were given within the first $4\frac{1}{2}$ weeks of hospitalization. The infant subsequently had an uneventful cardiac repair that was revised 2 days later because of stenosis. Six weeks after the first blood transfusion, alloantibody-E was found. The anti-E agglutinated R_2R_2 screening RBCs weakly at 37°C and sensitized the RBCs to react with anti-IgG. The infant's RBCs were type E−. The negative antibody screening tests of each donor unit and the absence of RBC alloantibodies in the mother's blood ruled out passive transfer of alloantibody-E. Stored samples of the boy's blood were tested. Anti-E was found about 11 days after exposure to a known E+ RBC unit.

Conclusion.—In this case, the timing of the appearance of alloantibody-E is consistent with a secondary immune response. Primary immunization probably occurred in the first 4 weeks of transfusion therapy.

▶ Current blood-banking practices do not require crossmatching of blood for transfusions of infants younger than 4 months of age if their initial antibody detection testing is negative. These practices are based on the observation that infants in this age group do not become sensitized by blood transfusions. This exceptional case demonstrates that antibody formation can occur in this pediatric setting and may provoke a reassessment of our pretransfusion practices for similar children.—P.M. Ness, M.D.

Platelet Immunology and Transfusion

Detection and Significance of Alpha Granule Membrane Protein 140 Expression on Platelets Collected by Apheresis

Triulzi DJ, Kickler TS, Braine HG (Johns Hopkins Univ, Baltimore, Md)

Transfusion 32:529–533, 1992

5–14

Purpose.—The study of platelet activation has been facilitated by the development of monoclonal antibodies (MoAbs) directed at antigens expressed on activated platelets. The MoAb S12 can be used to detect alpha–granule membrane protein 140 (GMP-140) antigen, which is expressed only on activated platelets. This technique was used to study the activation state of fresh platelets collected by apheresis and the effect of activation on platelet recovery.

Methods.—Flow cytometry was used to measure platelet activation with S12 MoAb in 20 apheresis platelet concentrates. Eleven concentrates were obtained with the CS-3000 system and 9 with the Spectra system. Six concentrates obtained by the Spectra system were filtered. All concentrates were measured 4 hours after collection. Twelve of the concentrates were subsequently transfused to 8 patients who were not refractory from a clinical or alloimmune standpoint.

Findings.—A mean of 25% of platelets were activated in concentrates obtained by the CS-3000 system and 29% in concentrates obtained by the Spectra system. In the filtered concentrates, the mean total number of platelets recovered after filtration decreased 18%. However, no difference was noted in the proportion of activated platelets measured immediately before and after filtration. The 1-hour post-transfusion platelet count increment in the transfused patients showed a significant inverse correlation between the platelet count increment and the proportion of activated platelets in the component.

Conclusion.—Measurement with the MoAb S12 suggests that apheresis platelet concentrates with more activated platelets have a reduced 1-hour recovery. Activation is not enhanced and activated platelets are not removed by filtration. Expression of GMP-140 could be a useful technique for evaluating the quality of platelet components.

▶ It is fairly common for the hematologist to transfuse platelets to patients who fail to respond to an appropriate transfusion dose. When this apparent platelet refractoriness occurs, alloimmunization to HLA factors or other clinical events, such as sepsis or disseminated intravascular coagulation, are the common causes. Another potential cause of platelet transfusion failure could be platelets that were inadequately prepared or stored. Platelets will not survive or function normally if the Ph decreases below 6; this knowledge is used in quality control procedures in blood banks, but it is not common practice to measure the Ph in all transfused platelet concentrates. Other means to assess whether platelets to be transfused are likely to survive and provide hemostasis would allow the hematologist to maximize therapy and to minimize the potential for transfusion complications such as alloimmunization or infection. One candidate test is described in this article where platelet activation can be detected using a monoclonal antibody with a flow cytometer. Whether these methods will be shown to be adequately predictive of transfusion outcome and technically feasible for routine implementation will require subsequent studies.—P.M. Ness, M.D.

Effects of Leukocyte Depletion and UVB Irradiation on Alloantigenicity of Major Histocompatibility Complex Antigens in Platelet Concentrates: A Comparative Study

Kao KJ (Univ of Florida, Gainesville)
Blood 80:2931–2937, 1992   5–15

Background.—Random-donor platelet concentrates have improved the outcome in patients receiving chemotherapy or undergoing marrow transplantation or open heart surgery, but as many as half of those given multiple transfusions become alloimmunized to HLA antigens and fail to respond to platelet therapy. Depleting leukocytes from donor blood components or allografts has prevented the development of alloantibodies to major histocompatibility complex antigens. Syngeneic mouse strains were used to determine the effects of leukocyte depletion and ultraviolet B (UVB) radiation on the alloantigenicity of platelet concentrates. Gamma-irradiation was also done.

Results.—The frequency of alloimmunization was halved by transfusing platelets containing 2 or fewer leukocytes per microliter. Irradiation of platelet concentrates with 1,200 mJ/cm² of UVB prevented alloimmunization. Ultraviolet B radiation was effective even when concentrates contained more than a fully immunogenic number of leukocytes. Irradiation with UVB was more effective than a 3-log leukocyte depletion in preventing primary alloimmunization to major histocompatibility complex antigens.

Conclusion.—Because most patients who require platelet transfusions have compromised immune function, antigenic differences between UBV-irradiated and leukocyte-depleted platelet concentrates may be less marked than those noted in healthy mice.

▶ A number of animal and human studies suggest that alloimmunization to HLA antigens in platelet concentrates can be limited by leukocyte depletion or irradiation of the platelet concentrate with ultraviolet light. A large multicenter study of adult leukemia is in progress to determine whether the alloimmunization and platelet refractoriness can be limited by these techniques. Although the ultimate answer can only be delivered from patient studies, the animal studies cited in this article can lead to treatment modifications that can be tested later in humans and will help investigators dissect the mechanisms by which alloimmunization occurs and treatment interventions block these immunologic responses.—P.M. Ness, M.D.

Selection of Platelets for Refractory Patients by HLA Matching and Prospective Crossmatching
Moroff G, Garratty G, Heal JM, MacPherson BR, Stroncek D, Huang ST, Ho W, Petz LD, Leach MF, Lennon SS, Rowe JM, Saleh MN, Arndt P, Foley K, Masel D, Postoway N (Jerome H Holland Lab, Rockville, Md; American Red Cross Blood Services, Los Angeles, Rochester, NY; et al)
Transfusion 32:633–640, 1992   5–16

Introduction.—The selection of compatible platelets for thrombocytopenic patients who are refractory to random-donor platelets continues to be a perplexing problem, the most common approach to which is matching donor platelets at the HLA-A and HLA-B loci. There is interest in platelet crossmatching, although correlations between crossmatching results and post-transfusion platelet increments have been variable. A comparison of the use of prospective platelet crossmatching using stored donor platelets and HLA-based selection was conducted.

Methods.—The study sample comprised 73 patients at 5 sites who were refractory to random-donor platelets. All received 2 plateletpheresis components, 1 chosen according to HLA criteria and the other by crossmatching. Results were interpreted with careful attention to exclude nonimmune factors that could adversely affect transfusion results. Each center used a familiar crossmatching experience.

Findings.—Using an HLA-based method of donor selection, including all grades of matching and mismatching, yielded a similar overall rate of successful transfusion as a crossmatch-based method of donor selection. Restricting HLA-based selection to grade A and BU matches was better

Percentage of Patients With Successful Transfusions

	Transfusion type		
	HLA*	CXM†	p values
1-hour CCI ≥ 7500/μL			
Set 1 (n = 73)	51	45	>0.05
Set 2 (n = 35)	60	54	>0.05
Set 1 and Set 2	54	48	>0.05
24-hour CCI ≥ 4500/μL			
Set 1 (n = 50)	36	26	<0.05
Set 2 (n = 27)	48	19	<0.05
Set 1 and Set 2	42	23	<0.05

* Platelets selected by HLA criteria.
† Platelets selected by crossmatching.
(Courtesy of Moroff G, Garratty G, Heal JM, et al: *Transfusion* 32:633–640, 1992.)

than crossmatching alone. This type of matching was also better than selection based on any degree of HLA mismatching. Basing the selection of HLA-cross-reactive groups was no more successful than basing it on grades C and D mismatches or crossmatching alone. Even though patients with nonimmune factors were eliminated from the study, few patients demonstrated lymphocytotoxic and platelet antibodies.

Conclusion.—This study finds that selecting platelets for refractory patients on the basis of grade A and BU HLA compatibility yields a higher success rate than crossmatching (table). This method is expensive, however, and hospitals without access to the necessary resources can use platelet crossmatching. Logistically, it is feasible to perform prospective crossmatching using stored platelets, either liquid or frozen, and subsequent drawing of blood from compatible donors.

▶ In hematologic patients who become alloimmunized to HLA antigens in platelets and refractory to transfusions, successful transfusion therapy can often be maintained by using HLA-matched platelets. This therapy is usually successful, but some patients fail to respond to HLA-matched transfusions. Many patients have uncommon HLA types, making them difficult to match, and blood centers require substantial time to locate a matched donor, perform a hemapheresis collection, test the component, and deliver it to the patient. Another approach uses platelet crossmatching where a sample of the patient's blood can be crossmatched with the donor platelets that may be available already or stored by a method acceptable for prospective crossmatching. This study attempted to compare the 2 methodologies and found HLA-matching to be slightly more successful than crossmatching. Unfortunately, the study design was somewhat flawed because the data pooled patients from a number of centers who used standardized HLA-matching protocols but different platelet crossmatching techniques. Another problem in these types of studies is the variable clinical evaluation that can occur so that cases where nonimmune factors cause the refractoriness can be missed. A single-institution study where HLA matching and platelet crossmatching are compared in a blind, prospective fashion would be of major interest.—P.M. Ness, M.D.

Autologous Transfusion

Factors Associated With Successful Autologous Blood Donation for Elective Surgery

McVay PA, Hoag MS, Lee SJ, Toy PTCY (Univ of California, San Francisco; Blood Bank of the Alameda-Contra Med Assoc, Oakland, Calif; Northern California Cancer Ctr, Belmont)
Am J Clin Pathol 97:304–308, 1992   5–17

Background.—Not all patients can donate as much autologous blood units as needed before surgery. Some factors associated with the ability to donate the number of units required have been studied, but a more thorough examination of these factors is needed.

Methods.—A total of 368 autologous blood donors at 1 community blood center was studied. These patients had been requested to give 4 or more units during the 6 weeks before their surgery.

Findings.—More men (86%) than women (42%) were able to donate 4 units of blood with no deferrals for anemia. Also, patients with an initial hemoglobin level exceeding 125 g/L, patients weighing more, and older patients were better able to donate the required amount. According to a multiple logistic regression analysis, only higher initial hemoglobin levels and male sex independently predicted successful donation of 4 or more units.

Conclusion.—Successful autologous blood donation is significantly associated with higher predonation hemoglobin levels and being male. Correcting iron deficiency in women may permit them to donate more units. As surgery is often considered several months before it is done electively, it may be helpful to determine hemoglobin levels and the iron reserves of women. If needed, supplemental iron should be given months before blood donation is anticipated.

▶ This study assessed a series of autologous blood donations and determined that patients with higher hemoglobin levels are typically more successful in donating 4 units preoperatively. Equally unsurprising is the observation that women are less successful in the autologous enterprise than men, probably because of limited iron stores. The results suggest that early iron replacement may be important for women contemplating predeposit autologous donation, especially if 4 units are desired, as required in this study. Because many patients need less than 4 units of blood, failure to complete an autologous program may be less common in more routine clinical practice.—P.M. Ness, M.D.

Predeposit Autologous Blood Transfusion in Patients With Colorectal Cancer: A Feasibility Study

Harrison S, Steele RJC, Johnston AK, Jones JA, Morris DL, Hardcastle JD (Univ Hosp, Nottingham, England)
Br J Surg 79:355–357, 1992   5–18

Background.—Although clinical and immunologic evidence are convincing, the effect of transfusion on cancer recurrence in humans has only been shown retrospectively. The feasibility of autologous transfusion in patients with colorectal cancer needs to be determined to establish whether enough patients can be recruited in a realistic period.

Methods and Findings.—During 2 years, a predeposit autologous blood transfusion service was provided for patients having elective surgery for left-sided colonic or rectal cancer. Of 129 patients eligible for the service, 28 were suitable for autologous donation. Eight of these patients received autologous blood only, and 13 needed no transfusion. Seven patients needed additional homologous blood. Thus, only a very small proportion of this group derived any benefit from the predeposit autologous blood transfusion service.

Conclusion.—Predeposit autologous blood transfusion for patients with colorectal cancer is possible but may not be feasible. If an autologous blood transfusion service is available, there is no reason why patients with cancer should not take advantage of it, as long as strict precautions are taken to prevent their blood from entering the random-donor pool. However, autologous transfusion primarily for patients with cancer would be difficult to justify on the basis of the present evidence.

▶ Armed with the growing pile of retrospective studies that suggest that tumor recurrence can be promoted by bank blood, these investigators attempted to use autologous transfusion support for patients with colorectal cancer. Patients with colon cancer have been most prominently featured in reports of cancer recurrence after blood transfusion. It is no great surprise that most patients with colorectal cancer cannot be autologous donors for a number of administrative and medical reasons affecting this elderly population. On the other hand, these authors identified 28 suitable autologous candidates (about 25% of their study population) who were able to participate in an autologous program. There is no contraindication to autologous donation in patients with cancer.—P.M. Ness, M.D.

Safety and Efficacy of Autologous Blood Donation Before Elective Aortic Valve Operation

Dzik WH, Fleisher AG, Ciavarella D, Karlson KJ, Reed GE, Berger RL (New England Deaconess Hosp, Boston; Harvard Med School, Boston; Westchester County Med Ctr, Valhalla, NY; et al)
Ann Thorac Surg 54:1177–1181, 1992   5–19

Introduction.—Patients scheduled for elective cardiac surgery increasingly receive autologous blood preoperatively, but those awaiting aortic valve replacement traditionally are denied access to autologous blood collection programs. An experience with 79 patients with serious aortic valve disease who donated 1 to 3 units of autologous blood before valve surgery was reviewed.

Methods.—The criterion for acceptance was a predonation hematocrit level of .33 or more. Blood was collected into citrate-phosphate-dextrose-adenine anticoagulant preservative bags 35 to 3 days before scheduled surgery and was stored as whole blood. Transfusion requirements were compared with those of 298 other patients having elective aortic valve replacement in the same period without donating autologous blood.

Blood Donor Exposures During Aortic Valve Replacement

Donor Exposures	Autologous Group (n = 78)	Nonautologous Group (n = 298)
No transfusions	4 (5)[b]	91 (31)
Autologous only	49 (63)[b]	. . .
1–2 homologous unit	12 (15)	76 (25)
3–10 homologous units	7 (9)	83 (28)
>10 homologous units	6 (8)	48 (16)

Note: The number of patients exposed to donor blood components (exposure to all components including whole blood, packed red cells, fresh frozen plasma, platelets, and cryoprecipitate during entire hospitalization) is shown. Values in parentheses are percentages.

[b] Proportion of patients with either no transfusion exposures or autologous-only transfusions is significantly different from nonautologous group (P < .0001).

(Courtesy of Dzik WH, Fleisher AG, Ciavarella D, et al: Ann Thorac Surg 54:1177–1181, 1992.)

Results.—A total of 129 units of blood were collected from the 79 participants. One patient with a history of exertional syncope had a syncopal episode 2 hours after donation. All but 1 of the patients underwent aortic valve replacement. More than 60% of patients received only autologous blood while hospitalized (table). Homologous blood was given to 69% of the 298 comparison patients. Patients predepositing their own blood received mainly autologous whole blood, whereas those who did not predeposit received chiefly packed red cells.

Conclusion.—Further experience is needed to gauge morbidity from preoperative blood donation, but the present findings suggest that autologous blood donation be considered for patients awaiting elective aortic valve replacement.

▶ It is fairly common for blood banks to establish policies that exclude patients or blood donors on very meager evidence. For this reason, I always enjoy studies, such as this cited article, that challenge dogma based largely on opinion rather than on fact. This article suggests that it is indeed safe to include patients with aortic stenosis as autologous blood donors; only 1 donor of 79 had a donor reaction. An invited commentary from Dr. Robert Thurer, a cardiac surgeon and known advocate of autologous blood donation, expresses appropriate cautions about the potential referral bias in this study and the need to corroborate the data elsewhere. I hope that other centers will accept this challenge and attempt to verify these intriguing findings.—P.M. Ness, M.D.

An Analysis of 9,918 Consecutive Perioperative Autotransfusions

Giordano GF, Giordano DM, Wallace BA, Giordano KM, Prust RS, Sandler SG (Southern Arizona Regional Red Cross Blood Program, Tucson; American

Red Cross, Washington, DC)
Surg Gynecol Obstet 176:103–110, 1993

5–20

Introduction.—Although the benefits of increased use of perioperative autotransfusion (PAT) are well established, the accompanying reduction in use of homologous blood does not necessarily result from increased use of PAT. Other possible factors include a change in indications for transfusion, predeposit of autologous blood, and more careful surgical technique. Another way to evaluate the efficacy of PAT would be to analyze the amount of blood salvaged and retransfused.

Methods.—The quality of autologous blood obtained by PAT and reinfused to patients in 9,918 consecutive procedures was studied. The amount of blood salvaged and the volume of autologous erythrocytes reinfused per procedure were recorded and converted to packed cell equivalents (PCEs). The analysis also included the use of postoperative salvage and salvage PAT.

Results.—The total percentage of standby patients was 11%, with the lowest number occurring in cardiac operations and the highest rate in orthopedic operations. The average return of autologous blood was equivalent to 2.61 units of PCE. The return was greatest in cardiac procedures and the least in orthopedic procedures, 3.98 and 1.05 units, respectively. For trauma patients, the mean figure was 3.59 units. Sixty-two percent of patients undergoing cardiopulmonary bypass operations received 2 units or more of PCE.

Conclusion.—Substantial quantities of blood can be salvaged by PAT in patients undergoing a variety of surgical procedures. The results of this analysis coincide with those reported previously. The data presented will serve as a general guide to the number of units likely to be salvaged during various surgical procedures.

▶ With the widespread growth of perioperative autologous transfusion, in particular the use of intraoperative autologous transfusion, this article provides a useful single-institution experience. A number of medical, legal, financial, and ethical concerns have driven the expansion of this procedure, in some cases leading to use that may not be medically rational or financially expedient. As shown in this article, the mean salvage for cardiac procedures of 4.65 units can be readily justified, but the mean salvage of 1.05 units in orthopedic operations suggests overuse in low-risk situations. More specific case analysis in orthopedic procedures showed that in redo procedures for total hip arthroplasty, cell salvage makes sense. With increasing public scrutiny of medical costs, these types of data are useful for directing expensive technology for reasonable purposes.—P.M. Ness, M.D.

Impact of Autologous Blood Transfusions on Patients Undergoing Radical Prostatectomy Using Hypotensive Anesthesia

Yamada AH, Lieskovsky G, Skinner DG, Shulman I, Groshen S, Chen S-C (Univ of Southern California, Los Angeles; Kenneth Norris Jr Comprehensive Cancer Ctr, Los Angeles)

J Urol 149:73–76, 1993   5–21

Background.—Patients undergoing major pelvic surgery have substantial transfusion requirements. The use of autologous blood, collected from the patient and stored before and used during the operation, has been successful in a variety of settings. The impact of preoperative autologous blood collection in 71 consecutive patients undergoing radical retropubic prostatectomy was reviewed.

Methods.—The patients underwent bilateral pelvic lymph node dissection and radial retropubic prostatectomy for adenocarcinoma of the prostate during an 8-month period. All operations were under controlled hypotensive anesthesia to decrease blood loss. Thirty-four patients, composing group 1, opted not to have autologous blood collected for use during surgery, whereas 37 patients, composing group 2, did deposit autologous blood. The 2 groups were operated on concurrently and compared retrospectively.

Results.—There were no significant differences in operative time and estimated blood loss. Of patients in group 1, 21% used a total of 20 units of homologous blood. In group 2, 41 units were transfused; all but 4 units were autologous, with only 8% of patients receiving homologous blood. Autologous blood deposition was associated with a decrease in blood concentration at admission; thus, 21 of 37 patients in group 2 were anemic during hospitalization (table). The anemia resulting from phlebotomy did not appear to resolve preoperatively in all cases.

Conclusion.—For patients undergoing radical retropubic prostatectomy, autologous blood collection reduces exposure to homologous blood. However, the effectiveness of this program is decreased by preoperative anemia. Measures should be taken to increase the EPO re-

Effect of Storing Autologous Blood on Preoperative
Hematocrit in Group 2

No. Units Stored	No. Pts.	Hematocrit (mean ± SD)	P Value
0—pre-phlebotomy	30	44.7 ± 2.5	0.02*
1	8	40.6 ± 3.0	0.05†
2	27	38.2 ± 3.0	
3	2	36.0	

(Courtesy of Yamada AH, Lieskovsky G, Skinner DG, et al: *J Urol* 149:73–76, 1993.)

sponse to this anemia. The study also suggests that autologous blood collection is expensive and wasteful, with an alarming 46% discard rate.

A Randomized Trial of Perioperative Hemodilution Versus Transfusion of Preoperatively Deposited Autologous Blood in Elective Surgery

Ness PM, Bourke DL, Walsh PC (Johns Hopkins Med Insts, Baltimore, Md)
Transfusion 31:226–230, 1992   5–22

Background.—Hemodilution is 1 of several methods proposed to reduce homologous blood transfusion in elective surgery. However, this method has not been tested prospectively to determine its success. Whether hemodilution is a viable alternative to preoperative autologous blood donation was determined.

Methods.—By random assignment, 50 patients either deposited 3 units of autologous blood before surgery or had hemodilution just before elective radical retropubic prostatectomy. All patients were treated with a standard protocol. One surgeon performed all operations.

Findings.—The preoperative deposit group received a mean of 2.44 blood units. Two of 25 patients needed homologous blood transfusion for blood loss of 2,600 mL and 1,700 mL, respectively. Patients undergoing hemodilution needed a mean of 2.88 units of autologous blood. None of those patients received homologous blood. Mean hematocrits at discharge were 35.5 for the preoperative deposit group and 31.8 for the hemodilution group. The treatment groups were comparable in perioperative morbidity. The initial patient hematocrit was the best predictor of the discharge hematocrit (Fig 5–2).

Conclusion.—Hemodilution can safely replace or at least augment preoperative autologous donation to reduce homologous blood transfusion. These findings apply to any elective surgical procedure in which a

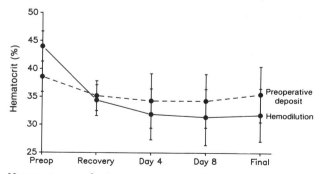

Fig 5–2.—Hematocrit course for preoperative deposit and hemodilution patients shown as mean percentage ± 1 SD before surgery, in the recovery room, on postoperative days 4 and 8, and at discharge. (Courtesy of Ness PM, Bourke DL, Walsh PC: *Transfusion* 31:226–230, 1992.)

1,000-mL blood loss is expected. The other advantages of hemodilution are convenience, lower cost, and better preservation of all components of autologous blood. This practice probably deserves wider application.

▶ Radical retropubic prostatectomy (RRP) is a procedure being performed more often in view of its efficacy in improving survival with limited tumor recurrence and its low rate of postoperative problems with urinary function or potency. Because most patients have a surgical blood loss exceeding 1,000 mL and are otherwise in good health, autologous blood donation is often performed in this setting.

The first article (Abstract 5–21) suggests that there is some benefit in reducing homologous blood exposure in these patients, but preoperative anemia, which is induced, may limit the technique; in addition, a high rate of autologous blood units collected in these patients was not transfused in this study, leading the authors to question the efficiency of this procedure. They also suggest that EPO may be a useful adjunct to correct the perioperative anemia. They conclude that the modest benefit seen may not be worth the highest cost induced.

We have considerable experience with RRP and autologous blood at Johns Hopkins and have had similar problems. Although most of the units that are collected are used, they may not meet strict blood transfusion criteria. We, therefore, performed a study (Abstract 5–22) comparing predeposit autologous donation to perioperative hemodilution and found that homologous blood use and discharge hematocrit were similar. Because some patients in both groups have anemia develop, a role for EPO could be found for both procedures. That the costs of performing hemodilution should be much less than the costs of predeposit donation and that hemodilution can be offered without recurrent visits to the blood bank are additional advantages. Although the apparent waste cited by Yamada et al. has not been a major problem for us, both of these studies suggest that there may be simpler solutions with less expense for RRP and many other elective surgery procedures. We may be going too far with our current autologous programs, because many patients with 1,000-mL surgical blood loss can clearly tolerate the mild anemia induced without requiring autologous or homologous blood.—P.M. Ness, M.D.

Autotransfusion of Potentially Culture-Positive Blood (CPB) in Abdominal Trauma: Preliminary Data From a Prospective Study
Ozmen V, McSwain NE Jr, Nichols RL, Smith J, Flint LM (Tulane Univ, New Orleans, La)
J Trauma 32:36–39, 1992   5–23

Background.—The increased use of autotransfusion for trauma-induced bleeding may decrease the amounts of banked blood needed for severe injuries. Although autotransfusion is standard for traumatic hemothorax, its use has been limited in patients with abdominal injuries. Autotransfusion of potentially culture-positive blood (CPB) in patients with abdominal injuries was assessed.

Methods.—Microbiological data on 152 patients with intestinal trauma were used. When blood loss was anticipated to be greater than 1,000 mL, blood from the peritoneal cavity was cultured, washed, concentrated, and recultured for reinfusion. The Penetrating Abdominal Trauma Index (PATI) was used to stratify infection rates. Fifty patients with PATIs exceeding 20 who received a mean of 1,800 mL of banked blood were compared with 20 patients receiving a mean of 3,900 mL of autotransfused, potentially CPB.

Results.—Wound infection occurred in 25% of patients in both groups. When the severity of injury was stratified according to PATI, there were no significant increases in site-specific infection risk. Bacteria cultured from autotransfused blood did not cause bacteremias, pulmonary infections, or urinary infections.

Conclusion.—Autotransfusion of blood aspirated from the peritoneal cavity is feasible and can reduce the need for banked blood in trauma victims. Blood washing removes bacteria from most of the units. Infusion of CPB does not increase the risk of subsequent infection in seriously injured patients. Further research is needed to assess the use of this technique in a larger group of patients.

▶ Intraoperative autologous transfusion (IAT) is a valuable procedure in many elective surgery procedures, but its widespread use is limited because potentially contaminated cases or cancer resection cases are usually excluded. These authors used IAT in patients with intestinal trauma and could not demonstrate a difference in the infection rate with IAT compared with patients receiving bank blood. The IAT blood did not cause bacteremias or other distant infections that would be spread by a hematogenous route. This study may stimulate others to reevaluate whether IAT is contraindicated in contaminated cases. An important qualification listed by the authors suggests that patients with implanted foreign devices should be excluded from these protocols in view of the known risk of infection at these sites.—P.M. Ness, M.D.

Adult Transfusion Practices

Red Cell Transfusions in Coronary Artery Bypass Surgery (DRGs 106 and 107)

Surgenor DM, Wallace EL, Churchill WH, Hao SHS, Chapman RH, Collins JJ Jr (Brigham and Women's Hosp, Boston; State Univ of New York at Buffalo; Ctr for Management Systems, Williamsville, New York)
Transfusion 32:458–464, 1992   5–24

Background.—An unique data base was recently used to explore how transfusions of RBCs are used to support hospital patients. The data base includes information on RBC component transfusion with abstracted patient discharge records coded by diagnosis-related group (DRG) and International Classification of Diseases, 9th revision, Clinical Modification (ICD-9-CM) diagnosis and procedure codes. The previous work was extended to explore the ways in which transfusions of RBCs were used to support patients undergoing coronary artery bypass graft (CABG) surgery.

Methods and Results.—A total of 3,216 CABG patients in 11 hospitals in the United States in 1988 formed the data base. Abstracted patient records were stratified by DRG and ICD-9-CM surgical procedure code. Patients in DRG 106—coronary artery bypass without catheterization—had significantly greater mean units per transfused patient, age, length of stay, and inhospital mortality compared with patients in DRG 107—coronary artery bypass with catheterization. Gender was a significant variable in transfusion outcomes. Women were more likely to undergo transfusion and, when transfused, received more units of RBCs than men. For a given DRG/ICD-9-CM procedure class, there were significant differences among hospitals in the percentage of patients transfused but not in mean units of RBCs per transfused patient. Within individual hospitals, however, the proportion of transfused patients and number of units per transfused patient did not significantly vary across DRG/ICD-9-CM procedure classes.

Conclusion.—Unidentified circumstances within hospitals appear to have more influence on transfusion decisions than the nature of the surgical intervention. Factors influencing the transfusion decision need to be better defined if hospitals are to limit exposure of patients undergoing CABG to the blood of allogeneic donors and to conserve blood.

▶ This article documented that the blood usage in similar procedures can vary substantially among institutions. It uses a transfusion data system developed by Surgenor and colleagues that is likely to produce data to answer questions in transfusion practice that have been addressed previously only by anecdotal methods. This data base will be a very important tool for blood bank physicians and quality assurance review groups to influence transfusion practices in their own institutions.—P.M. Ness, M.D.

Oxygen Extraction Ratio: A Valid Indicator of Transfusion Need in Limited Coronary Vascular Reserve?

Levy PS, Chavez RP, Crystal GJ, Kim S-J, Eckel PK, Sehgal LR, Sehgal HL, Salem MR, Gould SA (Humana Hosp–Michael Reese, Chicago; Univ of Illinois, Chicago)
J Trauma 32:769–774, 1992   5–25

Introduction.—Myocardial lactate production (-LACT), which indicates anaerobic metabolism, does not occur in normal hearts until the extraction ratio (ER) is more than 50% and the hematocrit is less than 10%. It remains to be seen, however, whether ER is a reliable indicator

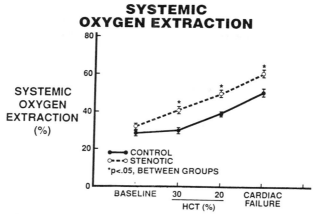

SYSTEMIC OXYGEN EXTRACTION

Fig 5–3.—Systemic oxygen extraction vs. hematocrit. (Courtesy of Levy PS, Chavez RP, Crystal GJ, et al: *J Trauma* 32:769–774, 1992.)

of the need for transfusion in patients with coronary stenosis. The effect of critical left anterior descending (LAD) coronary stenosis on compensation to acute blood loss anemia was assessed using dogs.

Methods.—Fourteen adult mongrel dogs were anesthetized, paralyzed, and mechanically ventilated. Half of the animals then underwent creation of a critical LAD stenosis; the rest were controls. Isovolemic exchange transfusion with 6% hetastarch in .9% NS was done until cardiac failure occurred. Measurements were made via catheters in the aorta, pulmonary artery, and anterior interventricular coronary vein.

Results.—Cardiac failure developed at a hematocrit of 9% in the control group vs. 17% in the stenosis group. The control animals had an increase in cardiac output, but the stenosis group did not. In both groups, -LACT began at a hematocrit of less than 20% and coincided with an ER of greater than 50% (Fig 5–3).

Conclusion.—These experimental findings suggest that cardiac failure occurs at a higher hematocrit in the presence of a critical LAD stenosis. Even in the presence of limited coronary vascular reserve, a whole-body ER of greater than 50% remains a valid indicator of myocardial metabolism in anemia and may be a useful guide to transfusion therapy.

▶ To reduce unnecessary blood transfusions, a consensus conference at the NIH on perioperative transfusion practices suggested that most patients do not require transfusions until their hematocrit decreases to less than 21%. One purpose of this meeting was to deflate the myth that transfusions were appropriate for all patients with hematocrits less than 30%. As part of the ensuing discussions, an intermediate group of patients has been identified with other medical factors that may make the lower limit of 21% unreasonably dangerous. Because most of these discussions of appropriate transfusion trigger were conducted from old data or anecdotes, studies such as the current citation are a welcome infusion of fact on which to base clinical practice. Using a dog model, these investigators occluded a portion of the coronary circulation to determine when biochemical determinations of cardiac function become abnormal. Using the ER of oxygen as a measure, they showed that cardiac failure developed at a hematocrit of 9% in healthy animals vs. 17% in animals with coronary stenosis. In clinical transfusion practice, the transfusion trigger should be established to allow for an additional margin of safety, so that most physicians would not allow patients to decrease to the low levels of 9% or 17%; however, this type of study may help to establish reasonable cutoffs that would minimize transfusions without jeopardizing patient care.—P.M. Ness, M.D.

Reevaluation of Current Transfusion Practices in Patients in Surgical Intensive Care Units
Babineau TJ, Dzik WH, Borlase BC, Baxter JK, Bistrian BR, Benotti PN (Harvard Med School, Boston)
Am J Surg 164:22–25, 1992

5–26

Background.—Wide concern over complications from packed red cell transfusion has prompted reassessment of conventional transfusion practices. Despite recent attempts to more clearly define indications for transfusion, especially for critically ill patients, transfusions still are ordered whenever the hemoglobin level is less than 10 g/dL. The impact of red cell transfusion on oxygen consumption was examined in 30 criti-

Red Cell Transfusion and Oxygen Metabolism			
	Pretransfusion* (n = 33)	Posttransfusion (n = 33)	p Value (*t*-test)
Hgb (g/dL)	9.4 ± 0.2	10.4 ± 0.3	<0.001
DO2 (mL/min/m²)	401 ± 20	433 ± 21	0.01
VO2 (mL/min/m²)	117 ± 4	115 ± 5	NS
SaO2 (%)	96 ± 1	95 ± 1	0.005
SvO2 (%)	67 ± 1	70 ± 1	0.005
Extract (%)	31 ± 1	28 ± 1	0.003
CI (L/min/m²)	3.2 ± 0.2	3.2 ± 0.2	NS
MAP (torr)	78 ± 3	81 ± 3	NS
SVR (dynes · s)	956 ± 49	1026 ± 63	NS
Heart rate (beats/min)	94 ± 3	92 ± 3	NS

Abbreviations: Hgb, hemoglobin; *CI,* cardiac index; *MAP,* mean arterial pressure; *SVR,* systemic vascular resistance; *SaO₂,* arterial oxygen saturation; *SvO₂,* venous oxygen saturation; *DO₂,* oxygen delivery; *VO₂,* oxygen consumption; *Extract,* oxygen extraction ratio.
* All transfusion values are mean ± SE.
(Courtesy of Babineau TJ, Dzik WH, Borlase BC, et al: *Am J Surg* 164:22–25, 1992.)

cally ill postoperative patients who received 33 transfusions because their hemoglobin level was less than 10 g/dL.

Results.—In the group, red cell transfusion did not appreciably alter oxygen consumption (table). Only one fourth of transfusions increased oxygen consumption by more than 20%. Oxygen consumption increased an average of 7% in septicemic patients but declined 9% on average in those who were not septic. Oxygen consumption increased after transfusion in all but 2 of 18 septic patients.

Conclusion.—The findings challenge the policy of transfusing patients solely on the basis of a hemoglobin level less than 10 g/dL. With such a policy, many transfused patients, especially nonseptic patients, will have no substantial rise in oxygen consumption.

▶ This article evaluated patients in intensive care with hematocrits slightly less than 30% to determine whether raising the hematocrit would increase oxygen consumption. Most of the transfusions in this setting had less than a 10% increase in oxygen consumption, with the exception of patients known to be septic. The study provides further evidence that the magical hematocrit of 30% should not be a rigid target for transfusions and that many patients, including those receiving intensive care, can tolerate lower hematocrits.—P.M. Ness, M.D.

Comparison of Two Transfusion Strategies After Elective Operations for Myocardial Revascularization
Johnson RG, Thurer RL, Kruskall MS, Sirois C, Gervino EV, Critchlow J, Weintraub RM (Beth Israel Hosp, Boston; Harvard Med School, Boston)
J Thorac Cardiovasc Surg 104:307–314, 1992   5–27

Background.—Strategies have been developed to limit transfused blood because of its limited availability and the risk of infection. Hemodilution is an accepted part of these strategies, but the degree of tolerable anemia has not been established. A liberal and a conservative postoperative transfusion strategy were compared in patients undergoing elective surgery.

Study Design.—A prospective, randomized trial was performed in 39 patients undergoing elective surgery and receiving autologous blood transfusions. The liberal group received transfusions to achieve a hematocrit value of 32% and the conservative group to achieve a value of less than 25%.

Outcome.—The 2 groups had significantly different mean hematocrit values from the fourth postoperative hour through the fifth postoperative day. However, there were no significant differences in fluid requirement, hemodynamic parameters, hospital complications, or length of stay in the intensive care unit or hospital (table). There were no significant differences in postoperative characteristics or management. How-

Postoperative Complications and Length of Stay

	Liberal transfusion	Conservative transfusion
No. of patients	18	20
Perioperative myocardial infarction	1	0
Pulmonary edema	1	0
Pneumothorax	0	2
Cerebrovascular accident	0	1
Postpericardiotomy syndrome	1	1
Arrhythmias	6	4
Mean length of stay (days)		
Intensive care	3.3 ± 3.4	3.2 ± 0.7
Total postop.	7.6 ± 1.9	7.9 ± 4.3

(Courtesy of Johnson RG, Thurer RL, Kruskall MS, et al: J Thorac Cardiovasc Surg 104:307–314, 1992.)

ever, significantly fewer units of packed cells were required in the conservative group. Exercise tests were performed on the fifth and sixth postoperative days. There were no significant differences between the 2 groups in duration or degree of exercise on either day.

Summary.—No adverse consequence could be ascribed to increased hemodilution. In fact, there was no direct relationship between the hematocrit value and exercise tolerance. Therefore, no arbitrary value can serve as an indication for transfusion. Instead, surgeons should accept whatever level of hemodilution their patients can tolerate, as determined by clinical indications. The benefits of increased hemodilution lie in the decreased requirement for total postoperative blood.

▶ This well-designed randomized study compared 2 transfusion strategies in patients undergoing cardiac surgery; 1 group of patients was liberally transfused to achieve hematocrits of 32%, whereas the other group was transfused to reach a target hematocrit of 25%. No differences in adverse events, postoperative exercise tolerance, or any parameter other than units of blood transfused in the perioperative period could be demonstrated. These studies reinforce the evolving data base that suggests that transfusion therapy should be individually directed by clinical symptomatology and not by arbitrary laboratory data.—P.M. Ness, M.D.

Fresh Blood Units Contain Large Potent Platelets That Improve Hemostasis After Open Heart Operations

Mohr R, Goor DA, Yellin A, Moshkovitz Y, Shinfeld A, Martinowitz U (The Chaim Sheba Med Ctr, Tel Hashomer, Israel)

Ann Thorac Surg 53:650–654, 1992

5–28

Introduction.—Platelets are the determinant of quality of hemostasis after open heart operations. Why fresh whole blood (FWB) is superior to platelet concentrates in aiding recovery of platelet function after these procedures was determined. It was assumed that the larger and more potent platelets are sedimented together with the packed cell fraction during centrifugation for separation of the platelet concentrate.

Patients and Methods.—Forty patients who were to undergo coronary bypass grafting were randomized to receive either platelet-rich plasma (PRP) separated from FWB (group A) or freshly packed RBCs (PC) after removal of PRP (group B). The PC and PRP were transfused to the patients immediately after bypass grafting. Postoperative hematologic variations studied included bleeding time, platelet count, mean platelet volume, and platelet aggregation in response to collagen, adenosine diphosphate, and epinephrine.

Results.—Platelet number in the PRP group was greater than in the PC group, but the difference was not significant. Group A patients bled more postoperatively than those in group B and received more RBC units and a larger number of blood products. Although transfusion of PRP to group A increased the platelet count, platelet functions did not improve. In group B, administration of PC increased the platelet count, improved platelet aggregation with collagen and epinephrine, and corrected the prolonged bleeding time.

Conclusion.—During preparation of platelet concentrates, fresh blood is separated into PC and PRP. The larger, more potent platelets are sedimented during centrifugation and are not included in the PRP. Thus, the platelets contained in FWB are more effective than those in platelet concentrates.

▶ One of the historic teachings in transfusion practice in that platelets will not survive cold storage; therefore, refrigerated whole blood will not support platelet function. A number of clinical investigations in the past few years by these authors (1) and others (2) have shown that clinical hemostatic benefits can be obtained in FWB or blood stored for as long as 48 hours. In this article, Mohr and his colleagues have extended their previous work by showing that the larger, more potent platelets are often not recovered in platelet concentrates made from whole blood; the platelets remaining after platelet harvesting will function even in red cell concentrates stored for several days. The implications of this type of study are profound. First, concentrates of platelets made from buffy coats, a practice common in Europe, may provide better hemostasis than our current platelet-harvesting procedures. Second, we may need to reconsider our attempts to discourage the use of fresh blood components in some cases where early hemostasis is important. One means of providing fresh red cells with platelets may be perioperative hemodilution, a procedure that is currently underused in the United States.—P.M. Ness, M.D.

References

1. Mohr R, et al: *J Thorac Cardiovasc Surg* 96:530–534, 1988.
2. Manno CS, et al: *Blood* 77:930–936, 1991.

Electrolyte and Acid-Base Changes With Massive Blood Transfusions
Wilson RF, Binkley LE, Sabo FM Jr, Wilson JA, Munkarah MM, Dulchavsky SA, Diebel LN (Detroit Receiving Hosp; Wayne State Univ, Detroit)
Am Surg 58:535–545, 1992   5–29

Introduction.—A high rate of complications and death has been indicated in patients given 10 or more units of blood within 24 hours. An increasing number of injured and critically ill patients require large amounts of blood.

Series.—Complications were surveyed in 471 patients who, from 1980 to 1991, received 10 or more units of blood within 24 hours. Trauma was responsible for blood loss in 370. The average number of blood units given in 24 hours was 21.

Results.—The mortality in 185 patients whose arterial pH was less than 7.15 during transfusion therapy was 71%. Surviving patients had less severe acidosis and higher bicarbonate values. Combined metabolic and respiratory acidosis (which often followed bicarbonate therapy) was associated with a mortality of 83%. Serum potassium levels were higher in patients who died within 48 hours of transfusion therapy. An ionized calcium level less than .7 mmol/L carried a mortality of 71%, compared with 40% in those with more normal values. Seven of 16 nontrauma patients who died were hypomagnesemic.

Conclusion.—It is very important to control bleeding rapidly and to restore the blood volume in patients given massive transfusions. The arterial pH, partial pressure of carbon dioxide, potassium, and ionized calcium levels should be monitored closely. Bicarbonate should not be given unless necessary, and, if it is, care is needed to avoid hypercarbia.

▶ This paper, an excellent discussion of the metabolic effects of massive transfusions, provides guidelines for the management of these patients and should be an excellent reference for those with interest in this complex problem.—P.M. Ness, M.D.

Clinical Trial of a Hemoglobin Based Blood Substitute in Patients With Sickle Cell Anemia

Feola M, Simoni J, Angelillo R, Luhruma Z, Kabakele M, Manzombi M, Kaluila M (Texas Tech Univ, Lubbock; Univ of Naples' II Polyclinico, Italy; Inst de Recherche en Sciences de la Sante—Ctr del'Anemie SS, Kinshasa, Zaire)

Surg Gynecol Obstet 174:379–386, 1992   5–30

Background.—Sickle cell anemia (SCA) is a serious problem in Zaire and the surrounding area. A hemoglobin-based "blood substitute," developed at Texas Tech University during the past 10 years, was used in a group of children with SCA admitted to a center in Zaire.

Patients and Methods.—Nine children were treated with the blood substitute. Five children were seen because of "aplastic crisis," and 4 were hospitalized because of unremitting severe pain from a "vaso-occlusive crisis." The blood substitute, containing 10% hemoglobin, was infused in a volume corresponding to 25% of blood volume, calculated for each child as equal to 7% of the body weight in kilograms.

Outcome.—None of the children suffered adverse reactions. All showed beneficial effects. The hemoglobin solution stimulated bone marrow to a significant erythropoietic effect in the patients with aplastic crisis. The number of reticulocytes in the peripheral blood of those patients increased from 0 to 47%. In the children with vaso-occlusive crisis, pain was alleviated quickly.

Conclusion.—This is the first report of a blood substitute administered to patients in large volumes and obtaining a beneficial rather than a toxic effect. Further research is needed to elucidate the mechanisms of the effects.

▶ Hemoglobin-based blood substitutes are a topic of major commercial and clinical interest. Several potential toxicities have inhibited their development, including renal toxicity and vasoconstrictive effects. Because these toxicities have slowed clinical evaluation in the United States with the Food and Drug Administration showing appropriate caution, this evaluation of a blood substitute in Africa presents some intriguing results and medical-ethical concerns. The feared toxicities did not seem to materialize, but the number of patients studied and the methods used were probably inadequate for evaluation. Was the described erythropoietic effect real or just the timely resolution of aplastic crisis? Whether it is ethical to study a potentially toxic treatment in patients for whom it will ultimately be too expensive to receive is a troubling question.—P.M. Ness, M.D.

A Human Recombinant Haemoglobin Designed for Use as a Blood Substitute

Looker D, Abbott-Brown D, Cozart P, Durfee S, Hoffman S, Mathews AJ, Miller-Roehrich J, Shoemaker S, Trimble S, Fermi G, Komiyama NH, Nagai K, Stetler GL (Somatogen Inc, Boulder, Colo; MRC Lab of Molecular Biology, Cambridge, England)
Nature 356:258–260, 1992   5–31

Background.—The need to develop a blood substitute is now more important than ever. Cell-free hemoglobin solutions and human hemoglobin synthesized in *Escherichia coli* and *Saccharomyces cerevisiae* as potential oxygen-carrying substitutes for RBCs have been studied. However, these hemoglobins cannot be used as a blood substitute for 2 reasons. The oxygen affinity in the absence of 2,3-bisphosphoglycerate is too high to allow unloading of enough oxygen in the tissues, and they dissociate into α-β-dimers cleared rapidly by renal filtration, which could lead to long-term kidney damage. A human recombinant hemoglobin designed for use as a blood substitute was described.

Methods and Results.—An *E. coli* expression vector was constructed containing 2 copies of the α-globin gene fused in tandem by a single codon encoding a glycine residue. This produced a fusion junction with the sequence Arg(141α) GlyVal(1α2). A single operon encoding a di-α-globin and a β-globin chain in this construct are transcribed from a single TAC promoter. An additional Asn-108β→Lys mutation was introduced to reduce the oxygen affinity of this engineered hemoglobin. The fusion of the 2 α-globin subunits lengthens the half-life of this hemoglobin molecule in vivo by preventing its dissociation into α-β-dimers, thus eliminating renal toxicity.

Conclusion.—This engineered hemoglobin is a strong candidate for a safe blood substitute. Genetically fused di-α-hemoglobin can be made in large quantities by simple microbial fermentation and purified without further modification, unlike hemoglobins that have been cross-linked chemically.

▶ Several approaches are used in the attempt to produce hemoglobin-base blood substitutes. One approach uses outdated red cells, removes the red cell membrane, and polymerizes the hemoglobin to arrive at a product with improved in vitro persistence, adequate viscosity, and useful oxygen delivery characteristics; another approach uses recombinant technology to produce human hemoglobin, but the costs of scaling up this methodology may be huge. This article described an innovative recombinant that was used to produce a mutant hemoglobin that will not require polymerization steps for potential efficacy. Whether this interesting method comes to the marketplace as a usable clinical product remains to be seen.—P.M. Ness, M.D.

A Randomized Trial Comparing Intravenous Immune Globulin and Plasma Exchange in Guillain-Barré Syndrome

van der Meché FGA, Schmitz PIM, Dutch Guillain-Barré Study Group (Academic Hosp Rotterdam, The Netherlands; Daniel den Hoed Cancer Ctr, Rotterdam, The Netherlands)
N Engl J Med 326:1123–1129, 1992   5–32

Background.—Treatment of patients with Guillain-Barré syndrome using plasma exchange results in faster improvement and significantly shorter periods of artificial ventilation than using supportive care alone. This treatment is generally agreed to be indicated for patients with major deficits in the first weeks of their disease. Treatment with immune globulin might also be effective for this syndrome. The latter treatment is more simply, more easily, and more quickly administered; more readily available; and is considered safe, especially with respect to viral transmission. The efficacy of treatment with immune globulin therapy was compared with that of plasma exchange for patients with Guillain-Barré syndrome.

Methods and Results.—Patients were eligible for this multicenter study if they had acute Guillain-Barré syndrome for less than 2 weeks, could not walk independently, and were age 4 years or older. They were randomly assigned to receive either 5 sessions of exchange of 200–250 mL of plasma per kg, or .4 g of immune globulin daily for 5 days. At entry and 16 times during 6 months of follow-up, patients were tested by motor functional score and Medical Research Council scores for 6 bilateral muscle groups. At each data collection after randomization, the proportion of patients who did not improve on the functional scale was shown

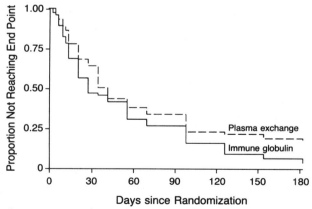

Fig 5–4.—Kaplan-Meier curves indicating the proportion of patients who did not have improvement by 1 or more functional grades during 182 days of follow-up, according to treatment group (P = .05). (Courtesy of van der Meché FGA, Schmitz PIM, Dutch Guillain-Barré Study Group: N *Engl J Med* 326:1123–1129, 1992.)

in a Kaplan-Meier curve (Fig 5–4). The main outcome measure was improvement by at least 1 grade on the functional scale by 4 weeks after randomization; secondary outcome measures included the time required for improvement of at least 1 functional grade and to regain the capacity for independent walking.

Results.—Of the first 150 evaluable, randomized patients, 53% of those who received immune globulin had improved their functional score—significantly more than 34% of those who received plasma exchange. The median time for improvement was 27 days for patients who received immune globulin—significantly less than the 41 days for patients who received plasma exchange. The median time to the recovery of independent walking was shorter for patients who received immune globulin than for those who received plasma exchange. Differences in functional score between the 2 treatments were most obvious earlier in the follow-up, when artificial ventilation was often required and most complications occurred. Five incidents of adverse effects were associated with administration of 380 infusions of immune globulin, but none was serious enough to interrupt treatment.

Conclusion.—Treatment with immune globulin seems to be safe and at least as efficacious as treatment with plasma exchange for patients with acute Guillain Barré syndrome.

▶ Patients with Guillain-Barré syndrome have benefited from plasmapheresis as documented by reduced ventilator support and shortened hospital stays. Because plasmapheresis is expensive, invasive, and not always available, other means to treat this disease would be useful. Anecdotal reports suggest that intravenous gamma-globulin may be useful treatment by a mechanism that remains unknown. This carefully performed, randomized clinical trial showed that intravenous gamma-globulin was safe and at least as effective as plasmapheresis in patients with Guillain-Barré syndrome. The use of a blinded observer of neurologic function adds additional confidence in the study's conclusions.—P.M. Ness, M.D.

Controlled Trial of Plasma Exchange and Leukapheresis in Polymyositis and Dermatomyositis
Miller FW, Leitman SF, Cronin ME, Hicks JE, Leff RL, Wesley R, Fraser DD, Dalakas M, Plotz PH (NIH, Bethesda, Md)
N Engl J Med 326:1380–1384, 1992   5–33

Introduction.—The commonly occurring polymyositis and dermatomyositis appear resistant to corticosteroid treatment. Clinicians have tried other therapies (e.g., the costly plasma exchange and leukapheresis) to alleviate the many symptoms related to these 2 conditions. Although reportedly beneficial, plasma exchange and leukapheresis have not been tested in patients with either condition. Each therapy in 39 patients was evaluated.

Methods.—Patients with either definite polymyositis or dermatomyositis after muscle biopsy participated in the study. The selected candidates were randomly assigned to undergo 1 of the follwing procedures: plasma exchange, leukapheresis, or sham apheresis.

Results.—The 3 groups had similar demographic and clinical characteristics after randomization. After the procedures, the 3 treatment groups demonstrated no significant difference in muscle strength or functional capacity. Most muscle biochemistry tests were similar for all patients except that the patients with plasma exchange and leukapheresis had significantly higher serum creatine kinase levels than sham-operated patients, but this outcome did not correlate with any clinical parameters. Adverse effects from the apheresis procedure were encountered. Nine patients improved (2 leukapheresis, 1 plasma exchange, and 6 sham procedure) so that their prednisone dose could be tapered. Even after aggressive therapy, 9 patients died of disease complications.

Conclusion.—Leukapheresis and plasma exchange rank with sham apheresis in treating corticosteroid-resistant polymyositis or dermatomyositis and, therefore, are not recommended as treatment for patients with these disorders.

▶ Clinical trials that are performed with care can be of great value in identifying therapies that clearly do not work as well as those with efficacy. This double-blind, sham-controlled study of plasma exchange and leukapheresis showed no benefit in patients with polymyositis and dermatomyositis. Because these therapies are expensive and have some adverse effects, this study should be of use to ensure that limited plasmapheresis capabilities and health care dollars are not spent for treatments not likely to be of therapeutic benefit.—P.M. Ness, M.D.

Experience With Autologous Bone Marrow Harvesting and Transfusion of Marrow-Derived Red Cells
Ciobanu N, Weinberg V, Sparano JA, Zervos G, Walewski J, Spivack M, Wiernik PH (Albert Einstein Cancer Ctr, New York; Montefiore Med Ctr, New York)
Transfusion 32:231–234, 1992   5–34

Background.—Autologous bone marrow transplantation is used with increasing frequency and success to treat a variety of malignancies. Autologous RBC transfusions are, for several reasons, an attractive alternative to homologous blood administration after marrow harvest. The results of marrow-derived RBC (MRBC) transfusions in patients undergoing marrow harvests were evaluated.

Patients and Methods.—Fifty-five consecutive patients undergoing 56 marrow harvests at 2 centers from 1987 to 1989 were studied. The

MRBCs from the autologous bone marrow harvests were rescued after processing and transfused as the sole transfusion support after surgery.

Findings.—The volume of harvest was uncorrelated with the total mononuclear cell count. The marrow collection induced a significant reduction in hematocrit values that was unrelated to diagnosis, patient age, or patient gender. Marrow processing resulted in a mean transfused MRBC mass of 258 mL, or 78% of the MRBC mass collected. There was a correlation between the amount of MRBCs transfused and the total mononuclear cell count. The patients tolerated MRBC transfusions well.

Conclusion.—In this series, all autologous MRBC transfusions were tolerated well and resulted in normalization of vital signs. Thus, patients undergoing marrow harvest for autologous use or for transfusion to unrelated bone marrow recipients should not need homologous blood transfusions. Preoperative autologous blood donation may be beneficial to prevent the transient, unstable vital signs that are sometimes associated with the procedure.

▶ Autologous bone marrow transplant procedures typically involve the harvesting of the bone marrow from the patient/donor with the marrow being processed and stored in the frozen state for subsequent infusion. The processing procedures and conditions for storage maximize hematopoietic cell recovery, and the red cells are a byproduct that is typically discarded. If the processing of the marrow can be performed rapidly, the red cells can be harvested and returned to the donor/patient who is often anemic because of chemotherapy or disease. These authors have shown that this procedure can work and can limit exposure to homologous blood components that may otherwise be necessary at harvest. The same technology can be applied to nonrelated bone marrow donors or ABO-incompatible bone marrow donors so that the donor's red cells can be returned if the marrow is subjected to cell processing. If the procedures are set up with care, the use of MRBCs is worthwhile.—P.M. Ness, M.D.

Pediatric Transfusion Practices

Red Blood Cell Transfusion and Cesarean Section

Dickason LA, Dinsmoor MJ (Med College of Virginia/Virginia Commonwealth Univ, Richmond)

Am J Obstet Gynecol 167:327-332, 1992   5–35

Background.—Preoperative autologous blood transfusions can reduce the risk of infection in some patients. However, in the obstetric patient, transfusion requirements are difficult to predict. Patients who required blood transfusions at the time of cesarean section were described, and factors that might predict transfusion need were identified.

Patients and Methods.—The charts of 61 cesarean patients who had received a packed red cell transfusion either intraoperatively or postop-

Comparison of Cesarean Section Characteristics in Patients
With and Without Blood Transfusions

Variable	Blood transfusion (n = 61)		No blood transfusion (n = 69)		p Value
	No.	%	No.	%	
Indication for cesarean section					
Elective repeat cesarean section	6	10	9	13	NS
Arrest of labor	7	12	16	23	NS
Fetal distress	16	26	16	23	NS
Placenta previa	8	13	0	0	0.002
Arrest of descent	8	13	2	3	0.045
Abnormal presentation	9	15	18	26	NS
Other	4	7	5	7	NS
Type of cesarean section					
Low transverse	41	67	65	94	0.004*
Vertical	14	23	4	6	0.005*
Cesarean hysterectomy	6	10	0	0	0.009*
Anesthesia					
General	32	53	20	29	0.007**
Epidural	21	34	39	57	0.014**
Spinal	3	5	6	9	NS
Other	5	8	4	6	NS
Preoperative hemoglobin (gm/dl, mean ± SD)	10.8 ± 1.7		11.6 ± 1.4		0.005

Abbreviation: NS, not significant.
*When compared with all other types of cesarean section combined.
† When compared with all other forms of anesthesia combined.
(Courtesy of Dickason LA, Dinsmoor MJ: Am J Obstet Gynecol 167:327–332, 1992.)

eratively were reviewed. An identical number of cesarean patients who had not received transfusions served as controls. Both groups were well matched regarding maternal age, prior cesarean section, neonatal birth weight, or intrauterine growth retardation.

Results.—Cesarean section indications included elective surgery, active-phase arrest, fetal distress, placenta previa, arrest of descent, and abnormal presentation. The 2 most often cited significant factors for cesarean section among the study group were placenta previa and arrest of descent (table). Lower gestational ages, antepartum bleeding, arrest of descent, and longer hospital stays correlated with transfusions. However, stepwise logistic regression analysis revealed that only antepartum bleeding and preoperative hemoglobin levels were significant independent predictors of the blood transfusion need.

Conclusion.—Although RBC transfusion is frequently performed during cesarean section, it is difficult to predict exactly which patients would benefit most from autologous donation. Therefore, the role of autologous donation in obstetric care remains to be defined.

▶ The appropriate patients who should be offered autologous donation are difficult to determine. Transfusions in the setting of labor and delivery with cesarean section were documented to occur in 6.8% of patients in this study with a mean transfusion exposure of 2.8 units. Because the majority of labor and delivery patients do not require transfusions, even if cesarean section becomes necessary, these authors attempted to find out whether any predictors could be determined. The only significant predictors were antepartum bleeding and low preoperative hemoglobin levels. Although it might be feasible to offer autologous donation to patients with high-risk conditions such as placenta previa, these authors reinforce other published studies that suggest that autologous donation has minimal use and a high potential for wasted services in the setting of labor and delivery.—P.M. Ness, M.D.

Delivery of Infants With Glanzmann Thrombasthenia and Subsequent Blood Transfusion Requirements: A Follow-Up of 39 Patients
Awidi AS (Jordan Univ, Amman)
Am J Hematol 40:1–4, 1992   5–36

Background.—Glanzmann's thrombasthenia (GT), an autosomal recessive condition, is characterized by lifelong mucosal bleeding, prolonged bleeding time, and no platelet aggregation with physiologic aggregating agents. The condition is common in some Middle Eastern countries. With prenatal diagnosis, fetuses with GT can now be detected in utero. It is not known whether cesarean section should be done in a heterozygous mother carrying a GT fetus. It is also important to determine bleeding complications to establish the safety of vaginal delivery and to study blood transfusion requirements in patients with GT.

Patients and Findings.—All patients between 1981 and 1989 who had a diagnosis of GT at a hospital in Jordan were included in the study. Thirty-nine patients from 22 families were confirmed to have GT. Type I thrombasthenia was found in 21 females and 12 males. Four females and 2 males had type II thrombasthenia. Twenty-one of the patients were born in the hospital, and 18 were born at home. All deliveries were vaginal. Neonates affected with thrombasthenia had no excessive hemorrhagic symptoms. The patients, followed for a total of 220 patient-years, received a total of 276 units of blood. The main reason for transfusion in the females was menorrhagia followed by gum bleeding and epistaxis. In the males, the transfusion was done most commonly for epistaxis, gum bleeding, and circumcision.

Conclusion.—Because GT is rare in the West, physicians caring for patients with this disorder must face many unanswered questions. In this series, there was no major bleeding in neonates with GT delivered vaginally. Some minor bleeding occurred, but it was not life-threatening and required no specific therapy. None of the neonates died. After puberty, the major bleeding problem in girls is menorrhagia.

▶ Most hematologists have taken care of very few patients with GT, a hereditary condition arising from the deficiency of glycoprotein IIb/IIIa from platelets. In families with this disorder, affected fetuses can now be detected in utero. The question of how to deliver the fetus then arises, and our limited clinical experience usually results in an elective cesarean section to protect the infant. The disorder is more common in the Middle East where Dr. Awidi was able to collect information from 39 patients (22 families) with GT. He found that none of the neonates had hemorrhagic symptoms, despite the fact that all underwent vaginal delivery, often at home. In subsequent follow-up studies, most of the patients did require transfusions later. We owe thanks to Dr. Awidi for helping us to answer this question.—P.M. Ness, M.D.

Prevention of Transfusion-Associated Cytomegalovirus Infection in Neonatal Patients by the Removal of White Cells From Blood

Eisenfeld L, Silver H, McLaughlin J, Klevjer-Anderson P, Mayo D, Anderson J, Herson V, Krause P, Savidakis J, Lazar A, Rosenkrantz T, Pisciotto P (Hartford and St. Francis Hosps, Conn; John Dempsey Hosp, Farmington, Conn)
Transfusion 32:205–209, 1992   5–37

Introduction.—Very-low-birth-weight (VLBW) neonates frequently receive many blood transfusions. These infants are at high risk for transfusion-associated cytomegalovirus (CMV) disease because they do not receive their mother's CMV antibodies. The death rate from transfusion-associated CMV among these young patients has been reported at 38%. A test of the WBC reduction of donor blood using a modified spin-cool-filter (SCF) method to remove about 95% of the WBCs and then using this filtered blood in VLBW neonates was done.

Methods.—The VLBW infants were born to CMV-seronegative women who had received at least 1 CMV-seropositive RBC transfusion. One group of neonates received RBCs prepared from whole blood using the SCF technique after centrifugation. Another neonate group received a transfusion of blood filtered with a WBC-induction filter that reportedly removed 98% of WBCs.

Results.—Of the 369 VLBW neonates born in the testing facility, 321 were eliminated. Of the remaining 48, 26 neonates received the SCF-filtered transfusions and 22 received the WBC-reduced transfusions. The CMV antibody prevalence in the blood from donors was about 37%. At discharge, the clinical and laboratory data demonstrated that 47 of 48 infants had no transfusion-associated CMV infection. One infant had transiently seroconverted because of passive transfer of the antibody.

Conclusion.—White blood cell and platelet reduction of donor blood may lower, or even prevent, the transfusion-associated CMV infections found in high-risk neonatal patients, particularly in situations when testing the blood supply for CMV would greatly delay or compromise the infant's chances of survival.

▶ With the expansion of indications for CMV-negative blood components from neonates to immunosuppressed oncology patients and transplant recipients, it has become even more difficult to find adequate supplies of seronegative blood. Because CMV is a cell-associated virus, techniques to remove white cells are also likely to reduce the risk of CMV transmission. This study of neonates used 2 techniques to remove white cells, in the range of 1 to 2 logs. Both techniques were successful in a small sample of patients. More extensive leukocyte depletion techniques are now available with other filters to reduce residual white cell levels to less than 10^6. Because these techniques have been effective in reducing CMV in bone marrow transplant recipients, the newer filter techniques for leukocyte depletion should be equally effective in neonatal medicine. The SCF technique would not be as reliable but might be used in an occasional emergency situation.—P.M. Ness, M.D.

Autologous Transfusions for Orthopaedic Procedures at a Children's Hospital
Simpson MB, Georgopoulos G, Orsini E, Eilert RE (Brake Army Med Ctr, Fort Sam Houston, Tex; The Children's Hosp, Denver)
J Bone Joint Surg [Am] 74-A:652–658, 1992   5–38

Introduction.—Although autologous blood donation is the preferred method of providing blood components for patients undergoing elective operations, underuse of programs to collect autologous blood remains a problem. The autologous blood program at a tertiary-care children's hospital was reviewed to determine its success in avoiding exposure to homologous blood in children undergoing orthopedic procedures.

Methods and Findings.—During a 5-year period, 198 children scheduled for an orthopedic admission donated blood. Twenty-three of these patients never received a transfusion and were eliminated from the analysis. The remaining 175 patients, who underwent a total of 202 procedures, needed autologous blood. The average number of units requested was 3.8, and the average number of units obtained and transfused was 3.4. Requirements were lower for the 25% of children with low body weight. Autologous blood only was given in 73% of cases. Intraoperative salvage was also used in 70 patients, but no benefit of this procedure could be proved. Problems arose in the preoperative donation of autologous blood in 40 patients, most commonly inability to obtain a sufficient amount of blood for storage. These problems were rarely serious, however. In a surprisingly high 7% of patients, human error results in them receiving homologous transfusion when autologous blood was available. Generally accepted criteria for transfusion were not met in 40% of all transfusions and in 38% of postoperative transfusions, homologous as well as autologous.

Conclusion.—Preoperative donation of autologous blood is a successful means of limiting exposure to homologous blood in children undergoing elective orthopedic procedures. Problems may arise, but most are not serious. Human errors and complications can occur, however. Surgeons should observe the standard indications for transfusion rather than administering homologous units just because they are available.

▶ This article reminds us that autologous programs benefit children undergoing elective surgery procedures as well as adults. That 7% of their patients received homologous blood as a result of human error when autologous blood was available may be startling to the non–blood bank audience; those of us who work in blood centers and transfusion services know that autologous services are difficult to provide and become very complicated interactions involving many individuals and organizations. A 7% failure rate is clearly unacceptable, but its documentation in this study may prompt others to examine their systems and improve them.—P.M. Ness, M.D.

Transplantation

Efficacy of a Single Pretransplant Donor-Specific Transfusion and Cyclosporin A Administered 24 to 48 Hours Before One-Haplotype–Mismatched Living Related Donor Kidney Transplant

Davies CB, Alexander JW, Cofer BR, First MR, Schroeder TJ (Univ of Cincinnati, Ohio)
Ann Surg 215:618–626, 1992   5–39

Background.—Elimination of multiple donor-specific blood transfusion (DST) sensitization is a concern for one-haplotype–mismatched living related transplant recipients. A single pretransplant DST immediately followed by cyclosporine infusion may aid in alleviating sensitization.

Patients and Methods.—A total of 86 one-haplotype–mismatched living related donor kidney recipients participated in 1 of 3 DST transfusion and cyclosporine treatment protocols. Thirty-four received multiple pretransplant DSTs and cyclosporine after the transplant (group 1); 31 received multiple pretransplant DSTs and pretransplant cyclosporine (group 2); and 21 received a single DST 24 to 48 hours before the transplant and intravenous cyclosporine initiation after the transfusion (group 3). Triple immunosuppression (prednisone, azathioprine, and cyclosporine) was continued in each group postoperatively.

Results.—At 1 year, patient and graft survival were comparable for the 3 groups; patient survival was 97%, 97%, and 93%, and graft survival was 91%, 90%, and 87% in groups 1, 2, and 3, respectively. In addition, no significant differences were found in rejection incidence or infectious complications at 1 year. Rejections occurred in 61%, 45%, and 60%, and infectious complications in 26%, 42%, and 47% of groups 1, 2, and 3, respectively.

Conclusion.—A single DST given 24 to 48 hours preoperatively followed by pretransplant cyclosporine is an effective alternative to traditional DST conditioning using either pre- or post-transplant cyclosporine. The single DST protocol is also less expensive and easier to administer. Finally, donors will not be eliminated because of sensitization with the single DST procedure. Further studies are suggested to determine the long-term benefits of combined DST and cyclosporine treatment.

▶ The use of blood transfusions from living related kidney donors has been a valuable adjunct to renal transplantation. Most of these protocols involved 3 transfusions during 1 month, and most of the studies took place before cyclosporine became widely available. The cited study showed that a single pretransplant donor-specific transfusion with pretransplant or post-transplant cyclosporine was as effective as a series of DSTs and was clearly much easier for the patient and the donor.—P.M. Ness, M.D.

Immunohematologic Complications of ABO-Unmatched Liver Transplants

Triulzi DJ, Shirey RS, Ness PM, Klein AS (Johns Hopkins School of Medicine, Baltimore, Md)
Transfusion 32:829–833, 1992   5–40

Introduction.—A limited supply of donor organs has led to the use of ABO-"unmatched" livers in as many as one third of liver transplant procedures. Recipients of such organs are at risk of having immune hemolysis caused by isohemagglutinins produced by passenger lymphocytes in the graft.

Patients and Methods.—The implications of using ABO-unmatched liver transplants were examined in a series of 41 patients having primary liver transplantation from 1989 to 1991. Six of the patients received a second transplant in the same period. Donor-derived antibody (DDAb) was detected by a positive direct antiglobulin isohemagglutinins of donor type.

Findings.—Nine of the 41 patients (22%) received 10 ABO-unmatched livers. Most of them were group O to A_1 mismatches. Five of 9 recipients of mismatched livers had DDAbs and hemolysis; all 5 of them were group A_1 and received group O livers. Hemolysis preceded the first positive direct antiglobulin test in 4 of 5 patients by a mean of nearly 2 days. The mean decrease in hemoglobin was 4.8 g/dL. Patients received a mean of 7.8 units of group O red cells. One patient had exchange transfusion for acute renal failure. Patients given unmatched grafts required twice as many red cell transfusions postoperatively as those given ABO-matched transplants.

Conclusion.—Recipients of ABO-unmatched livers are at high risk of having hemolysis, warranting the prophylactic use of donor-type red cells during and after liver transplantation.

▶ The use of group O livers, considered to be the universal donor type in blood transfusion, is complicated in as many as one half of group A liver recipients by hemolytic anemia developing 1–2 weeks after transplantation. This complication is caused by the production of isohemagglutinins by passenger lymphocytes in the graft. The hemolysis can last for several weeks before resolving spontaneously. This article failed to show any pretransplant donor characteristics that can identify a donor organ more likely to cause hemolysis. The suggestion that group O blood be used during the transplant procedure to reduce the red cell targets for subsequent hemolysis seems reasonable, although in some cases, group O cells also appear to be destroyed.—P.M. Ness, M.D.

Adverse Effects of Transfusion

Absence of Human Immunodeficiency Virus (HIV) Proviral Sequences in Seronegative Hemophilic Men and Sexual Partners of HIV-Seropositive Hemophiliacs

Bailly E, Kleim JP, Schneweis KE, van Loo B, Hammerstein U, Brackmann HH (Univ of Bonn, Germany)
Transfusion 32:104–108, 1992   5–41

Background.—Recent reports indicate that HIV-1 provirus may be detected by PCR in high-risk, seronegative individuals. Exposed but seronegative persons can be infected with HIV and apparently can pass through a long antibody-negative phase of latent infection. The possible occurrence of undiscovered HIV infection at a large hemophilia center was investigated.

Methods.—The PCR was used to examine specimens of peripheral blood leukocytes from patients with HIV-seronegative hemophilia and from the sexual partners of patients with HIV-seropositive hemophilia. The assessment involved the primer pair SK 38/39 derived from the gag region and/or the primer pair SK 68/69 corresponding to a conserved region of the *env* gene.

Findings.—The HIV proviral DNA was detected by PCR in 97% of the samples from 89 patients with HIV-seropositive hemophilia. However, no HIV-DNA was found in sera from 198 patients with HIV-seronegative hemophilia at risk. None of the 40 HIV-seronegative sexual partners of patients with HIV-infected hemophilia was PCR positive.

Conclusion.—The PCR is proving to be a sensitive way to confirm infection in patients with seropositive hemophilia. The negative findings in patients with HIV-seronegative hemophilia and HIV-seronegative sexual partners of patients with HIV-seronegative hemophilia suggest that a prolonged seronegative period of latent HIV infection is not typical.

▶ The 1989 publication of an article by Imagawa et al. (1) and the widespread media publicity about its findings led to this and other similar studies. Imagawa and his co-workers studied a group of homosexual men who appeared to remain HIV-seronegative for long periods during which HIV could be detected by more sensitive techniques such a PCR. These results suggested that transfusion recipients remained at risk despite HIV screening of the blood supply, and high-risk individuals with negative HIV antibody status might still be infected and infectious. This article failed to show HIV infection by PCR in seronegative men or their sex partners; many similar studies have been published for other publications. The findings of Imagawa have actually been retracted in subsequent correspondence. Despite all of this evidence to the contrary, the impression that HIV seroconversion is not a reliable determinant of HIV infection has been difficult to remove from the minds of the public and their physicians.—P.M. Ness, M.D.

Reference

1. Imagawa DT, et al: *N Engl J Med* 320:1458–1462, 1989.

Allogeneic Leukocytes But Not Therapeutic Blood Elements Induce Reactivation and Dissemination of Latent Human Immunodeficiency Virus Type 1 Infection: Implications for Transfusion Support of Infected Patients

Busch MP, Lee T-H, Heitman J (Irwin Mem Blood Ctrs, San Francisco; Univ of California, San Francisco)
Blood 80:2128–2135, 1992   5–42

Background.—Immune stimulation appears to facilitate both primary infection of cells by HIV-1 and the induction of HIV-1 replication in latently infected cells. Transfusing allogeneic blood components from heterologous donors is a strong immunologic stimulus and a potential route of lymphotropic virus transmission.

Methods.—The kinetics of HIV-1 expression and dissemination were examined in peripheral blood mononuclear cells from HIV-1–infected individuals after coculture with various transfused blood components. Cells from 3 anti–HIV-1–positive subjects were cultured with allogeneic donor blood mononuclear cells and with partially purified populations of various donor cell types.

Findings.—Allogeneic peripheral blood mononuclear cells led to dose-related activation of HIV-1 expression in cells infected in vivo and dissemination of virus to previously uninfected cells. Donor lymphocytes, monocytes, and granulocytes all activated HIV-1 replication, but leukocyte-depleted red cells, platelets, and plasma were ineffective. Allogeneic donor mononuclear cells upregulated expression of HIV-1 in a latently infected cell line and also made heterologous donor cells more susceptible to acute HIV-1 infection.

Conclusion.—Confirmation of these findings would suggest that HIV-1–infected patients be transfused as infrequently as possible and that leukocyte-depleted blood components be administered. Autologous transfusions or EPO therapy would be preferable.

▶ This important article demonstrates that HIV-infected cells become activated when exposed to allogeneic white cells. These in vitro data suggest that latent HIV infection or perhaps other latent viruses can be activated through blood transfusions and lead to more rapid disease progression. The data also suggest that removal of these white cells by a number of leukocyte depletion techniques could reduce the risk of viral activation from latency. Confirmation in patients by controlled clinical trials is being aggressively sought by a number of investigators, with the eager assistance of commercial vendors of leukocyte depletion technology. If this type of adverse effect of allogeneic white cells can be confirmed in patient experiments, the impetus for leukocyte depletion of all blood components will be difficult to deny.—P.M. Ness, M.D.

Transmission of Retroviruses From Seronegative Donors by Transfusion During Cardiac Surgery: A Multicenter Study of HIV-1 and HTLV-I/II Infections

Nelson KE, Donahue JG, Muñoz A, Cohen ND, Ness PM, Teague A, Stambolis VA, Yawn DH, Callicott B, McAllister H, Reitz BA, Lee H, Farzadegan H, Hollingsworth CG (Johns Hopkins Univ, Baltimore, Md; St Luke's Episcopal Hosp, Houston; Baylor College of Medicine, Houston; et al)
Ann Intern Med 117:554–559, 1992   5–43

Background.—The use of an enzyme-linked immunosorbent assay (ELISA) to detect HIV-1 antibodies has reduced, but not eliminated, inadvertent transmission of AIDS during transfusions. The prolonged interval between infection and seroconversion in blood donors has heightened concerns of continual retroviral infection from tested blood supplies. The incidence of HIV-1 and HTLV-I/II transmissions in cardiac patients receiving screened transfusions was monitored.

Patients and Methods.—A total of 9,294 cardiac patients receiving 120,312 units of blood components was examined. Serum samples were obtained and screened by ELISA for HIV-1 and HTLV-I/II antibodies before and 6 months after surgery.

Results.—Two new HIV-1 infections were found in these patients. In each case, a donor was identified who had been HIV-negative at the time of collection but had subsequently seroconverted. This represents an incidence of .0017% (1/60,000 units). Seven patients became infected with either HTLV-I or -II. Six of these patients were infected before blood screening processes were instituted. The combined rate of HTLV-I/II infection before testing was 1 in 8,500 units, which decreased to 1 in 69,272 units after screening. However, these differences were not statistically significant.

Conclusion.—Three factors have contributed to a low incidence of HIV-1 and HTLV-I/II transfusion-transmitted infections: antibody testing for HIV-1 and HTLV-1 (ELISA), high-risk donor exclusion via questionnaire results, and confidential unit exclusion. However, continued efforts to improve and monitor the safety of blood transfusions are necessary.

The Declining Risk of Post-Transfusion Hepatitis C Virus Infection

Donahue JG, Muñoz A, Ness PM, Brown DE Jr, Yawn DH, McAllister HA Jr, Reitz BA, Nelson KE (Johns Hopkins Univ, Baltimore, Md; Baylor College of Medicine, Houston; St Luke's Episcopal Hosp, Houston)
N Engl J Med 327:369–373, 1992
5–44

Introduction.—In the 1970s and early 1980s, the risk of transfusion-associated hepatitis C virus (HCV) was estimated at 5% to 18%. In late 1986, blood collection agencies began screening donated blood for surrogate markers of non-A, non-B hepatitis and antibodies to HCV. The current risk of transfusion-transmitted HCV infection was evaluated.

Rates of HCV Seroconversion, According to the Method Used to Screen Donated Blood

TYPE OF SCREENING	NO. OF SERO- CONVERSIONS	NO. OF PATIENTS AT RISK	NO. OF UNITS TRANSFUSED	SEROCONVERSION RATE	
				PER PATIENT	PER UNIT
				percent	
Routine only	35	912	7810	3.84	0.45
Routine plus surrogate markers	15	976	8015	1.54†	0.19‡
Routine plus surrogate markers and anti-HCV	3	522	9916	0.57§	0.03¶

† P = .001 for the comparison with routine screening only.
‡ P = .002 for the comparison with routine screening only.
§ P = .080 for the comparison with routine screening plus screening for surrogate markers.
¶ P = .001 for the comparison with routine screening plus screening for surrogate markers.
(Courtesy of Donahue JG, Muñoz A, Ness PM, et al: *N Engl J Med* 327:369–373, 1992.)

Patients and Methods.—In 1985–1991, blood samples and medical information were obtained prospectively from patients before and at least 6 months after cardiac surgery. Stored serum samples were tested for antibodies to HCV by an enzyme-linked immunosorbent assay (ELISA); samples positive on at least 2 of 3 ELISA tests were tested by a recombinant immunoblot assay (4-RIBA). The study included 912 patients transfused before donors were screened for surrogate markers, 976 who received transfusions with blood screened for surrogate markers, and 522 transfused since the addition of screening for antibodies.

Results.—The risk of seroconversion was 3.84% per patient in the first group, 1.54% per patient in the second group, and .57% per patient in the third group. The observed trend toward decreasing risk was statistically significant (table). After adjustment for the type of screening used, the risk of seroconversion to HCV increased with the number of units transfused. The 3 patients who seroconverted in the most recent period had transfusions involving 10–54 units of blood.

Conclusion.—The introduction of donor screening for surrogate markers and antibodies to HCV has substantially reduced the incidence of post-transfusion HCV. The current risk is about 3 per 10,000 units transfused.

▶ These 2 articles (Abstracts 5–43 and 5–44) come from a prospective study in 3 medical centers of cardiac surgery patients who received transfusions of blood from 1985 to 1991. The study was initially conceived to determine the risk of receiving blood that was screened and found to be negative for HIV but the patients still became HIV infected; the risk of HIV seroconversion was determined to be 1:60,000 units based on the exposure of almost 10,000 patients to 120,000 blood components. The risk of AIDS after transfusion is smaller. Current Centers for Disease Control estimates are 1 in 225,000. This discrepancy arises because many transfusion recipients will die of their primary illness or of natural causes before having symptomatic AIDS.

The study was initially designed to measure HIV, but the serum repository and data established led to studies of the risk of HCV seroconversion, when the agent causing most of the cases of non-A, non-B hepatitis was discovered in 1988 and tests for its identification became available in 1990. The study showed the value of various modifications of blood donor screening such as HIV serology, the so-called surrogate tests alanine aminotransferase and anti–hepatitis B core, and finally the first generation of anti-HCV tests. The resulting estimate of a current risk of 3 per 10,000 transfusions is not necessarily the correct current answer, because newer tests for anti-HCV will eliminate more infectious donors but would also detect more cases of seroconversion. Unfortunately, the study was terminated in 1991; its use as a continuing window on the safety of the blood supply would have provided the answer to the current status of HCV infection and the results of future modifications of donor screening protocols.—P.M. Ness, M.D.

Long-Term Mortality After Transfusion-Associated Non-A, Non-B Hepatitis

Seeff LB, Buskell-Bales Z, Wright EC, Durako SJ, Alter HJ, Iber FL, Hollinger FB, Gitnick G, Knodell RG, Perrillo RP, Stevens CE, Hollingsworth CG, The National Heart, Lung, and Blood Inst Study Group (Georgetown Univ, Washington, DC; Westat, Inc, Rockville, Md; NIH Blood Bank, Bethesda, Md; et al)
N Engl J Med 327:1906–1911, 1992   5–45

Background.—Non-A, non-B hepatitis appears to be clinically mild in its acute stage, but the disease often progresses to chronic hepatitis, and it is now linked to cirrhosis and hepatocellular carcinoma. Most cases of non-A, non-B hepatitis are transfusion associated. Using data from transfusion-associated non-A, non-B hepatitis cases seen between 1967 and 1980, long-term mortality in these patients was determined.

Patients and Methods.—The study group included 1,552 of the 6,438 non-A, non-B hepatitis patients and transfused controls included in the original 5 reports. The 5 studies were conducted in the United States. All enrolled subjects were monitored with serum aminotransferase measurements for at least 5 months. Each patient with hepatitis was matched with 2 control subjects who had received transfusions but did not have hepatitis. Death certificates, obtained from 97% of the 788 deceased subjects, were reviewed for cause-specific mortality; the National Death Index and Social Security Death Tapes provided data for mortality rates in the 3 groups (non-A, non-B hepatitis patients; first controls; and second controls).

Results.—At an average follow-up of 18 years, 51% of those with non-A, non-B hepatitis; 52% of first-control subjects; and 50% of second-control subjects had died (Fig 5–5). Mortality related to liver disease was 3.3%, 1.1%, and 2%, respectively, for the 3 groups (table). The survival

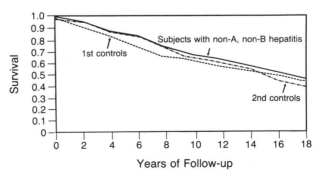

Fig 5–5.—Mortality from all causes among subjects with non-A, non-B hepatitis, first controls, and second controls. (Courtesy of Seeff LB, Buskell-Bales Z, Wright EC, et al: N Engl J Med 327:1906–1911, 1992.)

Mortality From All Causes and From Liver Disease

GROUP	ALL CAUSES		LIVER DISEASE AS UNDERLYING CAUSE *			ANY MENTION OF LIVER DISEASE		
	NO./TOTAL	%	NO.	%	P VALUE	NO.	%	P VALUE
Subjects with non-A, non-B hepatitis	287/568	51	19	3.3	—	35	6.2	—
1st controls	273/526	52	6	1.1	0.022	16	3.0	0.028
2nd controls	228/458	50	9	2.0	0.26	16	3.5	0.095
Combined controls	501/984	51	15	1.5	0.033	32	3.2	0.016

Note: The P values are for the comparison of the survival curves between the subjects with non-A, non-B hepatitis and the controls. Data for subjects who died of causes other than liver disease were censored at the time of death.
* Equivalent to the primary cause.
(Courtesy of Seeff LB, Buskell-Bales Z, Wright EC, et al: N Engl J Med 327:1906–1911, 1992.)

curve for patients with non-A, non-B hepatitis was significantly different from that for the first controls and for the 2 sets of controls combined. Detailed records were available for 28 of 34 subjects for whom the primary cause of death was liver disease; 20 (71%) had chronic alcoholism.

Conclusion.—Mortality was not increased from all causes after transfusion-associated non-A, non-B hepatitis. However, a small but statistically significant increase in the number of deaths was related to liver disease. This study cohort will continue to be observed for the possibility of increased mortality in later years.

▶ Transfusion-associated non-A, non-B hepatitis (NANBH), a disease now known to be caused by the hepatitis C virus, has been an elusive target with unclear medical significance. Historically, most patients were seen with minimal symptomatology as persistent but fluctuating elevations of alanine aminotransferase. Although an occasional case of fulminant hepatitis lacking hepatitis A or B serologic findings was attributed to hepatitis C, the long-term significance of infection was questioned and considered by many experts to be a laboratory entity referred to as transaminitis. Later studies by Alter and Hoofnagle at the NIH demonstrated that many patients with transfusion-associated NANBH had findings on liver biopsy compatible with chronic active hepatitis or cirrhosis with the long-term potential for hepatocellular carcinoma development. Based on this evolution of thinking about NANBH, aggressive testing programs using surrogate markers followed by specific tests have been used in blood donor screening. This history makes the results of this study very surprising because these investigators were not able to identify any increased mortality compared with controls after an average follow-up of 18 years. The cohort had a small increase in deaths related to liver disease, which may require even longer periods to become lethal in other patients. Although these data will not suggest to any knowledgeable observer that we discontinue hepatitis C screening of blood donors, they raise another series of questions in the development of our understanding of this unusual disease.—P.M. Ness, M.D.

Creutzfeldt-Jakob Disease and Blood Transfusion

Esmonde TFG, Will RG, Slattery JM, Knight R, Harries-Jones R, de Silva R, Matthews WB (Western Gen Hosp, Edinburgh, Scotland; Radcliffe Infirmary, Oxford, England; Poole Hosp)
Lancet 341:205–207, 1993   5–46

Background.—A few cases of Creutzfeldt-Jakob disease (CJD) in the United Kingdom have been a result of iatrogenic transmission during neurosurgery or corneal transplantation, or of peripheral inoculation during treatment with hormones derived from the human pituitary. The possibility of transmitting CJD by blood products has been considered.

Survey.—Evidence of blood product transfusion was sought among definite and probable causes of CJD identified in a prospective survey done in England and Wales from 1980 to 1984, as well as in a current prospective United Kingdom national surveillance project.

Findings.—A definite history of blood transfusion was found in 16 of 202 definite/probable cases of CJD. In 5 other cases, transfusion was a possibility. The mean time from transfusion to the onset of symptoms of CJD was nearly 15 years. Twenty-nine patients with CJD had donated blood. Neither transfusion nor donation was significantly different in frequency than in an age- and sex-matched control population. The clinical features of CJD resembled those of classic disease but differed from those in patients given human growth hormone.

Conclusion.—Every effort should be made not to acquire blood or blood products from individuals with CJD or those at high risk for the disease. The same warning applies to those who have received hormones extracted from human pituitary glands.

▶ After several cases of CJD were attributed to human growth hormone preparations from human pituitary glands that were recovered from patients with CJD, the concern has been raised that asymptomatic blood donors could transmit this disease to a blood recipient. Donors are disqualified if they give a history of receiving growth hormone from a pituitary source, which is now uncommon with the availability of the recombinant hormone. This study found a history of blood transfusion in about 10% of CJD cases and blood donation in 15% of cases. No secondary cases could be associated from blood transfusion, and the frequencies of receiving or donating blood among CJD cases were not different from age-matched controls. Although blood collections will continue their current programs, these studies question the need for this type of donor surveillance.—P.M. Ness, M.D.

Transfusion Associated Graft Versus Host Disease in an Immunocompetent Patient

O'Connor NTJ, Mackintosh P (Royal Shrewsbury Hosp, England; Regional Blood Transfusion Service, Birmingham, England)
J Clin Pathol 45:621–622, 1992

5–47

Background.—Transfusion-associated graft-vs.-host disease (GVHD), a rare disorder, usually occurs in immunosuppressed patients. The disorder developed in a woman who was presumed to be immunocompetent.

Case Report.—Woman, 77, was undergoing elective right knee replacement for rheumatoid arthritis. The surgery was uneventful. Two units of blood were given during the procedure. Thirteen days later, she reported malaise, a diffuse rash, and a wound infection. Oral flucloxacillin and fusidic acid treatment was begun for the *Staphylococcus aureus* infection. Her condition did not improve during the next 10 days. She had a persistent rash and low-grade fever. Twenty-three days after surgery, she had moderate anemia but otherwise normal hematologic findings. Another 3 units of blood was transfused. Two days later, she had profuse diarrhea and a widespread maculopapular erythrodermatous rash. She was jaundiced, confused, and feverish. Examinations revealed pancytopenia and grossly deranged liver function. Aplastic anemia was diagnosed. The aplasia worsened despite full supportive care, and 10 days after aplastic anemia was diagnosed, the patient died of renal failure. Further investigations aimed at discovering the cause of her anemia depended on the clinical suspicion of transfusion-associated GVHD. One unit of blood used in transfusion was from an individual homozygous for the same HLA haplotype as the patient.

Conclusion.—The diagnosis of transfusion-associated GVHD should be considered in patients with aplastic anemia within a month of blood product transfusion. Blood donations from first-degree relatives should not be allowed unless the donation is irradiated to prevent lymphocyte proliferation.

Transfusion-Associated Graft-Versus-Host Disease: Do Transfusions From Second-Degree Relatives Pose a Greater Risk Than Those From First-Degree Relatives?

Kanter MH (Kaiser Found Hosp, Los Angeles)
Transfusion 32:323–327, 1992

5–48

Background.—Patients receiving blood from a closely related donor have the potential for development of transfusion-associated graft-vs.-host disease (TA-GVHD). A mathematical model was developed and applied to assess the potential risk of TA-GVHD for 6 classes of related donors.

Methods and Findings.—The risk of TA-GVHD was considered to be present when an HLA-heterozygous patient received blood from a donor homozygous for 1 of the patient's haplotypes. According to calculations, second-degree related donors posed a greater risk of TA-GVHD than some first-degree relatives—siblings—but not all first-degree relatives, such as parents and children. In general, there was no sharp cutoff of risk among the different classes of donors.

Conclusion.—Transfusing blood from second-degree relatives may be more hazardous than transfusing blood from some first-degree relatives. The risk of a homozygous donor and heterozygous recipient pair is higher when blood is taken from a second-degree relative than from siblings, but not from parents or children. The risk declines continuously as the degree of relatedness decreases. It does not allow clear separation of donor blood that should be irradiated from blood that does not need irradiation. Some blood banks may wish to consider irradiating blood from all related donors.

▶ The TA-GVHD, a devastating complication of transfusion therapy, causes skin rash, liver disease, and gut disease and typically results in the death of the patient as a result of aplastic anemia. It can be prevented by irradiation of blood components, a routine practice for bone marrow transplant recipients, low-birth-weight neonates, and patients with congenital immunodeficiency. The first article (Abstract 5–47) described a case of TA-GVHD in a patient not fitting into any of these groups. The blood donor was retrospectively recognized to be homozygous for an HLA haplotype that he shared with the patient; the donor cells were not recognized as foreign and, thus, engrafted, causing TA-GVHD. On a statistical basis, this scenario can occur as often as 1 in 500 patients, particularly when the donor and patient represent a highly inborn population. The most common setting for this event is among blood relatives serving as the donor and recipient; it is now recommended that directed blood donations from first-degree relatives be irradiated to prevent TA-GVHD, whether or not the recipient is immunocompromised. The second article (Abstract 5–48) makes the case that the second-degree relatives can occasionally pose a greater risk than first-degree relatives, leading to broader recommendations that any family member donation should be irradiated. On a practical basis, it is probably prudent to irradiate all directed donor blood, because family histories of donors can be difficult to ascertain, especially when the donor blood is sent to the hospital from a distant site.—P.M. Ness, M.D.

A Case of Transfusion-Associated Graft-Versus-Host Disease Not Prevented by White Cell-Reduction Filters

Akahoshi M, Takanashi M, Masuda M, Yamashita H, Hidano A, Hasegawa K, Kasajima T, Shimizu M, Motoji T, Oshimi K, Mizoguchi H (Tokyo Women's

Medical College)
Transfusion 32:169–172, 1992

Background.—Transfusion-associated graft-vs.-host disease (TA-GVHD) usually occurs in immunocompromised transfusion recipients. Some have recently reported its occurrence in immunocompetent recipients. In most reported cases, TA-GVHD has been fatal. A patient having TA-GVHD despite the use of WBC-reduction filters was described.

Case Report.—Woman, 67, had diagnosis of diffuse, mixed-type non-Hodgkin's lymphoma at stage IIIA. Her treatment included combination chemotherapy and multiple blood transfusions for anemia and thrombocytopenia. The WBCs were reduced in the transfused components using WBC-reduction filters. However, the patients still had TA-GVHD develop, confirmed by skin biopsy. Thirty-three days after her first transfusion, the patient died of acute renal failure. At autopsy, histologic liver findings included intrahepatic pericholangitis with mild periportal fibrosis, which is consistent with acute hepatic GVHD.

Conclusion.—The WBC reduction by filters apparently does not prevent TA-GVHD in immunocompromised patients. All blood components should be irradiated before they are transfused to such patients.

▶ The standard therapy to prevent TA-GVHD is irradiation, now recommended at a dose of 2500 centigray. Although most tertiary-care centers have radiation capability and most blood centers have established mechanisms for smaller hospitals that lack this equipment, the question of whether leukocyte depletion through a third-generation filter capable of reducing contaminating white cells to less than 10^6 would be adequate TA-GVHD prophylaxis has been raised. This case report shows a failure in 1 case. Because TA-GVHD remains an uncommon transfusion complication, other failures would be expected to be uncommon. Irradiation facilities are readily available throughout the country, making the arguments for clinical trials of leukocyte depletion as a substitute for irradiation to prevent TA-GVHD not particularly persuasive.—P.M. Ness, M.D.

The Association of Perioperative Blood Transfusion With Colorectal Cancer Recurrence

Tartter PI (Mount Sinai Med Ctr, New York)
Ann Surg 216:633–638, 1992

Introduction.—Blood transfusions have been associated with clinical events related to immune suppression, and it has been proposed that this suppression promotes early tumor recurrence. Blood transfusion generally is necessary in patients requiring extensive cancer surgery. Transfusion therapy was related to survival in 339 patients who had elective surgery for colorectal cancer without evidence of metastasis.

Results.—Recurrences were seen in 28% of patients after surgery. Surviving patients were followed for an average of 5½ years. Blood transfusion was significantly associated with recurrence; 40% of transfused patients and 22% of the others had recurrences. The respective 5-year disease-free survival rates were 57% and 77%, respectively. The inverse association of transfusion with disease-free survival persisted after adjusting for age, blood loss, tumor differentiation, and tumor size.

Conclusion.—Perioperative blood transfusion is a significant and independent factor for predicting disease-free survival in patients with colorectal cancer.

▶ A number of retrospective studies have implicated blood transfusion as an independent predictor of tumor recurrence. Dr. Tartter was one of the early proponents of a causal relationship and began this prospective evaluation of the transfusion effect, correctly predicting the criticisms of the multiple retrospective studies published to date. Transfusions have been shown to have an independent adverse effect on recurrence and survival after adjusting for age, stage, size, and operative blood loss. This study goes a long way toward meeting the criticisms of previous studies, but a truly randomized study with transfusions of autologous or homologous blood for equivalent medical indications will be necessary to resolve this issue.—P.M. Ness, M.D.

A Clinical and Immunologic Study of Blood Transfusion and Postoperative Bacterial Infection in Spinal Surgery

Triulzi DJ, Vanek K, Ryan DH, Blumberg N (Univ of Rochester, NY)
Transfusion 32:517–524, 1992   5–51

Background.—Clinical and experimental evidence suggests that allogeneic blood transfusion may be an independent risk factor for postoperative bacterial infection. No prospective laboratory measurements of immune function have been correlated with postoperative bacterial infections in transfused patients. The relationships among transfusion, quantitative immunologic factors, and infection in 102 patients undergoing spinal fusion were studied.

Methods.—The patients underwent a total of 109 procedures. Autologous blood only was given in 60 procedures, at least 1 unit of allogeneic blood was given in 24 procedures, and no transfusions were given in 25 procedures. There were 22 cases of bacterial infection, 8 developing while the patient was in the hospital and 14 afterwards.

Findings.—Of patients who received allogeneic blood, 21% acquired infections in the hospital, compared with 4% of those who received no allogeneic blood. The length of stay was 12 days vs. 10 days; the length of fever was 4 days vs. 3 days; the time taking antibiotics was 4 days vs. 3 days; the duration of surgery was 309 minutes vs. 231 minutes; and the blood loss was 1,343 mL vs. 887 mL. All of these were significant on univariate analysis, as were surgeon and postoperative decrease in natural killer (NK) cells, 174/μL vs. 42/μL. On multivariate logistic and linear regression, the only significant predictor of inhospital infection, days on antibiotics, and length of stay was the number of allogeneic units transfused. No variables were significantly associated with posthospital infection, although the patients who had posthospital infection develop had a significantly greater reduction in NK cells.

Conclusion.—Transfusion of allogeneic blood is probably a risk factor for inhospital bacterial infection in surgical patients; more research is needed to prove this hypothesis. Patients who receive allogeneic blood have greater decreases in the number of NK cells than those who receive autologous blood or no transfusion. Exposure to allogeneic blood should be limited by autologous blood donation, preoperative hemodilution, and intraoperative salvage.

Homologous Blood Transfusion as a Risk Factor for Postoperative Infection After Coronary Artery Bypass Graft Operations
Murphy PJ, Connery C, Hicks GL Jr, Blumberg N (Univ of Rochester, NY)
J Thorac Cardiovasc Surg 104:1092–1099, 1992   5–52

Background.—Homologous blood transfusions are suspected of having immunosuppressive effects on recipients. These effects may be beneficial in allograft survival but may lead to an increased risk of postoperative infection. Whether homologous blood transfusion is an independent risk factor for postoperative infection in patients having coronary artery bypass graft (CABG) was ascertained.

Relationship Between Number of Units of Red
Cells and Whole Blood Transfused and Prevalence
of Culture-Proved Postoperative Infection

Units transfused	*Proportion infected*	
	No.	*%*
0	2 of 76*	2.6
1	1 of 32	3.1
2	3 of 45	6.7
3	2 of 26	7.7
4	1 of 19	5.3
5	1 of 13	7.7
≥6	6 of 27	22.2

* Six patients received at least 1 unit of fresh frozen plasma (5) or 6 units of platelets (1) but *no* red cells or whole blood. None of these 6 patients had an infection.
(Courtesy of Murphy PJ, Connery C, Hicks GL Jr, et al: *J Thorac Cardiovasc Surg* 104:1092–1099, 1992.)

Patients and Methods.—Clinical and laboratory data related to post-operative infection (pulmonary, urinary, and wound site) in 238 patients with CABG were reviewed.

Results.—Culture-proven postoperative infection was found in 16 of 238 (6.7%) patients. Three of 16 had deep sternal wound infections. Seven infections at other sites suggest that nonsurgical variables contributed in part to some of the infections. Factors found to be closely and significantly associated with increased risk of postoperative infection included female gender, diabetes, and higher transfusion dose. Infections were noted in 6 of 153 (3.9%) patients who received as many as 2 units of red cells or whole blood, 4 of 58 (6.9%) patients who received 3 to 5 units, and 6 of 27 (22%) patients who received 6 or more units (table). The transfusion dose was the most significant variable associated with postoperative infection and morbidity.

Conclusion.—Despite the small numbers studied, it seems unlikely that the significant relationship noted between transfusion dose and infection was coincidental. A three- to eightfold increased risk of postoperative infections among patients with CABG is associated, in a dose-dependent fashion, with the number of homologous blood units transfused. These infections may be the direct outcome of the transfusion-induced immunosuppression found in the patients.

▶ These 2 studies attempt to show that the immunomodulatory effects of transfusions lead to a higher rate of postoperative infections in transfused patients. The first study (Abstract 5–51) compared patients undergoing spinal surgery who had received autologous or allogeneic blood but no randomization was performed. Patients receiving allogeneic blood had a higher incidence of infection and greater decreases in NK cells. This study provides suggestive evidence of increased risk, but the method of ascertainment of infection needs to be considered. The authors considered only positive cultures or purulent sputum as evidence of infection, but these methods may have missed infections or considered asymptomatic bacteriuria as an infection. The second study (Abstract 5–52) of cardiac surgery patients makes my concerns about how much infection is sought and diagnosed even more cogent.—P.M. Ness, M.D.

Postoperative Infection and Natural Killer Cell Function Following Blood Transfusion in Patients Undergoing Elective Colorectal Surgery
Jensen LS, Andersen AJ, Christiansen PM, Hokland P, Juhl CO, Madsen G, Mortensen J, Møller-Nielsen C, Hanberg-Sørensen F, Hokland M (Aarhus County Hosp, Denmark; Aarhus Municipal Hosp, Denmark; Randers County Hosp, Denmark; et al)
Br J Surg 79:513–516, 1992   5–53

Introduction.—Blood transfusions can pose specific risks to patients' immune systems, causing immunosuppression in general. The results of

Blood Transfusion and Infection

	Filtered blood ($n = 48$)		Whole blood ($n = 56$)		
	Uninfected	Infected	Uninfected	Infected	P*
Preoperative transfusion					
No. of patients	18	0	21	2	n.s.
Median (range) units of blood	1 (1–3)	–	2 (1–5)	2·5 (2–3)	
Intraoperative transfusion					
No. of patients	22	1	16	8	<0·05
Median (range) units of blood	2 (1–5)	2	2 (1–3)	2 (1–3)	
Postoperative transfusion					
No. of patients	24	0	18	11	<0·01
Median (range) units of blood	2 (1–4)	–	2 (1–5)	2 (1–3)	

Note: Filtered blood is blood free from leukocytes and platelets.
* χ^2 test; *n.s.*, not significant.
(Courtesy of Jensen LS, Andersen AJ, Christiansen PM, et al: *Br J Surg* 79:513–516, 1992.)

comparing the infection frequency in patients having elective colorectal surgery involving no transfusion with that in patients randomly selected to receive either whole blood or WBC-free blood were reported. All patients underwent assessments of their immune system function.

Patients and Methods.—Patients undergoing elective colorectal surgery between August 1989 and September 1990 were screened for study participation. A total of 197 patients participated in the study; 104 required a blood transfusion. Of the 104 patients, 48 received the leucocyte-free blood and 56 received a whole blood transfusion. All patients received cefuroxime and metronidazole as antibiotic prophylaxis. The follow-up data collection included daily wound inspection, blood chemistries, and immunoglobulin monitoring.

Results.—Sixty patients had a natural killer–cell function measurement comparable with other patients with similar clinical profiles; 13 patients having whole blood transfusion had wound sepsis develop, whereas only 1 patient with a filtered blood transfusion did so, a significant difference. During the first postoperative week, the natural killer–cell activity decreased in both the nontransfused and the filtered transfusion patients (table). The whole blood transfusion group had a significant decrease in natural killer–cell activity during the first week after surgery, which remained for at least 1 month afterward.

Conclusion.—These findings indicate that the natural killer–cell function decreased significantly as long as 30 days after surgery in patients receiving whole blood. This result argues against the routine use of whole blood transfusion treatment in patients having elective colorectal surgery because decreased natural killer–cell function may contribute to infection.

▶ This study of the effects of blood transfusions on postoperative infections meets most of the chronic objections about studies in this area. The patients were randomized to receive whole blood or leukocyte-depleted blood. Patients who received whole blood had significantly more infections than patients receiving no blood or leukocyte-depleted blood; moreover, the infections were well-characterized instances of wound sepsis, abscess, or septicemia, rather than difficult-to-explain infections such as urinary tract infections or bronchitis featured prominently in other studies. Profound and persistent declines in natural killer cells were also documented in whole blood recipients. Although confirmatory evidence from similar studies should be sought, this study moves me from a very skeptical background toward a willingness to accept these findings.—P.M. Ness, M.D.

Blood Transfusion Impairs the Healing of Experimental Intestinal Anastomoses

Tadros T, Wobbes T, Hendriks T (Univ Hosp, Nijmegen, The Netherlands)
Ann Surg 215:276–281, 1992   5–54

Background.—The cell-mediated immune response appears to be impaired by blood transfusion. Because patients undergoing gastrointestinal surgery commonly need transfusions as a result of anemia or blood loss, it is important to establish the effect of transfusions on intestinal repair.

Methods.—Both the ileum and colon were resected in a group of adult male Lewis rats, followed by construction of either an everted or end-to-end anastomosis. The animals were given either saline or heparinized blood from Lewis or Brown Norway rat donors, 3 mL intravenously, immediately after the operation. Three days or 1 week postoperatively, the rats were killed and the strength of their anastomoses was tested by measuring the bursting pressure.

Results.—None of the control animals had anastomotic abscesses or generalized peritonitis, but the incidence of those complications was increased in animals that received transfusions, especially allogeneic transfusions. Anastomotic strength was significantly reduced at 3 days in rats that received transfusion from either Lewis or Brown Norway rats. For inverted ileal anastomoses, average bursting pressures were 79 mm Hg in controls, 46 mm Hg in rats receiving Lewis rat blood transfusion, and 21 mm Hg in those receiving Brown Norway rat blood transfusion. At 1 week, rupture was significantly more common within the anastomotic line in transfused animals.

Conclusion.—Blood transfusion impairs the healing of experimental intestinal anastomoses in rats and increases their vulnerability to intra-abdominal sepsis. This may result from some alteration of the local or systemic immune response to the intestinal trauma of surgery. These findings could have important clinical effects that warrant further study.

▶ Because of immunomodulatory effects of transfusion are so difficult to establish in patients who have a wide variety of difficult-to-control variables in their clinical care, animal models offer potential study means to determine the presence or absence of these effects. This study developed a rat intestinal anastomosis model and showed that allogeneic transfusions impaired the healing of the anastomoses and increased the likelihood of intra-abdominal sepsis. Although untransfused controls were studied, no animals received autologous transfusions as another control group. This model should be useful for further studies to dissect these immunologic effects.—P.M. Ness, M.D.

Does Blood Transfusion or Hemorrhagic Shock Induce Immunosuppression?

Cué JI, Peyton JC, Malangoni MA (Univ of Louisville, Ky; Med College of Georgia, Augusta; Case Western Reserve Univ, Cleveland, Ohio)
J Trauma 32:613–617, 1992   5–55

Background.—Blood transfusions may predispose patients to infection by inducing immunosuppression. The effects of syngeneic (ST) and allogeneic (AT) blood transfusion with and without hemorrhagic shock (HS) were assessed in female Lewis and ACI rats to determine if transfusion or the accompanying bleeding affects certain components of the immune response.

Methods.—Syngeneic or AT transfusions were given to Lewis rats at 10%, 20%, or 30% of blood volume. Other rats were subjected to hemorrhagic shock and resuscitated with either shed blood or substituted 10%, 20%, or 30% ST or AT. Immune system responses were measured using intradermal staphylococcal abscess size, peritoneal leukocyte elicitation, and peritoneal macrophage immune response gene-associated antigen (Ia) receptor expression.

Findings.—Hemorrhage shock significantly increased abscess size. However, ST or AT alone or combined with HS has no effect. Both shock and transfusion raised macrophage Ia receptor expression, but there was no additive or synergistic effect. Peritoneal leukocyte elicitation was unchanged by HS, ST, or AT.

Conclusion.—These results strongly suggest that transfusion does not independently influence the variables of immune function examined in the study model. Although the global immunosuppressive effect of hemorrhagic shock on abscess containment was confirmed, peritoneal macrophage requirement and Ia receptor expression were apparently not adversely affected in the experimental model used. Other macrophage functions not examined in the current study may be changed by shock or transfusion.

▶ Because many patients who are transfused for surgical procedures are receiving their blood components to treat circulatory shock, this article asks the provocative question of whether the immunomodulatory effects are caused by shock or the transfusions. The authors studied rats who were transfused by syngeneic or allogeneic blood with or without induced shock and found larger abscesses in only the rats that were shocked. Although these results are intriguing, they would not explain the well-documented immunomodulatory effects of blood transfusions in dialysis patients awaiting kidney transplantation, in whom shock does not appear. Because these studies were specific for infection, however, they might offer an alternative explanation for why surgical patients may have infections develop when transfused whereas dialysis patients on transfusion are not known to be especially prone to infectious complications.—P.M. Ness, M.D.

Subject Index

A

M

Author Index

We've read 236,287 journal articles (so you don't have to).

The Year Books–
The best from 236,287 journal articles.

At Mosby, we subscribe to more than 950 medical and allied health journals from every corner of the globe. We read them all, tirelessly scanning for anything that relates to your field.

We send everything we find related to a given specialty to the distinguished editors of the **Year Book** in that area, and they pick out the best, the articles they feel every practitioner in that specialty should be aware of.

For the 1993 **Year Books** we surveyed a total of 236,287 articles and found hundreds of articles related to your field. Our expert editors reviewed these and chose the best, the developments you don't want to miss.

The best articles–condensed and organized.

Not only do you get the past year's most important articles in your field, you get them in a format that makes them easy to use.

Every article that the editors pick is condensed into a concise, outlined abstract, a summary of the article's most important points highlighted with bold paragraph headings. So you can quickly scan for exactly what you need.

Personal commentary from the experts.

If that was it, if all our editors did was identify the year's best articles, the **Year Book** would still be a great reference to have. (Can you think of an easier way to keep up with all the developments that are shaping your field?)

But following each article, the editors also write concise commentaries telling whether or not the study in question is a reliable one, whether a new technique is effective, or whether a particular trend you've heard about merits your immediate attention.

No other abstracting service offers this expert advice to help you decide how the year's advances will affect the way you practice.

No matter how many journals you subscribe to, the Year Book can help.

When you subscribe to a **Year Book**, we'll also send you an automatic notice of future volumes about two months before they publish. If you do not want the **Year Book**, this convenient advance notice makes it easy for you to let us know. And if you elect to receive the new **Year Book**, you need do nothing. We will send it upon publication.

No worry. No wasted motion. And, of course, every **Year Book** is yours to examine FREE of charge for thirty days.